Post-COVID Symptoms in Long-Haulers: Definition, Identification, Mechanisms, and Management—Part II

Post-COVID Symptoms in Long-Haulers: Definition, Identification, Mechanisms, and Management—Part II

Editors

César Fernández-de-las-Peñas
Domingo Palacios-Ceña

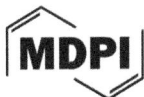

Basel • Beijing • Wuhan • Barcelona • Belgrade • Novi Sad • Cluj • Manchester

Editors
César Fernández-de-las-Peñas
Universidad Rey Juan Carlos
Madrid
Spain

Domingo Palacios-Ceña
Universidad Rey Juan Carlos
Madrid
Spain

Editorial Office
MDPI AG
Grosspeteranlage 5
4052 Basel, Switzerland

This is a reprint of articles from the Special Issue published online in the open access journal *Journal of Clinical Medicine* (ISSN 2077-0383) (available at: https://www.mdpi.com/journal/jcm/special_issues/XOHG0C9QX7).

For citation purposes, cite each article independently as indicated on the article page online and as indicated below:

Lastname, A.A.; Lastname, B.B. Article Title. *Journal Name* **Year**, *Volume Number*, Page Range.

ISBN 978-3-7258-1883-9 (Hbk)
ISBN 978-3-7258-1884-6 (PDF)
doi.org/10.3390/books978-3-7258-1884-6

© 2024 by the authors. Articles in this book are Open Access and distributed under the Creative Commons Attribution (CC BY) license. The book as a whole is distributed by MDPI under the terms and conditions of the Creative Commons Attribution-NonCommercial-NoDerivs (CC BY-NC-ND) license.

Contents

About the Editors vii

Kin Israel Notarte, Maria Helena Santos de Oliveira, Princess Juneire Peligro, Jacqueline Veronica Velasco, Imee Macaranas, Abbygail Therese Ver, et al.
Age, Sex and Previous Comorbidities as Risk Factors Not Associated with SARS-CoV-2 Infection for Long COVID-19: A Systematic Review and Meta-Analysis
Reprinted from: *J. Clin. Med.* **2022**, *11*, 7314, doi:10.3390/jcm11247314 1

Lisa Goudman, Ann De Smedt, Stijn Roggeman, César Fernández-de-las-Peñas, Samar M. Hatem, Marc Schiltz, et al.
Association between Experimental Pain Measurements and the Central Sensitization Inventory in Patients at Least 3 Months after COVID-19 Infection: A Cross-Sectional Pilot Study
Reprinted from: *J. Clin. Med.* **2023**, *12*, 661, doi:10.3390/jcm12020661 25

Marco Ranucci, Ekaterina Baryshnikova, Martina Anguissola, Sara Pugliese, Luca Ranucci, Mara Falco and Lorenzo Menicanti
The Very Long COVID: Persistence of Symptoms after 12–18 Months from the Onset of Infection and Hospitalization
Reprinted from: *J. Clin. Med.* **2023**, *12*, 1915, doi:10.3390/jcm12051915 39

Aysegul Bostanci, Umut Gazi, Ozgur Tosun, Kaya Suer, Emine Unal Evren, Hakan Evren and Tamer Sanlidag
Long-COVID-19 in Asymptomatic, Non-Hospitalized, and Hospitalized Populations: A Cross-Sectional Study
Reprinted from: *J. Clin. Med.* **2023**, *12*, 2613, doi:10.3390/jcm12072613 50

Tamara del Corral, Raúl Fabero-Garrido, Gustavo Plaza-Manzano, César Fernández-de-las-Peñas, Marcos José Navarro-Santana and Ibai López-de-Uralde-Villanueva
Minimal Clinically Important Differences in Inspiratory Muscle Function Variables after a Respiratory Muscle Training Programme in Individuals with Long-Term Post-COVID-19 Symptoms
Reprinted from: *J. Clin. Med.* **2023**, *12*, 2720, doi:10.3390/jcm12072720 60

Gerardo Salvato, Elvira Inglese, Teresa Fazia, Francesco Crottini, Daniele Crotti, Federica Valentini, et al.
The Association between Dysnatraemia during Hospitalisation and Post-COVID-19 Mental Fatigue
Reprinted from: *J. Clin. Med.* **2023**, *12*, 3702, doi:10.3390/jcm12113702 74

Stefan Malesevic, Noriane A. Sievi, Dörthe Schmidt, Florence Vallelian, Ilijas Jelcic, Malcolm Kohler and Christian F. Clarenbach
Physical Health-Related Quality of Life Improves over Time in Post-COVID-19 Patients: An Exploratory Prospective Study
Reprinted from: *J. Clin. Med.* **2023**, *12*, 4077, doi:10.3390/jcm12124077 85

Mª Pilar Rodríguez-Pérez, Patricia Sánchez-Herrera-Baeza, Pilar Rodríguez-Ledo, Elisabet Huertas-Hoyas, Gemma Fernández-Gómez, Rebeca Montes-Montes and Marta Pérez-de-Heredia-Torres
Influence of Clinical and Sociodemographic Variables on Health-Related Quality of Life in the Adult Population with Long COVID
Reprinted from: *J. Clin. Med.* **2023**, *12*, 4222, doi:10.3390/jcm12134222 96

Joerg Lindenmann, Christian Porubsky, Lucija Okresa, Huberta Klemen, Iurii Mykoliuk, Andrej Roj, et al.
Immediate and Long-Term Effects of Hyperbaric Oxygenation in Patients with Long COVID-19 Syndrome Using SF-36 Survey and VAS Score: A Clinical Pilot Study
Reprinted from: *J. Clin. Med.* **2023**, *12*, 6253, doi:10.3390/jcm12196253 107

Einat Shmueli, Ophir Bar-On, Ben Amir, Meir Mei-Zahav, Patrick Stafler, Hagit Levine, et al.
Pulmonary Evaluation in Children with Post-COVID-19 Condition Respiratory Symptoms: A Prospective Cohort Study
Reprinted from: *J. Clin. Med.* **2023**, *12*, 6891, doi:10.3390/jcm12216891 120

Juan Luis Sánchez-González, Luis Almenar-Bonet, Noemí Moreno-Segura, Francisco Gurdiel-Álvarez, Hady Atef, Amalia Sillero-Sillero, et al.
Effects of COVID-19 Lockdown on Heart Failure Patients: A Quasi-Experimental Study
Reprinted from: *J. Clin. Med.* **2023**, *12*, 7090, doi:10.3390/jcm12227090 132

Dovilė Važgėlienė, Raimondas Kubilius and Indre Bileviciute-Ljungar
The Impact of Previous Comorbidities on New Comorbidities and Medications after a Mild SARS-CoV-2 Infection in a Lithuanian Cohort
Reprinted from: *J. Clin. Med.* **2024**, *13*, 623, doi:10.3390/jcm13020623 145

Anna Kim, Eun-yeob Kim and Jaeyoung Kim
Impact of the COVID-19 Pandemic on Obesity, Metabolic Parameters and Clinical Values in the South Korean Adult Population
Reprinted from: *J. Clin. Med.* **2024**, *13*, 2814, doi:10.3390/jcm13102814 155

About the Editors

César Fernández-de-las-Peñas

Dr. César Fernández-de-las-Peñas is a Physical Therapist (PT) with a PhD in Biomedical Sciences and a master's degree in Sciences (Dr. Med Sci.). He has 25 years of experience as a Professor at Universidad Rey Juan Carlos, Madrid, Spain. He previously served as the Head (Chief) of the Department of Physical Therapy, Occupational Therapy and Rehabilitation at Universidad Rey Juan Carlos for 10 years, creating the first chronic pain clinic in a public university in Spain; here, he combined clinical practice with teaching and research. He has published up to 760 publications in JCR journals, and a clinical researcher with a particular interest in chronic pain and more recently long-COVID. He has published more than 100 papers on long-COVID, the topic of this Special Issue.

Domingo Palacios-Ceña

Dr. Domingo Palacios-Ceña is a nurse with a PhD in Public Health. He has 15 years of experience as a Professor at Universidad Rey Juan Carlos, Madrid, Spain. He has published up to 200 publications in JCR journals, and is a researcher with a particular interest in qualitative research and more recently in long-COVID. He has published more than 20 papers on long-COVID, the topic of this Special Issue.

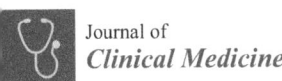

Review

Age, Sex and Previous Comorbidities as Risk Factors Not Associated with SARS-CoV-2 Infection for Long COVID-19: A Systematic Review and Meta-Analysis

Kin Israel Notarte [1], Maria Helena Santos de Oliveira [2], Princess Juneire Peligro [3], Jacqueline Veronica Velasco [3], Imee Macaranas [3], Abbygail Therese Ver [3], Flos Carmeli Pangilinan [3], Adriel Pastrana [3], Nathaniel Goldrich [4], David Kavteladze [5], Ma. Margarita Leticia Gellaco [3], Jin Liu [1], Giuseppe Lippi [6], Brandon Michael Henry [7] and César Fernández-de-las-Peñas [8],*

1. Department of Pathology, Johns Hopkins University School of Medicine, Baltimore, MD 21205, USA
2. Department of Biostatistics, State University of Maringa, Maringá 87020-900, Brazil
3. Faculty of Medicine and Surgery, University of Santo Tomas, Manila 1008, Philippines
4. New York Medical College, Valhalla, NY 10595, USA
5. Department of Biomedical Engineering, Johns Hopkins University, Baltimore, MD 21218, USA
6. Section of Clinical Biochemistry, University of Verona, 37129 Verona, Italy
7. Clinical Laboratory, Division of Nephrology and Hypertension, Cincinnati Children's Hospital Medical Center, Cincinnati, OH 45229, USA
8. Department of Physical Therapy, Occupational Therapy, Physical Medicine and Rehabilitation, Universidad Rey Juan Carlos, 28933 Madrid, Spain
* Correspondence: cesar.fernandez@urjc.es; Tel.: +34-91-488-88-84

Abstract: Identification of predictors of long COVID-19 is essential for managing healthcare plans of patients. This systematic literature review and meta-analysis aimed to identify risk factors not associated with Severe Acute Respiratory Syndrome Coronavirus 2 (SARS-CoV-2) infection, but rather potentially predictive of the development of long COVID-19. MEDLINE, CINAHL, PubMed, EMBASE, and Web of Science databases, as well as medRxiv and bioRxiv preprint servers were screened through 15 September 2022. Peer-reviewed studies or preprints evaluating potential pre-SARS-CoV-2 infection risk factors for the development of long-lasting symptoms were included. The methodological quality was assessed using the Quality in Prognosis Studies (QUIPSs) tool. Random-effects meta-analyses with calculation of odds ratio (OR) were performed in those risk factors where a homogenous long COVID-19 definition was used. From 1978 studies identified, 37 peer-reviewed studies and one preprint were included. Eighteen articles evaluated age, sixteen articles evaluated sex, and twelve evaluated medical comorbidities as risk factors of long COVID-19. Overall, single studies reported that old age seems to be associated with long COVID-19 symptoms (n = 18); however, the meta-analysis did not reveal an association between old age and long COVID-19 (n = 3; OR 0.86, 95% CI 0.73 to 1.03, $p = 0.17$). Similarly, single studies revealed that female sex was associated with long COVID-19 symptoms (n = 16); which was confirmed in the meta-analysis (n = 7; OR 1.48, 95% CI 1.17 to 1.86, $p = 0.01$). Finally, medical comorbidities such as pulmonary disease (n = 4), diabetes (n = 1), obesity (n = 6), and organ transplantation (n = 1) were also identified as potential risk factors for long COVID-19. The risk of bias of most studies (71%, n = 27/38) was moderate or high. In conclusion, pooled evidence did not support an association between advancing age and long COVID-19 but supported that female sex is a risk factor for long COVID-19. Long COVID-19 was also associated with some previous medical comorbidities.

Keywords: post-COVID-19 condition; long COVID-19 symptoms; risk factors; sex; age; co-morbidity

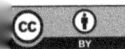

1. Introduction

Long COVID-19 is a term used for defining the persistence of signs and symptoms in people who recovered from an acute Severe Acute Respiratory Syndrome Coronavirus 2

(SARS-CoV-2) infection [1]. Long COVID-19 is defined by the World Health Organization (WHO) as: "post-COVID-19 condition, occurs in individuals with a history of probable or confirmed SARS-CoV-2 infection, usually 3 months from the onset, with symptoms that last for at least 2 months and cannot be explained by an alternative diagnosis [2]." Several meta-analyses investigating the prevalence of post-COVID-19 symptoms have been published, concluding that around 30–50% of subjects who recover from a SARS-CoV-2 infection develop persistent symptoms lasting up to one year [3,4]. A recent meta-analysis concluded that two years after the initial spread of coronavirus disease 2019 (COVID-19), up to 42% of infected patients experienced long COVID-19 symptoms [5].

Different narrative reviews have mentioned prognostic aspects, but no comprehensive synthesis has been provided so far [6–9]. Identification of potential risk factors associated with post-COVID-19 syndrome is important since identifying individuals at higher risk can guide management healthcare plans for these patients and reorganize healthcare accordingly. Iqbal et al. tried to pool data, but these authors were only able to pool prevalence data of post-COVID-19 symptomatology, but not risk factors [10]. All these narrative reviews have suggested that female sex, old age, higher number of comorbidities, higher viral load, and greater number of COVID-19 onset symptoms can be potential risk factors for long COVID-19 [6–10]. However, no systematic search or assessment of methodological quality was conducted in these reviews [6–10]. Two meta-analyses have recently focused on risk factors of long COVID-19. Maglietta et al. identified that female sex was a risk factor for long COVID-19 symptoms, whereas a more severe condition at the acute phase was associated just with long COVID-19 respiratory symptoms [11]. Thompson et al. found that old age, female sex, white ethnicity, poor pre-pandemic health, obesity, and asthma can predict long COVID-19 symptoms [12]. However, this analysis included just studies from the United Kingdom, and used the definition of long COVID-19 proposed by the National Institute for Health Care and Excellence (NICE) [13].

Accordingly, current evidence on risk factors associated with post-COVID-19 condition is heterogeneous. Risk factors can be classified as pre-infection (e.g., age, sex, previous comorbidities, and previous health status) and infection-associated (e.g., disease severity, symptoms at onset, viral load, hospitalization stay, and intensive care unit admission) factors. The current systematic review and meta-analysis aimed to identify factors not directly associated with acute SARS-CoV-2 infection (i.e., pre-infection factors) such as age, sex, and previous medical comorbidities, which may predict the development of long COVID-19 symptomatology.

2. Methods

This systematic literature review and meta-analysis aiming to identify the association of age, sex, and comorbidities as predictive factors for development of long COVID-19 was conducted following the Preferred Reporting Items for Systematic reviews and Meta-Analyses (PRISMA) statement of 2020 [14]. We also followed specific criteria recommended by Riley et al. to systematic reviews and the meta-analysis of prognostic factor studies [15]. The review study was prospectively registered in the Open Science Framework (OSF) database (https://osf.io/79pdg).

2.1. Search Strategy and Selection Criteria

Two different authors performed an electronic search for articles published up to 15 September 2022 MEDLINE, CINAHL, PubMed, EMBASE, and Web of Science databases, as well as on preprint servers medRxiv and bioRxiv, using the following search terms: "long COVID-19" OR "post-acute COVID" OR "post-COVID-19 condition" OR "long hauler" AND "age" OR "sex" OR "medical comorbidities" OR "transplant" OR "obesity" OR "diabetes" OR "hypertension" OR "pulmonary disease" OR "asthma" OR "chronic obstructive pulmonary disease". The search was focused on the medical comorbidities likely associated with a more severe COVID-19 condition. Combinations of these search terms using Boolean operators are outlined in Table 1.

Table 1. Database formulas during literature search.

PubMed Search Formula
#1 "post-acute COVID-19 syndrome" [MeSH Terms] OR "long COVID-19" [All Fields] OR "long COVID-19 symptoms" [All Fields] OR "long hauler" [All Fields] OR "post-COVID-19" [All Fields] OR "post-acute COVID-19 symptoms" [All Fields] OR "COVID-19 sequelae" [All Fields]
#2 "age" [All Fields]
#3 "sex" [MeSH Terms] OR "sex" [All Fields]
#4 "comorbidity" [MeSH Terms] OR ("transplants" [MeSH Terms] OR "transplantation" [MeSH Terms] OR transplant [All Fields]) OR ("obesity" [MeSH Terms] OR obesity [All Fields]) OR ("diabetes mellitus" [MeSH Terms] OR "diabetes insipidus" [MeSH Terms] OR diabetes [All Fields]) OR ("hypertension" [MeSH Terms] OR hypertension [All Fields]) OR ("lung diseases" [MeSH Terms] OR pulmonary disease [All Fields]) OR ("asthma" [MeSH Terms] OR asthma [All Fields]) OR ("pulmonary disease, chronic obstructive" [MeSH Terms] OR COPD [All Fields])
#5 #1 AND #2
#6 #1 AND #3
#7 #1 AND #4
MEDLINE/CINAHL (via EBSCO) Search Formula
#1 "post-acute COVID-19 syndrome" OR "long COVID-19" OR "long COVID-19 symptoms" OR "long hauler" OR "post-COVID-19" OR "post-acute COVID-19 symptoms" OR "COVID-19 sequelae"
#2 "age"
#3 "sex"
#4 "comorbidity" OR "transplants" OR "transplantation" OR "obesity" OR "diabetes mellitus" OR "diabetes" OR "hypertension" OR "pulmonary disease" OR "asthma" OR "chronic obstructive pulmonary disease"
#5 #1 AND #2
#6 #1 AND #3
#7 #1 AND #4
WOS (EMBASE)/Web of Science Search Formula
("post-acute COVID-19 syndrome" OR "long COVID-19" OR "long COVID-19 symptoms" OR "long hauler" OR "post-COVID-19" OR "post-acute COVID-19 symptoms" OR "COVID-19 sequelae" AND (("age") OR ("sex") OR ("comorbidity" OR "transplants" OR "transplantation" OR "obesity" OR "diabetes mellitus" OR "diabetes" OR "hypertension" OR "pulmonary disease" OR "asthma" OR "chronic obstructive pulmonary disease"))

The Population, Intervention, Comparison. and Outcome (PICO) principle was used to describe the inclusion and exclusion criteria:

Population: Adults (>18 years) infected by SARS-CoV-2 and diagnosed with real-time reverse transcription-polymerase chain reaction (RT-PCR) assay. Subjects could have been hospitalized or not by SARS-CoV-2 acute infection.

Intervention: Not applicable.

Comparison: People infected by SARS-CoV-2 who did not develop long COVID-19 symptoms.

Outcome: Collection of long COVID-19 symptoms developed after an acute SARS-CoV-2 infection by personal, telephone, or electronic interview. We defined post-COVID-19 condition according to Soriano et al. [2], where "post-COVID-19 condition occurs in individuals with positive history of probable or confirmed SARS-CoV-2 infection, usually 3 months from onset of COVID-19, with symptoms that last for at least 2 months and cannot be explained by alternative diagnosis." We considered any long COVID-19 symptom appearing after the infection, e.g., fatigue, dyspnea, pain, brain fog, memory loss, skin rashes, palpitations, cough, and sleep problems. Results should be reported as odds ratio (OR), hazards ratio (HR), or mean incidence of the symptoms.

2.2. Screening Process, Study Selection, and Data Extraction

This review included observational cohort, cross-sectional, and case-control studies whether presence of risk factors for development of symptoms appearing after an acute

SARS-CoV-2 infection were investigated in COVID-19 survivors, either hospitalized or non-hospitalized. The current review was limited to human studies and English language papers. Editorials, opinion, and correspondence articles were excluded.

Two authors screened title and abstract of publications obtained from database search and removed duplicates. Full text of eligible articles was retrieved and analyzed. The following data were extracted from each study: authors, country, design, sample size, age range, assessment of symptoms, long COVID-19 symptoms, and effect (measure) of risk factor studied. Discrepancies between reviewers in any part of the screening and data extraction process were resolved by a third author.

2.3. Risk of Bias

The Quality in Prognosis Studies (QUIPSs) tool was used to determine the risk of bias (RoB) of the studies [16]. The QUIPS consists of six domains such as study participation, study attrition, prognostic factor measurement, outcome measurement, adjustment for other prognostic factors, and statistical analysis. RoB was initially evaluated by two authors. If there is disagreement, a third researcher arbitrated a consensus decision. Risk of bias was scored as low, moderate, or high as follows: 1 if all domains are classified as having low RoB, or just one as moderate RoB, the paper was classified as low RoB (green); 2 if one or more domains are classified as having high RoB; or ≥3 if all domains have moderate RoB, the paper was classified as high RoB (red). All papers in between were classified as having moderate RoB (yellow) [17].

2.4. Data Synthesis

We conducted a qualitative synthesis of data for those risk factors where the heterogeneity of results did not permit to perform a meta-analysis. We only included articles in the meta-analysis that followed the Soriano et al. definition of post-COVID-19 condition [2], hence meta-analysis was possible for age and sex.

To synthesize the association between age and sex with post-COVID-19 condition, random-effects meta-analyses were performed using MetaXL software (https://www.epigear.com/index_files/metaxl.html) to estimate weighted mean differences (for age) and pooled odds ratios (ORs) with 95% confidence intervals (CIs) for sex and age above 60 years (old adults). A p-value < 0.05 was considered statistically significant. Given the heterogeneity expected, a random-effects model was employed. Measures of heterogeneity such as the I square statistics and Cochran's Q test statistic and p-value are also reported. When each age group was reported using median and interquartile range values, the method described by Wan was used for transformation in mean and standard deviation.

3. Results

3.1. Study Selection

The electronic search allowed to initially identify 1978 titles for screening. After removing duplicates (n = 154) and papers not directly related to risk factors (n = 1352), 472 studies remained for abstract examination. Four hundred and twenty-five (n = 425) were excluded after reading the abstract, thus leading to a total of 47 text articles for eligibility (Figure 1). Nine articles were excluded because there were no comparisons between subgroups (n = 2) [18,19], inappropriate methodology (n = 2) [12,20], data not extractable (n = 1) [21], unrelated to association of risk factors (n = 1) [22], and type of literature commentary, case reports, and case series (n = 3) [23–25]. A total number of 37 peer-reviewed studies and one pre-print study were finally included [26–63]. All papers could be included in qualitative analysis, whereas seven of these could also be pooled in the meta-analysis.

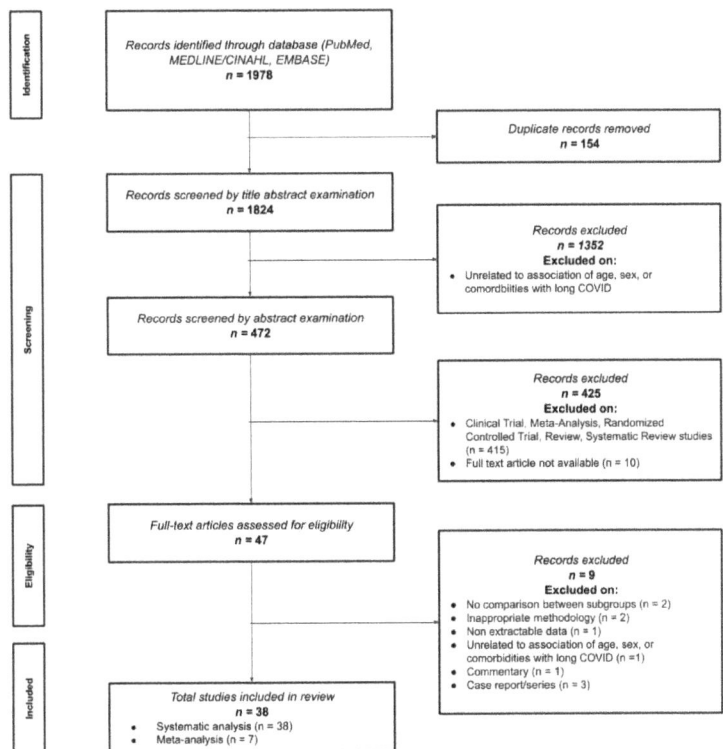

Figure 1. Preferred Reporting Items for Systematic reviews and Meta-Analyses (PRISMA) flow diagram.

3.2. Age and Post-COVID-19 Condition

A total of 18 articles, including 819,884 COVID-19 survivors analyzed age as a risk factor for developing long COVID-19 symptoms (Table 2) [26–43]. Four articles used percentages [27,33,34,38], five used means [26,31,40,41,43], seven OR [28–30,32,36,37,39], one adjusted OR (aOR) [35], and one adjusted hazard ratio (aHR) [42]. Eight articles included population samples aged ≥50 years old [27,28,32,35,37,38,40,41], eight individuals aged between 40 and 49 years [26,29,31,33,34,39,42,43], and one a population between 18 and 64 years [27]. Two studies included children aged 10–12 years [30,36], but data from these age groups were not considered in the main analyses.

Overall, most articles observed that old age was associated with long COVID-19 symptoms [26,28,29,31,33–35,37–41,43]. Contrastingly, Peghin et al. did not find an association between age and long COVID-19 symptoms [32]. Subramanian et al. stated that adults aged >70 years displayed lower risk of developing long COVID-19 symptoms than those aged 30–39 years [42].

Three articles (n = 30,371 patients) were included in the meta-analysis based on their similar study design, study outcomes, and long COVID-19 definition [32,42,44]. We grouped individuals aged over 60 years old, since this age group is considered to be at higher risk of severe COVID-19. The meta-analysis did not reveal a significant association between old age and long COVID-19 symptomatology (OR 0.86, 95% CI 0.73 to 1.03, Q = 3.54, p = 0.17, I2: 44%, Figure 2). Another three articles reporting data as mean (with their standard deviation) or median (interquartile range) were also pooled [42,45,46]. We pooled these data through a random effects model, resulting in a non-significant weighted mean difference (WMD) of −0.25 (95% CI −3.78 to 3.27, Q = 3.27, p = 0.19, I2: 39%, Figure 3).

Table 2. Studies investigating the effect of age in long COVID-19 symptomatology [10,26–33,35–43].

Author	Country Study Period	Study Design Sample Size	Age	Symptoms Assessment	Post-COVID-19 Symptoms	Main Findings
Buonsenso et al., 2022	Italy 1 April 2020–31 April 2021	Prospective cohort n = 507	Adults, 44 y	ISARIC Global COVID-19 protocol EQ-5D-5L	Headache, Malaise, Fatigue	Probability of being fully recovered: 1–3 months Adults 0.83 (0.38), $p = 0.001$ 6–9 months Adults 0.83 (0.38), $p = 0.016$
Yellumahanthi et al., 2022	USA 13 March 2020–12 March 2021	Prospective cohort n = 53	18–64 y (n = 38) ≥65 y (n = 15)	Self-reported questionnaire three months after	Fatigue, Brain fog Shortness of breath, Joint pain, Loss taste/smell, Anxiety/Depression, Hair loss, Sleep disturbances, Cough	18–64 y Symptoms present n = 20 Symptoms absent n = 18 >65 y Symptoms present n = 7 Symptoms absent n = 8 $p = 0.696$
Huang et al., 2021	China 16 June 2020–13 September 2020	Cohort study n = 1733	mean 57 y	EQ-5D-5L	Fatigue, Sleep difficulties, Anxiety/Depression	Per 10-year increase im age—Risk of Fatigue OR 1.17, 95% CI 1.07–1.27 *
Sudre et al., 2021	UK, USA, Sweden March 2020–December 2020	Prospective cohort n = 8364	Positive for SARS-CoV-2 42 y (IQR 32–53) Negative for SARS-CoV-2 42 y (IQR 32–53)	COVID-19 Symptoms Study app	Abdominal pain, Chest pain, Sore throat, Shortness of breath, Fatigue, Hoarse voice, Diarrhea, skipped meals, Cough, Muscle pain, Loss of smell, Headache	OR (95% CI)—18–30 y 30–40 y—OR from 2.11 to 4.12 * 40–50 y—OR from 2.24 to 4.35 * 50–60 y—OR from 6.65 to 11.49 * 60–70 y—OR from 6.53 to 14.0 * ≥70 y—OR from 5.46 to 18.56 *
Asadi-Pooya et al., 2021 #	Iran February 2020–February 2021	Cross-Sectional n = 58	Mean age 12.3 y (SD 3.3)	Telephone interview	Fatigue, Shortness of breath, Exercise intolerance, Walking intolerance, Cough, Sputum, Sleep difficulty, Muscle/Joint pain, Headache, Chest pain, Palpitation, Loss of smell, Sore throat, Dizziness	OR 1.314 (95% CI 1.043–1.656), $p = 0.002$ *
Taquet et al., 2021	USA January 2020–December 2020	Retrospective cohort n = 388,067	COVID-19 (unmatched) Mean age 46.3 y (SD 9.8) COVID-19 (matched) Mean age 39.4 y (SD 18.4) Influenza (matched) Mean age 38.3 y (SD 19.7)	Electronic health records	Breathlessness, Fatigue/malaise, Chest pain, Throat pain, Headache, Abdominal pain, Myalgia, Cognitive symptoms, Anxiety/depression	6-month incidence of long COVID-19 symptoms % (95% CI) 10–21 y—55.06 (54.34–55.77) 45–64 y—58.92 (58.24–59.59) ≥65 y—61.05 (60.29–61.81)
Peghin et al., 2021	Italy March 2020–November 2020	Cohort n = 599	Mean age 53 y (SD 15.8)	Questionnaire via telephone interview	Dyspnea, Cough, Fatigue, Chest pain, Anosmia/Dysgeusia, Headache, Sleep disorders, Neurological Disorders, Brain Fog, Anxiety/Depression, Skin lesion, Gastrointestinal Dis., Hair loss, Ocular involvement	41–60 vs.18–40 y OR 1.0 (95% CI 0.6–11.6), $p = 0.9$ >60 vs. 18–40 y OR 1.03 (95% CI 0.6–1.7), $p = 0.9$ >60 vs. 41–60 y OR 1.04 (95% CI 0.67–1.6), $p = 0.8$

Table 2. Cont.

Author	Country Study Period	Study Design Sample Size	Age	Symptoms Assessment	Post-COVID-19 Symptoms	Main Findings
Carvalho-Schneider et al., 2021	France March 2020–August 2020	Cohort n = 150	Mean age 49 y (IQR 34–64)	Telephone interviews	Dyspnea Chest pain Palpitations Anosmia/Ageusia Headache Cutaneous signs Arthralgia/Myalgia Digestive disorders Fever Sick leave	One or more long COVID-19 symptom n (%) D30 (n = 150) * <30 y—7 (6.8) 30–39 y—21 (20.4) 40–49 y—24 (23.3) 50–59 y—28 (27.2) 60–69 y—11 (10.7) $p = 0.06$ D60 (n = 130) * <30 y—4 (4.7) 30–39 y—19 (22.1) 40–49 y—23 (26.7) 50–59 y—21 (24.4) 60–69 y—10 (11.6) $p = 0.026$
Iqbal et al., 2021	Pakistan September 2020–December 2020	Cross Sectional n = 158	Mean age 40.1 y (SD 12.42)	Questionnaire	Fatigue, Sleep quality, Anxiety/Depression Dyspnea, Joint pain, Loss of smell/taste, Cough, Loss Hair, Headache, Chest pain, Brain fog, Blurred vision, Tinnitus	Relation of age with post-COVID-19 Dyspnea ($p = 0.007$) * Cough ($p < 0.001$) * Joint pain ($p < 0.001$) * Chest pain ($p < 0.001$) *
Tleyjeh et al., 2021	Saudi Arabia May 2020–January 2021	Prospective Cohort n = 222	Mean age 52.5 y (IQR 38.52–66.42)	Structured interview via phone call	Insomnia, Fever, Fatigue, Joint pain, Muscle pain, Memory loss, Headaches, Loss of taste, Abdominal pain, Nausea/Vomiting, Diarrhea, Loss of smell, Sore throat, Runny nose, Chest pain, Cough, Shortness of breath	Hazard model of new or persistent symptoms at follow-up (n = 222) Adjusted HR (95% CI) 0.99 (0.98–1.01), $p = 0.38$
Osmanov et al., 2022 #	Russia April 2020–February 2021	Prospective Cohort n = 518	Mean age 10.4 y (IQR 3–15.2)	Telephone Interview—1.0 ISARIC COVID-19 Health and Wellbeing Follow-Up Survey for Children	Respiratory symptoms, Neurological symptoms, Sleep problems, Gastrointestinal Dermatological Cardiovascular Fatigue Musculoskeletal	Presence of any persistent symptom at time of follow-up (n = 127) 2–5 y—OR 0.93 (95% CI 0.38–2.22) 6–11 y—OR 2.57 (95% CI 1.29–5.36) * 12–18 y—OR 2.52 (95% CI 1.34–5.01) *
Righi et al., 2022	Italy February 2020–February 2021	Prospective Cohort n = 465	Mean age 56 y (IQR 45–66)	Questionnaire	Cough, Diarrhea, Fatigue, Myalgia, Anosmia, Dysgeusia, Breathlessness	Persistence of symptoms at 9-month follow-up >50 y—OR 2.5 (95% CI 1.28–4.88), $p = 0.007$ * Persistence of fatigue at 9-month follow-up >50 y—HR 0.98 (95% CI 0.97–0.99)

Table 2. *Cont.*

Author	Country Study Period	Study Design Sample Size	Age	Symptoms Assessment	Post-COVID-19 Symptoms	Main Findings
de Miranda et al., 2022	Brazil March 2020–November 2021	Longitudinal study n = 646	Mean age 50.3 y (SD 15.8)	In person or virtual interview	Sore throat, Runny nose, Sputum, Skin lesion, Tachycardia, Vertigo, Chest pain, Joint pain, Diarrhea, Anxiety, Insomnia, Myalgia, Headache, Loss of smell/taste, Dyspnea, Fatigue	Mild COVID-19: 59.3% of 329 patients developed symptoms—<60 y: n = 162 (83.1%) Severe COVID-19: 33.1% of 260 patients developed symptoms ≤60 y old: n = 48 (55.8%) >60 y old: n = 38 (44.2%)
Loosen et al., 2022	Germany 1 March 2020–31 March 2021	Cross-sectional n = 50,402	Mean age 48.8 y (SD 19.3)	Medical record data from the Disease Analyzer database	Fatigue, Abnormalities of breathing, Disturbances of smell/taste, Disturbances in attention	≤30 years/COVID-19 patients: n = 10,443 Patients developing long COVID-19: n = 213 31–45 years/COVID-19 patients: n = 12,963 Patients developing long COVID-19: n = 379 46–60 years/COVID-19 patients: n = 14,424 Patients developing long COVID-19: n = 664 >60 years/COVID-19 patients: n = 12,572 Patients developing long COVID-19: n = 452
Messin et al., 2021	France March 2020–October 2020	Retrospective observational n = 74 With persistent symptoms: n = 53 Without persistent symptoms: n = 21	Mean age: 54.7 y (SD 16.9)	Telephone interview	Asthenia, Dyspnea, Anxiety, Anosmia, Ageusia, Nasal obstruction, Rhinorrhea, Sneezing, Odynophagia, Dysphonia, Chest pain, Palpitations, Headache, Dizziness, Drowsiness, Neuropathic pain, Depressive syndrome, Memory impairment, Attention deficit, Hair loss, Diarrhea, Cough, Pain, Erectile dysfunction	18–30 years—number (%) Symptoms: 5 (9.4)/No symptoms: 4 (19.1) 31–40 years—number (%) Symptoms: 8 (15.1)/No symptoms: 7 (33.3) 41–50 years—number (%) Symptoms: 8 (15.1)/No symptoms: 6 (28.6) 51–60 years—number (%) Symptoms: 9 (17)/No symptoms 0 61–70 years—number (%) Symptoms: 14 (26.4)/No symptoms: 0 >71 years—number (%) Symptoms: 9 (17)/No symptoms: 4 (19.1)
Kim et al., 2022	Korea 31 August 2020–2 March 2021	Prospective cohort n = 170 With persistent symptoms: n = 129 Without persistent symptoms: n = 41	Median age: 51 y (IQR 37–61)	Individualized questionnaire	Fever, Myalgia, Cough, Arthralgia, Fatigue, Sore throat, Rhinorrhea, Chest pain, Dyspnea, Palpitation, Arrhythmia, Headache, Cognitive dysfunction, Dizziness, Insomnia, Depression/Anxiety, Vomiting, Diarrhea Anosmia, Ageusia, Tinnitus, Alopecia, Skin rash, Paresthesia	20–29 years—number (%) Symptoms: 19 (14.7)/No symptoms: 10 (24.4) 30–39 years—number (%) Symptoms: 18 (14)/No symptoms: 6 (14.6) 40–49 years—number (%) Symptoms: 17 (13.2)/No symptoms: 9 (22) 50–59 years—number (%) Symptoms: 35 (27.1)/No symptoms: 9 (22) 60–70 years—number (%) Symptoms: 40 (31)/No symptoms: 7 (17.1)

Table 2. Cont.

Author	Country Study Period	Study Design Sample Size	Age	Symptoms Assessment	Post-COVID-19 Symptoms	Main Findings
Subramanian et al., 2022	United Kingdom 31 January 2020–15 April 2021	Retrospective matched cohort study Non-hospitalized COVID-19 survivors n = 486,149 Matched patients with no evidence of COVID-19 n = 1,944,580	Patients infected with SARS-CoV-2 Mean age 44.1 y (SD 17.0) Comparator cohort Mean age 43.8 y (SD 16.9)	Interviews and questionnaires	A total of 62 symptoms were significantly associated with SARS-CoV-2 infection after 12 weeks: Anosmia, Hair loss, Sneezing, Ejaculation difficulty, Reduced libido, Shortness of breath at rest, Fatigue, Chest pain, Hoarse voice, Fever	18–29 years (n = 95,969) With symptoms: n (%) 6932 (7.2) 30–39 years (n = 78,302) With symptoms: n (%) 5805 (7.4) 40–49 years (n = 75,349) With symptoms: n (%) 5784 (7.7) 50–59 years (n = 73,262) With symptoms: n (%) 5485 (7.5) 60–69 years (n = 35,932) With symptoms: n (%) 2790 (7.8) ≥70 years (n = 25,323) With symptoms: n (%) 3073 (12.1)
Helmsdal et al., 2022	Faroe Islands March 2020–January 2022	Cohort n = 180	Mean age 40 y (SD 19.4)	Standardized questionnaire via telephone interview	Fatigue, loss taste, loss smell, Headache, Skin rashes, Arthralgia, Dyspnea, Myalgia, Rhinorrhea, Chest tightness, Cough, Diarrhea, Nausea, Anorexia, Chills, Fever, Sore throat	Prevalence (%) of long COVID-19 (n = 170) at 23-months Mean (SD) Age at symptom onset * Symptoms (n = 65) age: 45.1 (18.5) No symptoms (n = 105) age: 36.9 (19.3) $p = 0.03$ Persistent symptoms vs. No symptoms—n (%) 0–17 y—4 (6.2) vs. 17 (16.2) 18–34 y—16 (24.6) vs. 34 (32.4) 35–49 y—17 (26.2) vs. 22 (21.0) 50–67 y—18 (27.7) vs. 25 (23.8) >67 y—10 (15.4) vs. 7 (6.7) $p = 0.1$

* Statistically significant ($p < 0.05$); # Data from children were not considered in the analyses. y: years; SD: standard deviation.

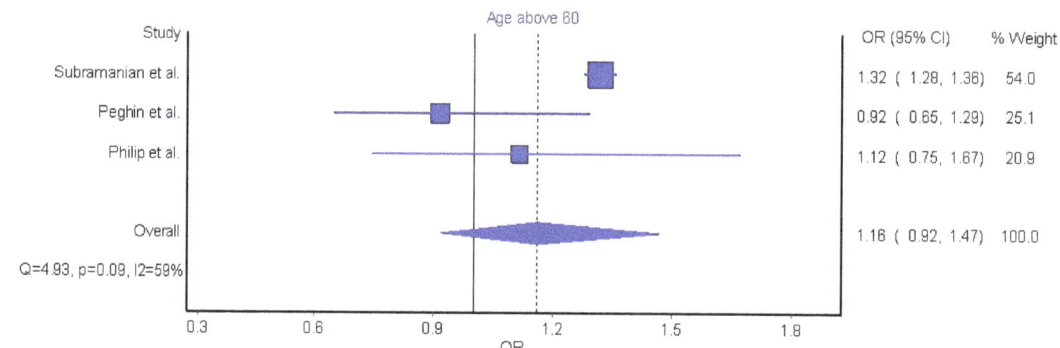

Figure 2. Pooled analysis of odds ratio (OR) for the association between age older than 60 years and the presence of long COVID-19 symptoms [32,42,44].

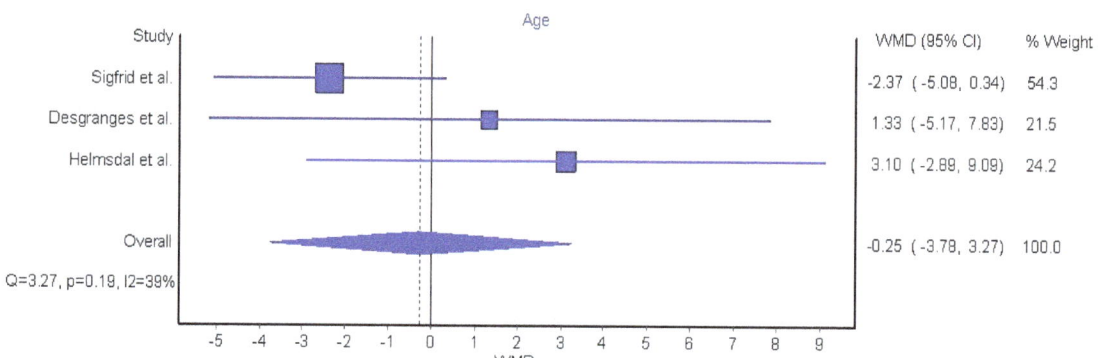

Figure 3. Pooled weighted mean difference (WMD) for the association between age as continuous variable and the presence of long COVID-19 symptoms [43,45,46].

3.3. Sex and Post-COVID-19 Condition

A total of 16 articles [32,42–56] including 504,044 COVID-19 survivors were used in the analysis of sex as a risk factor for developing long COVID-19 symptomatology (Table 3). Data were presented as OR, aOR, HR, aHR, and percentage. Seven articles used OR [32,47–52], two used aOR [45,53], another two used both OR and aOR [46,54], while three articles used percentage [43,44,55], one article used both percentage and OR [56], and one article used both HR and aHR [42].

Fourteen articles observed that female sex (n = 276,953) was associated with higher risk of long COVID-19 [32,42,45–56], whilst two articles (n = 475) reported that female sex was not associated with higher risk of long COVID-19 [43,44].

Seven articles (n = 386,234 COVID-19 patients who recovered from acute SARS-CoV-2 infection) were included in the meta-analysis due to their similarities in study design, definition of long COVID-19, as well as similarities in data presentation [32,42–46,50]. The meta-analysis revealed that female sex was significantly associated with nearly 50% higher risk (OR 1.48, 95% CI 1.17 to 1.86, Q = 17.2, p = 0.01, I2: 65%, Figure 4) of long COVID-19 symptomatology.

Table 3. Studies investigating the effect of sex in long COVID-19 symptomatology [32,42–55].

Author	Country Study Period	Study Design Sample Size	Age	Symptoms Assessment	Post-COVID-19 Symptoms	Main Findings
Bai et al., 2021	Italy 15 April 2020–15 December 2020	Prospective Cohort n = 377 Female 137	Median age 57 y (IQR 49–68)	Interview and physical examination Impact of Event Scale-Revised (IES-R)	Anosmia, Dysgeusia, Gastrointestinal symptoms, Fever, Joint pain, Myalgia, Dyspnea at rest, Exertional dyspnea, Fatigue, Brain fog, PTSD, Depression, Anxiety	Female Sex Risk Long COVID-19 OR 2.78 (95% CI 1.68–4.62) * Long COVID-19 AOR 3.32 (95% CI 1.78–6.17) *
Pela et al., 2022	Italy Follow-up: May 2020–March 2021	Cohort n = 223 Female 89	Mean age 59 y (SD 13)	Retrospective Medical records Prospective Long COVID-19 reevaluation	Dyspnea, Cough, Fatigue, Chest pain, Palpitations, Myalgia, Sleep disturbance	Female Sex Risk Dyspnea OR 2.35 (95% CI 1.12–4.94) * Fatigue OR 6.72 (95% CI 2.34–19.26) * Chest pain OR 2.04 (95% CI 1.00–4.15) * Palpitation OR 2.30 (95% CI 1.14–4.65) *
Sigfrid et al., 2021	UK NR	Prospective Cohort n = 327 Female 135	Media age 60 y (IQR 51.7–67.7)	Washington group short scale MRC Dyspnea Scale EQ5D-5L	Fatigue, Breathlessness, Sleep problems, Headache, Limb weakness, Muscle pain, Joint pain, Dizziness, Palpitations, Ocular problems, Stomach pain, Diarrhea, Cough, Chest pain, Loss of smell, Fever, Loss of taste, Nausea, Vomiting, Skin rashes	Female Sex < 50 years Risk Long COVID-19 (AOR 5.09, 95% CI 1.64–15.74) * Fatigue (AOR 2.06, 95% CI 0.81–3.31) Breathlessness (AOR 7.15, 95% CI 2.24–22.83) *
Fernandez-de-las-Peñas et al., 2022	Spain 10 March 2020–31 May 2020	Cross-sectional n = 1969 Female 915	Mean age 61 y (SD 16)	Telephone interview	Fatigue, Dyspnea at rest, Dyspnea at exertion, Pain, Memory loss, Brain fog, Concentration loss, Hair loss, Palpitations, Skin rashes, Diarrhea, Voice problems, Gastrointestinal problems, Ageusia, Anosmia, Ocular Problems, Throat pain, Anxiety/Depression, Sleep quality	Female Sex Risk Symptoms (AOR 2.54, 95% CI 1.67–3.86) * Fatigue (AOR 1.51, 95% CI 1.04–2.20) * Dyspnea rest (AOR 1.42, 95% CI 1.08–1.88) * Dyspnea exertion (AOR 1.4, 95% CI 1.10–1.79) * Pain (AOR 1.34, 95% CI 1.05–1.72) * Hair loss (AOR 4.52, 95% CI 2.78–7.36) * Ocular problems (AOR 1.98, 95% CI 1.18–3.31) * Depression (AOR 1.60, 95% CI 1.00–2.57) * Sleep quality (AOR 1.63, 95% CI 1.09–2.43) *
Gebhard et al., 2022	Switzerland February 2020–December 2020	Prospective cohort n = 2927 Female 1346	NR	Self-reported questionnaires	Dyspnea, Reduced exercise performance, Changes in smell and taste	Females reported at least one persistent symptom than males (43.5% vs. 32.0%, $p < 0.001$) The higher prevalence of PASC in females was observed in both outpatients (40.5% in females vs. 25.4% in males, $p < 0.001$) and hospitalized patients (63.1% in females vs. 55.2% in males, $p < 0.001$)
Tleyjeh et al., 2022	Saudi Arabia May 2020–July 2020	Cohort n = 222 Female 51	Range > 18 y	Medical research council (MRC) dyspnea scale Metabolic equivalent of task (MET) score Chronic fatigability syndrome questionnaire	Breathlessness, Exercise intolerance, Chronic fatigue, Poor mental well-being	Female Sex Risk Exertional Dyspnea OR 4.36 (95% CI 2.25–8.46) * Lower MET exercise tolerance score OR 0.19 (95% CI 0.09–0.42) * Chronic Fatigability Syndrome OR 3.97 (95% CI 1.85–8.49) *
Desgranges et al., 2022	Switzerland 26 February–27 April 2020	Prospective cohort n = 418 Female 261	Median age 41 y (IQR 31–54)	Structured and standardized phone survey	Fatigue, Smell or taste disorder, Dyspnea, Headache, Memory impairment, Hair loss, Sleep disorders	Female Sex Risk Symptoms AOR 1.67 (95% CI 1.09–2.56) * Dyspnea AOR 1.71 (95% CI 0.93–3.16) Smell/taste disorder AOR 1.9 (95% CI 1.09–3.22) * Fatigue AOR 1.61 (95% CI 1.00–2.59) *

Table 3. Cont.

Author	Country Study Period	Study Design Sample Size	Age	Symptoms Assessment	Post-COVID-19 Symptoms	Main Findings
Garcia-Abellán at al., 2021	Spain 10 March–30 June 2020	Prospective longitudinal study n = 146 Female 58	Median age 65 y (IQR 55–75)	Self-rated COVID-19 symptom questionnaire (CSQ)	Fatigue, Myalgia, Sweating, Headache, Cough, Difficulty breathing, Congestion, Sore throat, Anosmia, Diarrhea, Vomiting, Abdominal pain	Female Sex Risk Highest COVID-19 symptom questionnaire (CSQ) scores OR 2.41 (95% CI 1.20–4.82). *
Asadi-Pooya et al., 2021	Iran 19 February 2020–20 November 2020	Retrospective observational study n = 4681 Female 2203	Mean age 52 y (SD 15)	Telephone interview	Weakness, Muscle pain, Fatigue, Sleep difficulty, Palpitations, Cough, Brain fog, Walking intolerance	Female Sex Risk Long COVID-19 Symptoms OR1.26 (95% CI1.12–1.43) *
Munblit et al., 2021	Russia 8 April 2020–10 July 2020	Longitudinal cohort study n = 2649 Female 1353	Median age 56 y (IQR 46–66)	Study case report form (CRF) British Medical Research Council (MRC) dyspnoea scale EQ-5D-5L WHODAS 2.0	Fatigue, Breathlessness, Forgetfulness, Muscle weakness, Ocular problems, Hair loss, Sleeping problem	Female Sex Risk Symptoms OR1.83 (95% CI 1.55–2.17) * Fatigue OR1.67 (95% CI 1.39–2.02) * Neurological OR2.03 (95% CI 1.60–2.58) * Mood OR1.83 (95% CI 1.41–2.40) * Dermatological OR3.26 (95% CI 2.36–4.57) * Gastrointestinal OR2.50 (95% CI 1.64–3.89) * Sensory OR1.73 (95% CI 2.06–2.89) * Respiratory OR1.31 (95% CI 1.06–1.62) *
Chudzik et al., 2022	Poland 1 September 2020–30 September 2021	Retrospective cohort n = 2218 Female 1410	Mean age 54 y (SD 13.5)	Health questionnaire	Fatigue, Headache, Cough Brain fog, Dyspnoea, Hair loss, Olfactory dysfunction, Osteoarticular pain	Female Sex Risk Symptoms OR 1.44 (95% CI 1.20–1.72) * Brain fog OR1.15 (95% CI0.88–1.51) Fatigue OR1.06 (95% CI0.89–1.28)
Peghin et al., 2021	Italy March 2020–November 2020	Cohort n = 599 Female 320	Mean age 53 y (SD 15.8)	Questionnaire via telephone interview	Dyspnea, Cough, Fatigue, Myalgia, Chest Pain, Anosmia/Dysgeusia, Headache, Arthralgia, Neurological Disorders Anxiety/Depression, Sleep Disorders, Brain Fog, Skin Lesions, Gastrointestinal Disorders, Hair Loss, Nose Cold, Sneezing, Odynophagia, Ocular Problems	Female Sex Risk Long COVID-19 Symptoms OR 1.55 (95% CI 1.05–2.27) *
Philip et al., 2022	UK October 2020	Retrospective cohort n = 4500	Range age 50–59 y	Asthma UK and British Lung Foundation survey	Fatigue, Breathlessness, Pain (chest or whole body)	No association between female sex and long COVID-19 symptoms
Helmsdal et al., 2022	Faroe Islands March 2020–January 2022	Cohort n= 180 Female 93	Mean age 40 y (SD 19.4)	Standardized questionnaire via telephone interview	Fatigue, affected taste, affected smell, Headache, Arthralgia, Dyspnea, Myalgia, Skin rashes, Rhinorrhea, Chest tightness, Cough, Nausea, Diarrhea, Fever, Sore throat	No association between female sex and long COVID-19 symptoms
Subramanian et al., 2022	United Kingdom 31 January 2020–15 April 2021	Retrospective matched cohort study Non-hospitalized COVID-19 survivors n = 486,149 Matched patients with no evidence of COVID-19 n = 1,944,580	Patients infected with SARS-CoV-2 Mean age 44.1 y (SD 17.0) Comparator cohort Mean age 43.8 y (SD 16.9)	Interviews and questionnaires	Anosmia, Hair loss, Sneezing, Ejaculation difficulty, Reduced libido, Shortness of breath at rest, Fatigue, Chest pain, Hoarse voice, Fever	Female Sex Risk Long COVID-19 Symptoms HR 1.86 (95% CI 1.81–1.90) * aHR 1.52 (95% CI 1.48–1.56) *

WHODAS: Washington disability score and World Health Organization Disability Assessment Schedule. * Statistically significant ($p < 0.05$). NR: not reported; y: years; SD: standard deviation.

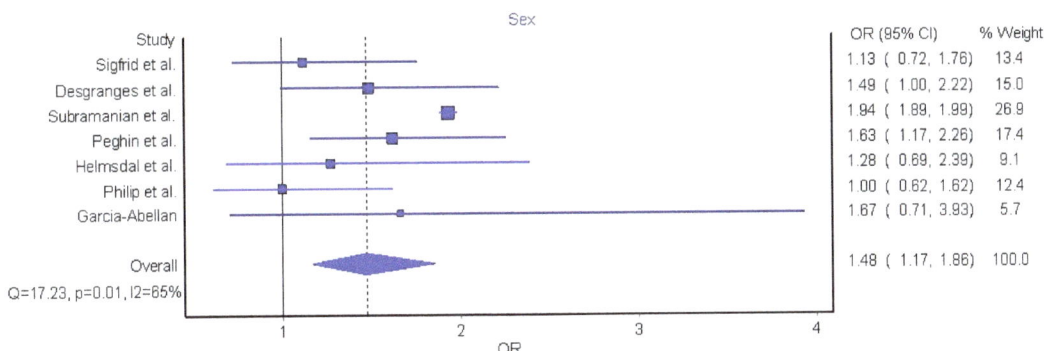

Figure 4. Pooled analysis of odds ratio (OR) for the association between sex and the presence of long COVID-19 [32,42–46,50].

3.4. Medical Comorbidities and Post-COVID-19 Condition

A total of 12 articles with 677,045 COVID-19 survivors were analyzed for association between long COVID-19 and comorbidities (Table 5) [29,39,44,52,56–63]. Four comorbidities were included: pulmonary disease (n = 4), diabetes (n = 1), obesity (n = 6), and organ transplantation (n = 1). Data were presented as means, medians, percentages, odds ratio (OR), and incident rate ratio (IRR). One study used mean [61], one used both median and percentage [59], three used percentage only [44], five used OR [29,39,52,55,60], and two used both OR and IRR [57,59].

Three articles on pulmonary disease revealed an association between asthma and longer symptom duration among patients recovering from COVID-19 [29,44,60]. However, both asthma and chronic pulmonary disease were not associated with long COVID-19 in one study [52]. For diabetes, no difference was found in the number of long COVID-19 symptoms among diabetic and non-diabetic patients [57]. For obesity, all six articles noted that this metabolic disease was associated with worse health due to increased number of long COVID-19 symptoms [39,59], longer persistence of symptoms [56,63], more presence of pathological pulmonary limitations [61], and metabolic abnormalities [58]. Meanwhile, one study on kidney transplant patients revealed that patients have higher susceptibility to developing long COVID-19 symptoms, although this did not affect mortality rate [62].

3.5. Risk of Bias

From out of 18 papers evaluating age as risk factor [26–43], three [35,41,43] were classified as low risk of bias (green), five [26,37–40] as moderate risk of bias (yellow), and the remaining ten [27–29,31–34,36,42,51] as high risk of bias (red). Figure 5 visually graphs that the most frequent risk of bias was adjustment for other prognostic factor (i.e., if important potential confounding factors were appropriately accounted for), which was properly performed in just one study [41].

On the other hand, from 16 papers evaluating sex as a risk factor [32,42–56], four studies [45,50,53,55] were classified as low risk of bias (green), five [46,49,52,54,56] as moderate risk of bias (yellow), and the remaining seven [32,42–44,47,48,51] as high risk of bias (red). Figure 6 visually graphs that the most frequent risk of bias in this group of studies were adjustment for other prognostic factors and study attrition (i.e., the representativeness of the participants with follow-up data with respect to those originally enrolled in the study, selection bias).

Table 4. Studies investigating the effect of previous medical comorbidities in long COVID-19 symptomatology [29,39,44,52,53,56,58–63].

Author	Country Study Period	Study Design Sample Size	Age	Symptoms Assessment	Post-COVID-19 Symptoms	Main Findings
				Diabetes		
Fernandez-de-las-Peñas et al., 2021	Spain 1 March–31 May 2020	Case-control n = 435 Patients n = 145 Control n = 290	Patients Mean age 70.2 y (SD 13.2) Controls Mean age 70.4 y (SD 13.4)	Hospital medical records Telephonic interview	Fatigue, Dyspnea on exertion and at rest, Pain, Memory loss, Skin rashes, Gastrointestinal dis., Brain fog, Concentration loss, Ageusia, Ocular disorder, Anosmia, Tachycardia, Cough, Headache, Sleep, Depression/Anxiety	Number of post-COVID-19 symptoms (IRR 1.06, 95% CI 0.92–1.24) Fatigue (OR 1.45, 95% CI 0.93–2.25) Dyspnea (OR 0.97, 95% CI 0.64–1.47) Pain (OR 0.951, 95% CI 0.76–1.18) Anxiety (OR 1.30, 95% CI 0.77–2.20) Depression (OR 1.31, 95% CI 0.79–2.17) Poor sleep (OR 1.34, 95% CI 0.89–2.03)
				Obesity		
Lacavalerie et al., 2022	France October 2020–June 2021	Retrospective observational n = 80 Patients n = 33 Controls n = 18 n = 29	Patients Mean age 60 y (SD 11) Controls Mean age 50 y (SD 13)	Clinical evaluation with spirometry, cardiopulmonary and exercise testing	Fatigue, Dyspnea, Chest pain, Pulmonary function test, Cardiopulmonary exercise testing	Non-obese vs. obese, p value Pulmonary function test Predicted FEV1 (%) 87 ± 13/75 ± 13 p = 0.002 * Predicted FVC (%) 82 ± 16/74 ± 14 p = 0.04 * TLC (%) 79 ± 9/69 ± 12 p = 0.003 * RV (%) 71 ± 25/86 ± 24 p = 0.04 * KCO (%)100 ± 11/108 ± 12 p = 0.03 * Cardiopulmonary exercise testing Peak VE/VO2 35 ± 5/39 ± 7 p = 0.011 * Ventilatory reserve (%) 40 ± 14/25 ± 21 p = 0.011 * VE VCO2 slope 34 ± 6/31 ± 4 p = 0.045 * Peak SpO2 (%) 98 ± 2/96 ± 3 p = 0.036 *
Fernandez-de-las-Peñas et al., 2022	Spain 1 March 2020–31 March 2021	Case-control n = 264 Patients n = 88 Controls n = 176	Patients Mean age 52 y (SD 14.5) Controls Mean age 52.2 y (SD 14.2)	Hospital medical records Telephonic interview	Fatigue, Dyspnea, Memory loss, Skin rashes, Brain Fog, Gastrointestinal disorders, Concentration loss, Ageusia, Ocular disorders, Tachycardia, Pain, Anosmia, Headache, Sleep, Depression/Anxiety	Number of post-COVID-19 symptoms (IRR 1.51, 95% CI 1.24–1.84) * Sleep quality (OR 2.27, 95% CI 1.34–3.86) * Fatigue (OR 1.39; 95% CI 0.79–2.43) Dyspnea (OR 1.41, 95% CI 0.79–2.53) Anxiety (OR 1.75, 95% CI 0.82–3.72) Depression (OR 0.83, 95% CI 0.40–1.73)
Loosen et al., 2022	Germany 1 March 2020–31 March 2021	Retrospective Observational n = 50,402	Mean age 48.8 y (SD 19.3)	Medical record	Fatigue, Abnormalities of breathing, Loss of smell and taste, disturbances in attention	Obesity (OR 1.25 95% CI 1.08–1.44) * Hypertension (OR 1.31, 95% CI 1.15–1.48) *
Shang et al., 2021	Wuhan, China 20 February–20 March 2020	Cohort Study n = 118 Patients n = 53 Controls n = 65	Patients Mean age 51 y (IQR 41–58) Controls Mean age 57 y (IQR 48–62)	Interview, Physical exam, Blood sample, Lung function test, CT scan	Shortness of breath, Fatigue, Sleep problems, Joint pain, Smell disorder, Diarrhea, Constipation	No differences in the prevalence of long COVID-19 Symptoms existed between obese and non-obese patients.
Whitaker et al., 2022	UK 15–28 September 2020 27 October–10 November 2020 25 January–8 February 2021 12–25 May 2021	Cohort n = 606,434	Age >18	Online/telephone survey	Tiredness, Tight chest, Sore throat, Sore eyes, Sneezing, Shortness of breath, Fatigue, Runny nose, Skin lesions, Cough, Pain symptoms, Nausea, Vomiting, Loss of taste or smell, Hoarse voice, Headache, Dizziness, Difficulty sleeping, Diarrhoea, Chest pain, Abdominal pain	Persistence of one or more symptoms for 12 weeks or more Obesity (OR 1.39, 95% CI 1.32–1.48) *

Table 5. Studies investigating the effect of previous medical comorbidities in long COVID-19 symptomatology [29,39,44,52,53,56,58–63].

Author	Country Study Period	Study Design Sample Size	Age	Symptoms Assessment	Post-COVID-19 Symptoms	Main Findings
				Obesity		
Chudzik et al., 2022	Poland 1 September 2020–30 September 2021	Retrospective observational n = 2218	Mean age = 53.8 ± 13.5 years	Health questionnaire	Cough, Dyspnea, Fatigue, Hair loss, Olfactory disturbances, Headache, Pain, Brain fog	Presence of overall persistent symptoms Obesity (OR1.16, 95% CI 0.96–1.41) Fatigue (OR 1.49, 95% CI 1.24–1.80) *
				Pulmonary Disease		
Sudre et al., 2021	UK 25 March–30 June 2020	Prospective cohort n = 8364 COVID-19 n = 4182 No COVID-19 n = 4182	Mean age 46 y	COVID-19 Symptom Study app1	Abdominal pain, Chest pain, Sore throat, Fatigue, Shortness of breath, Hoarse voice, Delirium, Diarrhea, Fever, Cough, Muscle pain, Anosmia, Headache	Presence of long COVID-19 symptoms Asthma (OR 2.14, 95% CI 1.55–2.96) *
Munblit et al., 2021	Russia 8 April–10 July 2020	Prospective cohort n = 2649	Median age 56 y	ISARIC Long-term Follow-up Study questionnaire	Fatigue, Shortness of breath, Forgetfulness	Asthma and chronic pulmonary disease were not associated with persistent symptoms overall, but asthma was associated with neurological (OR1.95, 95% CI 1.25–2.98) * and chronic pulmonary disease was associated with fatigue (OR 1.68, 95% CI 1.21–2.32) *
Philip et al., 2022	UK October 2020	Retrospective cohort n = 4500 COVID-19 n = 471 No COVID-19 n = 3036 COVID-19 n = 972	Range age 50–59 y	Asthma UK and British Lung Foundation survey	Fatigue, Breathlessness, Pain (chest or whole body)	For many people with asthma, COVID-19 is associated with prolonged symptoms and worsening asthma control
Jia et al., 2022	USA March 2020–February 2021	Prospective cohort n = 637 Patients n = 617 Controls n = 20	Patients Mean age 51 y Controls Mean age 54 y	Survey	Cough, Shortness of breath, Fever, Nausea, Vomiting	Comorbid lung disease, asthma and lower levels of initial IgG response to SARS-CoV-2 nucleocapsid antigen were associated with longer symptom duration (mean days: 55 versus 44 days; $p = 0.04$) *
				Transplant		
Oto et al., 2022	Turkey 15 March 2021–11 June 2021	Retrospective cohort n = 944 Patients n = 523 Control n = 421	Mean age 46 y	Survey	Respiratory symptoms	Persistence of respiratory symptoms without increased risk of acute rejection, BK and CMV infection, thromboembolic event or urinary tract infection

* Statistically significant ($p < 0.05$). y: years; SD: standard deviation.

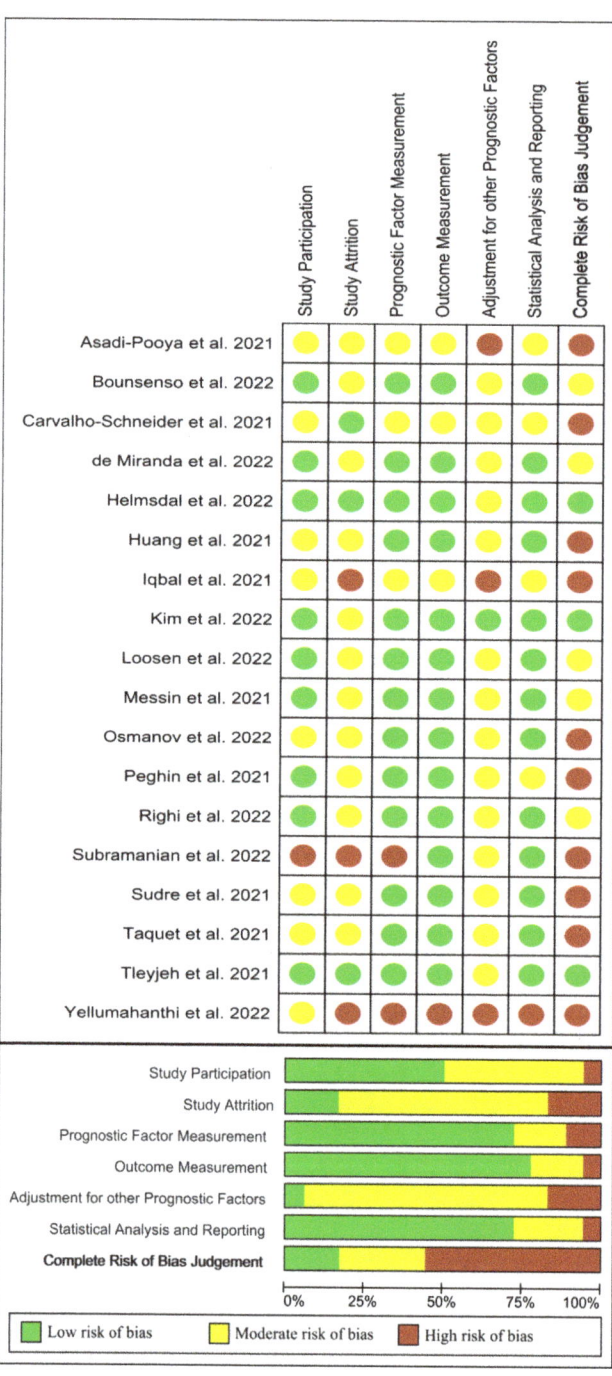

Figure 5. Plot of the risk of bias of those studies investigating age as a risk factor of long COVID-19 [10,26–33,35–43].

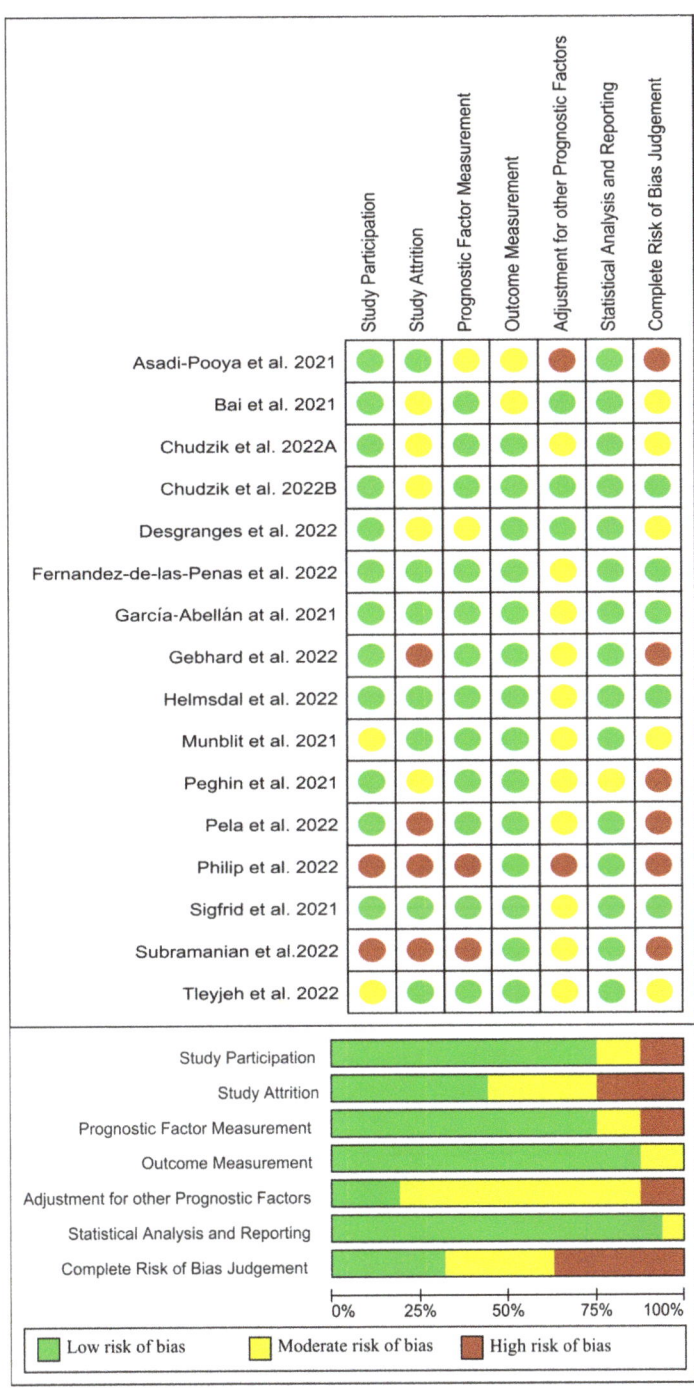

Figure 6. Plot of the risk of bias of those studies investigating sex as a risk factor of long COVID-19 [1,32,42–52,54–56].

Lastly, from 12 papers evaluating previous medical comorbidities as a risk factor [29,39,44,52,56–63], four [57–59,61] were classified as low risk of bias (green), two [52,62] as moderate risk of bias (yellow), and the remaining six [29,39,44,56,60,63] as high risk of bias (red). Figure 7 visually graphs that the most frequent risk of bias in this group of studies was concerned prognostic factor measurement (i.e., if the prognostic factors were measured in a similar way for all the participants).

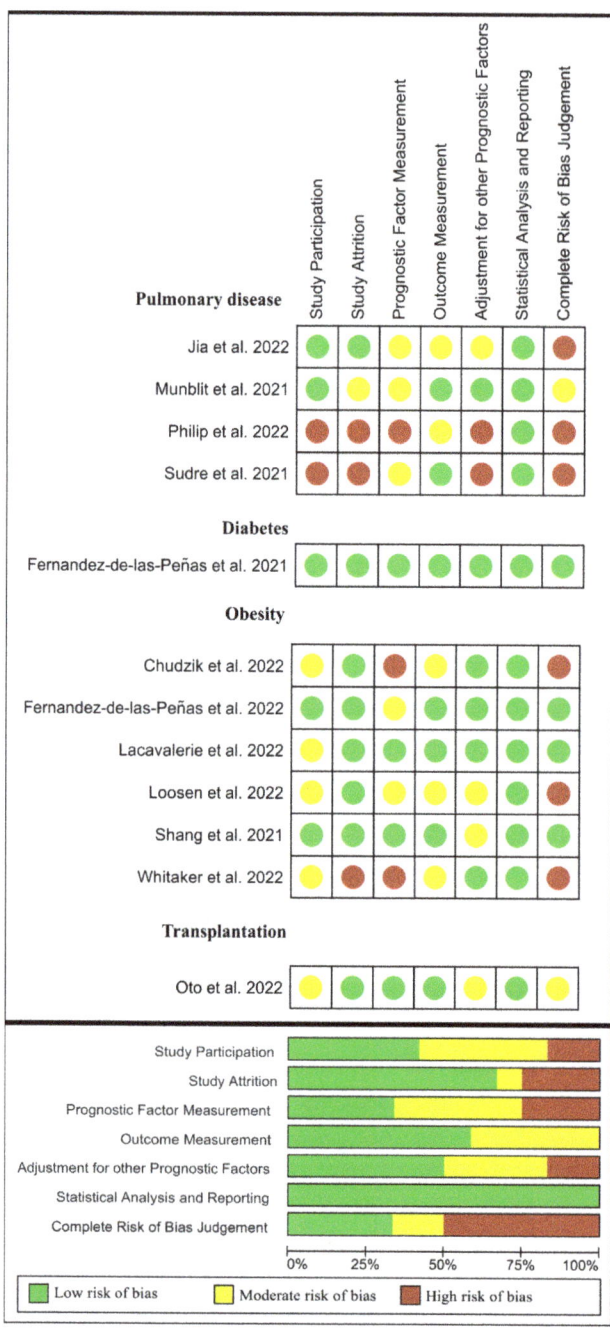

Figure 7. Plot of the risk of bias of those studies investigating medical comorbidities as a risk factor of long COVID-19 [4,29,39,44,52,53,56,58,60–63].

4. Discussion

This systematic review and meta-analysis explored the association of long COVID-19 with risk factors not directly related to an acute SARS-CoV-2 infection (i.e., pre-infection factors), including age, sex, or previous comorbidities. The results support that female sex may be a predictor of long COVID-19 while old age was reported to be associated with long COVID-19 in single studies; however, the pooled evidence was not significant. Finally, prior medical comorbidities can also be potential predictors of long COVID-19 symptoms. These results should be considered with caution because most studies exhibited moderate to high risk of bias.

4.1. Old Age and Long COVID-19

Old age is an important risk factor of poor outcomes in COVID-19 hospitalization [64]; however, the impact of age on long COVID-19 is controversial. Old age is associated with higher risk of long COVID-19 symptomatology in single studies and in two previous reviews [10,12], but not in the meta-analysis by Maglietta et al. [11]. Results from our qualitative analysis suggest that older adults can develop more long COVID-19 symptoms than younger adults; however, this assumption was not supported when pooling data into a meta-analysis. We conducted two meta-analyses, the first one categorizing those adults older than 60 years (Figure 2), and a second one considering age as a continuous variable (Figure 3); neither analysis revealed an association between old age and risk of developing long COVID-19. Nevertheless, the number of studies pooled in our analyses of age was notably limited (n = 3). Our data are consistent with the meta-analysis of Maglietta et al. [11] but disagree with Thompson et al. [12]. Several differences can explain the discrepancy with Thompson et al. [12]. It is possible that the use of a different definition of long COVID-19 by these authors [12] can lead to inconclusive comparisons of results. In addition, Thompson et al. [12] did not pool data of age and long COVID-19 into a meta-analysis, but only calculated regression of proportions of subjects at each age group developing long COVID-19 symptoms. The significance of old age as a risk factor for long COVID-19 development requires further investigation. In fact, just three out of eighteen papers (16%) analyzing age as prognostic factor showed low risk of bias. The most significant bias of these studies was the proper control of other cofounding factors observed in older people, i.e., higher presence of medical comorbidities, or longer hospitalization stay, which can also be associated with long COVID-19.

4.2. Female Sex and Long COVID-19

Sex is another important risk factor which has been studied in relation to COVID-19 and long COVID-19. Evidence supports that men and women exhibit the same probability of being infected by SARS-CoV-2; however, males are at a higher risk of worse outcomes and death than females during the acute phase of infection [65]. Results from our systematic review and meta-analysis support that female sex may be associated with higher risk of developing long COVID-19 (OR 1.48, 95% CI 1.17 to 1.86). Our results are similar to those previously observed by Maglietta et al. [11], who also reported that female sex was associated with long COVID-19 symptoms (OR1.52, 95% CI 1.27–1.82), and with results (OR1.60, 95% CI 1.23–2.07) previously reported by Thompson et al. [12]. Based on available data, females are more vulnerable to develop long COVID-19 than males. Hence, considering sex differences in diagnosis, prevention and treatment are necessary, and fundamental steps towards precision medicine in COVID-19 [66]. Biological (i.e., hormones and immune responses), and sociocultural (i.e., sanitary-related behaviors, psychological stress, and inactivity) aspects play a significant role in creating sex-differences in long COVID-19 symptoms [48], although mechanisms behind increased risk of long COVID-19 in females remain unknown and warrant investigation.

4.3. Medical Comorbidities and Long COVID-19

Such as with old age, the presence of prior medical comorbidities (e.g., hypertension, obesity, diabetes, chronic kidney disease, cerebrovascular disease, chronic obstructive pulmonary disease, or cardiovascular disease) is known to induce a more severe COVID-19 disease progression [67,68]. A potential reason is that such comorbidities can contribute to degradation of angiotensin-converting enzyme 2 (ACE2). Since the SARS-CoV-2 virus uses this receptor as entry pathway in host cells, higher degradation of ACE2 could lead to a long-lasting inflammatory cytokine storm, oxidative stress, and hemostasis activation, which are all hallmarks of severe/critical COVID-19 illness [69]. Nevertheless, this hypothesis is not yet supported by the literature.

The current qualitative analysis suggests that prior comorbidities may contribute the risk of developing long COVID-19. Among different comorbidities, obesity seems to be associated; however, this assumption should be considered with caution at this stage, since potential cofounding factors, particularly those related to hospitalization (obese patients have more severe COVID-19 disease and higher hospitalization rates than non-obese patients), were not properly controlled in these studies. Moreover, the association of long COVID-19 with other medical comorbidities such as diabetes or transplants was only investigated in one prior study.

4.4. Strengths and Limitations

The results of this systematic review and meta-analysis should be considered according to potential strengths and limitations. Among the strengths, we conducted a systematic search of all the currently available evidence on factor not related to an acute SARS-CoV-2 infection but associated with higher risk of developing long COVID-19. This led to identification of thirty-eight studies. Second, this is the first time that several medical comorbidities have been systematically investigated as risk factors of long COVID-19.

One of the limitations is the lack of a consistent definition of long COVID-19 in available literatures. We included all identified studies within the qualitative analysis, but only those using the definition by Soriano et al. [2] of long COVID-19 were included in the meta-analyses. This assumption led to a small number of studies in the meta-analyses. Future studies using a more consistent definition of long COVID-19 are needed for improved quantification of the results. Another limitation is the lack of differentiation of risk factors between hospitalized and non-hospitalized patients. Similarly, no study investigating risk factors considered the SARS-CoV-2 variants of concern. Therefore, studies identifying long COVID-19 risk factors not directly associated with SARS-CoV-2 infection differentiating between hospitalized and non-hospitalized patients, and among different SARS-CoV-2 variants of concern are now needed. Finally, it should be considered that this systematic review and meta-analysis only investigated risk factors not associated with an acute SARS-CoV-2 infection. Other potential SARS-CoV-2-associated factors, such as severity of disease during the acute phase of infection or the number of COVID-19-associated onset symptoms have also been preliminarily identified as risk factors associated with long COVID-19 symptoms, particularly with respiratory symptoms [11]. Similarly, it is possible that some long COVID-19 symptoms can also be related to hospitalization factors which were also not investigated in this review.

5. Conclusions

The current review demonstrates that female sex and previous medical comorbidities may be predisposing factors for the development of long COVID-19 symptomatology. The current literature does not conclusively confirm that old age would significantly influence long COVID-19 risk. These results should be considered with caution due to moderate to high risk of bias in most published studies. These findings highlight the need for further research with improved control of confounding factors and use of a consistent and validated definition of long COVID-19.

Author Contributions: All the authors cited in the manuscript had substantial contributions to the concept and design, the execution of the work, or the analysis and interpretation of data; drafting or revising the manuscript and have read and approved the final version of the paper. K.I.N.: conceptualization, visualization, methodology, validation, formal analysis, data curation, writing—original draft, writing—review and editing. conceptualization, formal analysis, data curation, writing—review and editing. M.H.S.d.O.: methodology, validation, formal analysis, data curation, writing—original draft, writing—review and editing. P.J.P.: methodology, validation, formal analysis, data curation, writing—original draft, writing—review and editing. J.V.V.: methodology, validation, formal analysis, data curation, writing—original draft, writing—review and editing. I.M.: methodology, validation, formal analysis, data curation, writing—original draft, writing—review and editing. A.T.V.: methodology, validation, formal analysis, data curation, writing—original draft, writing—review and editing. F.C.P.: methodology, validation, formal analysis, data curation, writing—original draft, writing—review and editing. A.P.: methodology, validation, formal analysis, data curation, writing—original draft, writing—review and editing. N.G.: writing—review and editing. D.K.: writing—review and editing. M.M.L.G.: writing—review and editing. J.L.: writing—review and editing. G.L.: writing—review and editing. B.M.H.: writing—review and editing. C.F.-d.-l.-P.: conceptualization, visualization, validation, formal analysis, writing—review and editing. All authors have read and agreed to the published version of the manuscript.

Funding: The project was supported by a grant associated to the Fondo Europeo De Desarrollo Regional—Recursos REACT-UE del Programa Operativo de Madrid 2014–2020, en la línea de actuación de proyectos de I+D+i en materia de respuesta a COVID-19 (LONG COVID-19-EXP-CM). The sponsor had no role in the design, collection, management, analysis, or interpretation of the data, draft, review, or approval of the manuscript or its content. The authors were responsible for the decision to submit the manuscript for publication, and the sponsor did not participate in this decision.

Data Availability Statement: All data derived from the study are included in the paper.

Conflicts of Interest: The authors declare no conflict of interest.

References

1. Fernández-de-Las-Peñas, C. Long COVID: Current Definition. *Infection* **2022**, *50*, 285–286. [CrossRef] [PubMed]
2. Soriano, J.B.; Murthy, S.; Marshall, J.C.; Relan, P.; Diaz, J.V. A Clinical Case Definition of Post-COVID-19 Condition by a Delphi Consensus. *Lancet Infect. Dis.* **2022**, *22*, e102–e107. [CrossRef] [PubMed]
3. Han, Q.; Zheng, B.; Daines, L.; Sheikh, A. Long-Term Sequelae of COVID-19: A Systematic Review and Meta-Analysis of One-Year Follow-Up Studies on Post-COVID Symptoms. *Pathogens* **2022**, *11*, 269. [CrossRef]
4. Fernández-de-Las-Peñas, C.; Palacios-Ceña, D.; Gómez-Mayordomo, V.; Florencio, L.L.; Cuadrado, M.L.; Plaza-Manzano, G.; Navarro-Santana, M. Prevalence of Post-COVID-19 Symptoms in Hospitalized and Non-Hospitalized COVID-19 Survivors: A Systematic Review and Meta-Analysis. *Eur. J. Intern. Med.* **2021**, *92*, 55–70. [CrossRef] [PubMed]
5. Chen, C.; Haupert, S.R.; Zimmermann, L.; Shi, X.; Fritsche, L.G.; Mukherjee, B. Global Prevalence of Post COVID-19 Condition or Long COVID: A Meta-Analysis and Systematic Review. *J. Infect. Dis.* **2022**, *226*, 1593–1607. [CrossRef] [PubMed]
6. Yong, S.J. Long COVID or Post-COVID-19 Syndrome: Putative Pathophysiology, Risk Factors, and Treatments. *Infect. Dis.* **2021**, *53*, 737–754. [CrossRef] [PubMed]
7. Crook, H.; Raza, S.; Nowell, J.; Young, M.; Edison, P. Long Covid-Mechanisms, Risk Factors, and Management. *BMJ* **2021**, *374*, n1648. [CrossRef]
8. Akbarialiabad, H.; Taghrir, M.H.; Abdollahi, A.; Ghahramani, N.; Kumar, M.; Paydar, S.; Razani, B.; Mwangi, J.; Asadi-Pooya, A.A.; Malekmakan, L.; et al. Long COVID, a Comprehensive Systematic Scoping Review. *Infection* **2021**, *49*, 1163–1186. [CrossRef]
9. Nalbandian, A.; Sehgal, K.; Gupta, A.; Madhavan, M.V.; McGroder, C.; Stevens, J.S.; Cook, J.R.; Nordvig, A.S.; Shalev, D.; Sehrawat, T.S.; et al. Post-Acute COVID-19 Syndrome. *Nat. Med.* **2021**, *27*, 601–615. [CrossRef]
10. Iqbal, F.M.; Lam, K.; Sounderajah, V.; Clarke, J.M.; Ashrafian, H.; Darzi, A. Characteristics and Predictors of Acute and Chronic Post-COVID Syndrome: A Systematic Review and Meta-Analysis. *eClinicalMedicine* **2021**, *36*, 100899. [CrossRef]
11. Maglietta, G.; Diodati, F.; Puntoni, M.; Lazzarelli, S.; Marcomini, B.; Patrizi, L.; Caminiti, C. Prognostic Factors for Post-COVID-19 Syndrome: A Systematic Review and Meta-Analysis. *J. Clin. Med.* **2022**, *11*, 1541. [CrossRef] [PubMed]
12. Thompson, E.J.; Williams, D.M.; Walker, A.J.; Mitchell, R.E.; Niedzwiedz, C.L.; Yang, T.C.; Huggins, C.F.; Kwong, A.S.F.; Silverwood, R.J.; Di Gessa, G.; et al. Long COVID Burden and Risk Factors in 10 UK Longitudinal Studies and Electronic Health Records. *Nat. Commun.* **2022**, *13*, 3528. [CrossRef] [PubMed]
13. Overview I COVID-19 Rapid Guideline: Managing the Long-Term Effects of COVID-19 I Guidance I NICE. Available online: https://www.nice.org.uk/guidance/ng188 (accessed on 17 October 2022).

14. Page, M.J.; McKenzie, J.E.; Bossuyt, P.M.; Boutron, I.; Hoffmann, T.C.; Mulrow, C.D.; Shamseer, L.; Tetzlaff, J.M.; Akl, E.A.; Brennan, S.E.; et al. The PRISMA 2020 Statement: An Updated Guideline for Reporting Systematic Reviews. *BMJ* **2021**, *372*, n71. [CrossRef] [PubMed]
15. Riley, R.D.; Moons, K.G.M.; Snell, K.I.E.; Ensor, J.; Hooft, L.; Altman, D.G.; Hayden, J.; Collins, G.S.; Debray, T.P.A. A Guide to Systematic Review and Meta-Analysis of Prognostic Factor Studies. *BMJ* **2019**, *364*, k4597. [CrossRef]
16. Hayden, J.A.; van der Windt, D.A.; Cartwright, J.L.; Côté, P.; Bombardier, C. Assessing Bias in Studies of Prognostic Factors. *Ann. Intern. Med.* **2013**, *158*, 280–286. [CrossRef]
17. Grooten, W.J.A.; Tseli, E.; Äng, B.O.; Boersma, K.; Stålnacke, B.-M.; Gerdle, B.; Enthoven, P. Elaborating on the Assessment of the Risk of Bias in Prognostic Studies in Pain Rehabilitation Using QUIPS-Aspects of Interrater Agreement. *Diagn. Progn. Res.* **2019**, *3*, 5. [CrossRef]
18. Tosato, M.; Carfi, A.; Martis, I.; Pais, C.; Ciciarello, F.; Rota, E.; Tritto, M.; Salerno, A.; Zazzara, M.B.; Martone, A.M.; et al. Prevalence and Predictors of Persistence of COVID-19 Symptoms in Older Adults: A Single-Center Study. *J. Am. Med. Dir. Assoc.* **2021**, *22*, 1840–1844. [CrossRef]
19. Vanichkachorn, G.; Newcomb, R.; Cowl, C.T.; Murad, M.H.; Breeher, L.; Miller, S.; Trenary, M.; Neveau, D.; Higgins, S. Post-COVID-19 Syndrome (Long Haul Syndrome): Description of a Multidisciplinary Clinic at Mayo Clinic and Characteristics of the Initial Patient Cohort. *Mayo Clin. Proc.* **2021**, *96*, 1782–1791. [CrossRef]
20. Sadat Larijani, M.; Ashrafian, F.; Bagheri Amiri, F.; Banifazl, M.; Bavand, A.; Karami, A.; Asgari Shokooh, F.; Ramezani, A. Characterization of Long COVID-19 Manifestations and Its Associated Factors: A Prospective Cohort Study from Iran. *Microb. Pathog.* **2022**, *169*, 105618. [CrossRef]
21. Xie, Y.; Bowe, B.; Al-Aly, Z. Burdens of Post-Acute Sequelae of COVID-19 by Severity of Acute Infection, Demographics and Health Status. *Nat. Commun.* **2021**, *12*, 6571. [CrossRef]
22. Ocsovszky, Z.; Otohal, J.; Berényi, B.; Juhász, V.; Skoda, R.; Bokor, L.; Dohy, Z.; Szabó, L.; Nagy, G.; Becker, D.; et al. The Associations of Long-COVID Symptoms, Clinical Characteristics and Affective Psychological Constructs in a Non-Hospitalized Cohort. *Physiol. Int.* **2022**, *109*, 230–245. [CrossRef] [PubMed]
23. Elhadedy, M.A.; Marie, Y.; Halawa, A. COVID-19 in Renal Transplant Recipients: Case Series and a Brief Review of Current Evidence. *NEF* **2021**, *145*, 192–198. [CrossRef] [PubMed]
24. Qui, L.; Zhang, J.; Huang, Y.; Cheng, G.; Chen, Z.; Ming, C.; Lu, X.; Gong, N. Long-Term Clinical and Immunological Impact of Severe COVID-19 on a Living Kidney Transplant Recipient—A Case Report. *Front. Immunol.* **2021**, *12*, 3687. [CrossRef]
25. Bhoori, S.; Rossi, R.E.; Citterio, D.; Mazzaferro, V. COVID-19 in Long-Term Liver Transplant Patients: Preliminary Experience from an Italian Transplant Centre in Lombardy. *Lancet Gastroenterol. Hepatol* **2020**, *5*, 532–533. [CrossRef] [PubMed]
26. Buonsenso, D.; Munblit, D.; Pazukhina, E.; Ricchiuto, A.; Sinatti, D.; Zona, M.; De Matteis, A.; D'Ilario, F.; Gentili, C.; Lanni, R.; et al. Post-COVID Condition in Adults and Children Living in the Same Household in Italy: A Prospective Cohort Study Using the ISARIC Global Follow-Up Protocol. *Front. Pediatr.* **2022**, *10*, 447. [CrossRef] [PubMed]
27. Yellumahanthi, D.K.; Barnett, B.; Barnett, S.; Yellumahanthi, S. COVID-19 Infection: Its Lingering Symptoms in Adults. *Cureus* **2022**, *14*, e24736. [CrossRef]
28. Huang, C.; Huang, L.; Wang, Y.; Li, X.; Ren, L.; Gu, X.; Kang, L.; Guo, L.; Liu, M.; Zhou, X.; et al. 6-Month Consequences of COVID-19 in Patients Discharged from Hospital: A Cohort Study. *Lancet* **2021**, *397*, 220–232. [CrossRef] [PubMed]
29. Sudre, C.H.; Murray, B.; Varsavsky, T.; Graham, M.S.; Penfold, R.S.; Bowyer, R.C.; Pujol, J.C.; Klaser, K.; Antonelli, M.; Canas, L.S.; et al. Attributes and Predictors of Long COVID. *Nat. Med.* **2021**, *27*, 626–631. [CrossRef]
30. Asadi-Pooya, A.A.; Nemati, H.; Shahisavandi, M.; Akbari, A.; Emami, A.; Lotfi, M.; Rostamihosseinkhani, M.; Barzegar, Z.; Kabiri, M.; Zeraatpisheh, Z.; et al. Long COVID in Children and Adolescents. *World J. Pediatr.* **2021**, *17*, 495–499. [CrossRef]
31. Taquet, M.; Dercon, Q.; Luciano, S.; Geddes, J.R.; Husain, M.; Harrison, P.J. Incidence, Co-Occurrence, and Evolution of Long-COVID Features: A 6-Month Retrospective Cohort Study of 273,618 Survivors of COVID-19. *PLoS Med.* **2021**, *18*, e1003773. [CrossRef]
32. Peghin, M.; Palese, A.; Venturini, M.; De Martino, M.; Gerussi, V.; Graziano, E.; Bontempo, G.; Marrella, F.; Tommasini, A.; Fabris, M.; et al. Post-COVID-19 Symptoms 6 Months after Acute Infection among Hospitalized and Non-Hospitalized Patients. *Clin. Microbiol. Infect.* **2021**, *27*, 1507–1513. [CrossRef] [PubMed]
33. Carvalho-Schneider, C.; Laurent, E.; Lemaignen, A.; Beaufils, E.; Bourbao-Tournois, C.; Laribi, S.; Flament, T.; Ferreira-Maldent, N.; Bruyère, F.; Stefic, K.; et al. Follow-up of Adults with Noncritical COVID-19 Two Months after Symptom Onset. *Clin. Microbiol. Infect.* **2021**, *27*, 258–263. [CrossRef] [PubMed]
34. Iqbal, A.; Iqbal, K.; Arshad Ali, S.; Azim, D.; Farid, E.; Baig, M.D.; Bin Arif, T.; Raza, M. The COVID-19 Sequelae: A Cross-Sectional Evaluation of Post-Recovery Symptoms and the Need for Rehabilitation of COVID-19 Survivors. *Cureus* **2021**, *13*, e13080. [CrossRef]
35. Tleyjeh, I.M.; Saddik, B.; AlSwaidan, N.; AlAnazi, A.; Ramakrishnan, R.K.; Alhazmi, D.; Aloufi, A.; AlSumait, F.; Berbari, E.; Halwani, R. Prevalence and Predictors of Post-Acute COVID-19 Syndrome (PACS) after Hospital Discharge: A Cohort Study with 4 Months Median Follow-Up. *PLoS ONE* **2021**, *16*, e0260568. [CrossRef]
36. Osmanov, I.M.; Spiridonova, E.; Bobkova, P.; Gamirova, A.; Shikhaleva, A.; Andreeva, M.; Blyuss, O.; El-Taravi, Y.; DunnGalvin, A.; Comberiati, P.; et al. Risk Factors for Post-COVID-19 Condition in Previously Hospitalised Children Using the ISARIC Global Follow-up Protocol: A Prospective Cohort Study. *Eur. Respir. J.* **2022**, *59*, 2101341. [CrossRef]

57. Righi, E.; Mirandola, M.; Mazzaferri, F.; Dossi, G.; Razzaboni, E.; Zaffagnini, A.; Ivaldi, F.; Visentin, A.; Lambertenghi, L.; Arena, C.; et al. Determinants of Persistence of Symptoms and Impact on Physical and Mental Wellbeing in Long COVID: A Prospective Cohort Study. *J. Infect.* **2022**, *84*, 566–572. [CrossRef] [PubMed]

58. de Miranda, D.A.P.; Gomes, S.V.C.; Filgueiras, P.S.; Corsini, C.A.; Almeida, N.B.F.; Silva, R.A.; Medeiros, M.I.V.A.R.C.; Vilela, R.V.R.; Fernandes, G.R.; Grenfell, R.F.Q. Long COVID-19 Syndrome: A 14-Months Longitudinal Study during the Two First Epidemic Peaks in Southeast Brazil. *Trans. R. Soc. Trop. Med. Hyg.* **2022**, *116*, 1007–1014. [CrossRef] [PubMed]

59. Loosen, S.H.; Jensen, B.-E.O.; Tanislav, C.; Luedde, T.; Roderburg, C.; Kostev, K. Obesity and Lipid Metabolism Disorders Determine the Risk for Development of Long COVID Syndrome: A Cross-Sectional Study from 50,402 COVID-19 Patients. *Infection* **2022**, *50*, 1165–1170. [CrossRef]

60. Messin, L.; Puyraveau, M.; Benabdallah, Y.; Lepiller, Q.; Gendrin, V.; Zayet, S.; Klopfenstein, T.; Toko, L.; Pierron, A.; Royer, P.-Y. COVEVOL: Natural Evolution at 6 Months of COVID-19. *Viruses* **2021**, *13*, 2151. [CrossRef]

61. Kim, Y.; Kim, S.-W.; Chang, H.-H.; Kwon, K.T.; Hwang, S.; Bae, S. One Year Follow-Up of COVID-19 Related Symptoms and Patient Quality of Life: A Prospective Cohort Study. *Yonsei Med. J.* **2022**, *63*, 499–510. [CrossRef]

62. Subramanian, A.; Nirantharakumar, K.; Hughes, S.; Myles, P.; Williams, T.; Gokhale, K.M.; Taverner, T.; Chandan, J.S.; Brown, K.; Simms-Williams, N.; et al. Symptoms and Risk Factors for Long COVID in Non-Hospitalized Adults. *Nat. Med.* **2022**, *28*, 1706–1714. [CrossRef] [PubMed]

63. Helmsdal, G.; Hanusson, K.D.; Kristiansen, M.F.; Foldbo, B.M.; Danielsen, M.E.; Steig, B.Á.; Gaini, S.; Strøm, M.; Weihe, P.; Petersen, M.S. Long COVID in the Long Run—23-Month Follow-up Study of Persistent Symptoms. *Open Forum. Infect. Dis.* **2022**, *9*, ofac270. [CrossRef] [PubMed]

64. Philip, K.E.J.; Buttery, S.; Williams, P.; Vijayakumar, B.; Tonkin, J.; Cumella, A.; Renwick, L.; Ogden, L.; Quint, J.K.; Johnston, S.L.; et al. Impact of COVID-19 on People with Asthma: A Mixed Methods Analysis from a UK Wide Survey. *BMJ Open Respir. Res.* **2022**, *9*, e001056. [CrossRef]

65. Sigfrid, L.; Drake, T.M.; Pauley, E.; Jesudason, E.C.; Olliaro, P.; Lim, W.S.; Gillesen, A.; Berry, C.; Lowe, D.J.; McPeake, J.; et al. Long Covid in Adults Discharged from UK Hospitals after Covid-19: A Prospective, Multicentre Cohort Study Using the ISARIC WHO Clinical Characterisation Protocol. *Lancet Reg. Health Eur.* **2021**, *8*, 100186. [CrossRef]

66. Desgranges, F.; Tadini, E.; Munting, A.; Regina, J.; Filippidis, P.; Viala, B.; Karachalias, E.; Suttels, V.; Haefliger, D.; Kampouri, E.; et al. Post-COVID-19 Syndrome in Outpatients: A Cohort Study. *J. Gen. Intern. Med.* **2022**, *37*, 1943–1952. [CrossRef] [PubMed]

67. Pelà, G.; Goldoni, M.; Solinas, E.; Cavalli, C.; Tagliaferri, S.; Ranzieri, S.; Frizzelli, A.; Marchi, L.; Mori, P.A.; Majori, M.; et al. Sex-Related Differences in Long-COVID-19 Syndrome. *J. Women's Health* **2022**, *31*, 620–630. [CrossRef] [PubMed]

68. Gebhard, C.E.; Sütsch, C.; Bengs, S.; Todorov, A.; Deforth, M.; Buehler, K.P.; Meisel, A.; Schuepbach, R.A.; Zinkernagel, A.S.; Brugger, S.D.; et al. Understanding the Impact of Sociocultural Gender on Post-Acute Sequelae of COVID-19: A Bayesian Approach. *medRxiv* **2021**. [CrossRef]

69. Tleyjeh, I.M.; Saddik, B.; Ramakrishnan, R.K.; AlSwaidan, N.; AlAnazi, A.; Alhazmi, D.; Aloufi, A.; AlSumait, F.; Berbari, E.F.; Halwani, R. Long Term Predictors of Breathlessness, Exercise Intolerance, Chronic Fatigue and Well-Being in Hospitalized Patients with COVID-19: A Cohort Study with 4 Months Median Follow-Up. *J. Infect. Public Health* **2022**, *15*, 21–28. [CrossRef]

70. García-Abellán, J.; Padilla, S.; Fernández-González, M.; García, J.A.; Agulló, V.; Andreo, M.; Ruiz, S.; Galiana, A.; Gutiérrez, F.; Masiá, M. Antibody Response to SARS-CoV-2 Is Associated with Long-Term Clinical Outcome in Patients with COVID-19: A Longitudinal Study. *J. Clin. Immunol.* **2021**, *41*, 1490–1501. [CrossRef]

71. Asadi-Pooya, A.A.; Akbari, A.; Emami, A.; Lotfi, M.; Rostamihosseinkhani, M.; Nemati, H.; Barzegar, Z.; Kabiri, M.; Zeraatpisheh, Z.; Farjoud-Kouhanjani, M.; et al. Risk Factors Associated with Long COVID Syndrome: A Retrospective Study. *Iran J. Med. Sci.* **2021**, *46*, 428–436. [CrossRef]

72. Munblit, D.; Bobkova, P.; Spiridonova, E.; Shikhaleva, A.; Gamirova, A.; Blyuss, O.; Nekliudov, N.; Bugaeva, P.; Andreeva, M.; DunnGalvin, A.; et al. Incidence and Risk Factors for Persistent Symptoms in Adults Previously Hospitalized for COVID-19. *Clin. Exp. Allergy* **2021**, *51*, 1107–1120. [CrossRef] [PubMed]

73. Fernández-de-las-Peñas, C.; Martín-Guerrero, J.D.; Pellicer-Valero, Ó.J.; Navarro-Pardo, E.; Gómez-Mayordomo, V.; Cuadrado, M.L.; Arias-Navalón, J.A.; Cigarán-Méndez, M.; Hernández-Barrera, V.; Arendt-Nielsen, L. Female Sex Is a Risk Factor Associated with Long-Term Post-COVID Related-Symptoms but Not with COVID-19 Symptoms: The LONG-COVID-EXP-CM Multicenter Study. *JCM* **2022**, *11*, 413. [CrossRef] [PubMed]

74. Bai, F.; Tomasoni, D.; Falcinella, C.; Barbanotti, D.; Castoldi, R.; Mulè, G.; Augello, M.; Mondatore, D.; Allegrini, M.; Cona, A.; et al. Female Gender Is Associated with Long COVID Syndrome: A Prospective Cohort Study. *Clin. Microbiol. Infect.* **2022**, *28*, e9–e611. [CrossRef] [PubMed]

75. Chudzik, M.; Lewek, J.; Kapusta, J.; Banach, M.; Jankowski, P.; Bielecka-Dabrowa, A. Predictors of Long COVID in Patients without Comorbidities: Data from the Polish Long-COVID Cardiovascular (PoLoCOV-CVD) Study. *JCM* **2022**, *11*, 4980. [CrossRef]

76. Chudzik, M.; Babicki, M.; Kapusta, J.; Kałuzińska-Kołat, Ż.; Kołat, D.; Jankowski, P.; Mastalerz-Migas, A. Long-COVID Clinical Features and Risk Factors: A Retrospective Analysis of Patients from the STOP-COVID Registry of the PoLoCOV Study. *Viruses* **2022**, *14*, 1755. [CrossRef]

77. Fernández-de-las-Peñas, C.; Guijarro, C.; Torres-Macho, J.; Velasco-Arribas, M.; Plaza-Canteli, S.; Hernández-Barrera, V.; Arias-Navalón, J.A. Diabetes and the Risk of Long-Term Post-COVID Symptoms. *Diabetes* **2021**, *70*, 2917–2921. [CrossRef]

58. Shang, L.; Wang, L.; Zhou, F.; Li, J.; Liu, Y.; Yang, S. Long-term Effects of Obesity on COVID-19 Patients Discharged from Hospital. *Immun. Inflamm. Dis.* **2021**, *9*, 1678–1685. [CrossRef]
59. Fernández-de-las-Peñas, C.; Torres-Macho, J.; Elvira-Martínez, C.M.; Molina-Trigueros, L.J.; Sebastián-Viana, T.; Hernández-Barrera, V. Obesity Is Associated with a Greater Number of Long-term Post-COVID Symptoms and Poor Sleep Quality: A Multicentre Case-control Study. *Int. J. Clin. Pract.* **2021**, *75*, e14917. [CrossRef]
60. Jia, X.; Cao, S.; Lee, A.S.; Manohar, M.; Sindher, S.B.; Ahuja, N.; Artandi, M.; Blish, C.A.; Blomkalns, A.L.; Chang, I.; et al. Anti-Nucleocapsid Antibody Levels and Pulmonary Comorbid Conditions Are Linked to Post–COVID-19 Syndrome. *JCI Insight* **2022**, *7*, e156713. [CrossRef]
61. Lacavalerie, M.R.; Pierre-Francois, S.; Agossou, M.; Inamo, J.; Cabie, A.; Barnay, J.L.; Neviere, R. Obese Patients with Long COVID-19 Display Abnormal Hyperventilatory Response and Impaired Gas Exchange at Peak Exercise. *Future Cardiol.* **2022**, *18*, 577–584. [CrossRef]
62. Oto, O.A.; Ozturk, S.; Arici, M.; Velioğlu, A.; Dursun, B.; Guller, N.; Şahin, İ.; Eser, Z.E.; Paydaş, S.; Trabulus, S.; et al. Middle-Term Outcomes in Renal Transplant Recipients with COVID-19: A National, Multicenter, Controlled Study. *Clin. Kidney J.* **2022**, *15*, 999–1006. [CrossRef] [PubMed]
63. Whitaker, M.; Elliott, J.; Chadeau-Hyam, M.; Riley, S.; Darzi, A.; Cooke, G.; Ward, H.; Elliott, P. Persistent COVID-19 Symptoms in a Community Study of 606,434 People in England. *Nat. Commun.* **2022**, *13*, 1957. [CrossRef] [PubMed]
64. Li, Y.; Ashcroft, T.; Chung, A.; Dighero, I.; Dozier, M.; Horne, M.; McSwiggan, E.; Shamsuddin, A.; Nair, H. Risk Factors for Poor Outcomes in Hospitalised COVID-19 Patients: A Systematic Review and Meta-Analysis. *J. Glob. Health* **2021**, *11*, 10001. [CrossRef] [PubMed]
65. Sahu, A.K.; Mathew, R.; Aggarwal, P.; Nayer, J.; Bhoi, S.; Satapathy, S.; Ekka, M. Clinical Determinants of Severe COVID-19 Disease—A Systematic Review and Meta-Analysis. *J. Glob. Infect. Dis.* **2021**, *13*, 13–19. [CrossRef] [PubMed]
66. Mauvais-Jarvis, F.; Bairey Merz, N.; Barnes, P.J.; Brinton, R.D.; Carrero, J.-J.; DeMeo, D.L.; De Vries, G.J.; Epperson, C.N.; Govindan, R.; Klein, S.L.; et al. Sex and Gender: Modifiers of Health, Disease, and Medicine. *Lancet* **2020**, *396*, 565–582. [CrossRef] [PubMed]
67. Abumweis, S.; Alrefai, W.; Alzoughool, F. Association of Obesity with COVID-19 Diseases Severity and Mortality: A Meta-Analysis of Studies. *Obes. Med.* **2022**, *33*, 100431. [CrossRef]
68. Chen, Z.; Peng, Y.; Wu, X.; Pang, B.; Yang, F.; Zheng, W.; Liu, C.; Zhang, J. Comorbidities and Complications of COVID-19 Associated with Disease Severity, Progression, and Mortality in China with Centralized Isolation and Hospitalization: A Systematic Review and Meta-Analysis. *Front. Public Health* **2022**, *10*, 923485. [CrossRef]
69. Liu, D.; Yuan, X.; Gao, F.; Zhao, B.; Ding, L.; Huan, M.; Liu, C.; Jiang, L. High Number and Specific Comorbidities Could Impact the Immune Response in COVID-19 Patients. *Front. Immunol.* **2022**, *13*, 899930. [CrossRef]

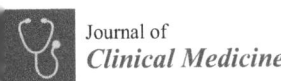

Article

Association between Experimental Pain Measurements and the Central Sensitization Inventory in Patients at Least 3 Months after COVID-19 Infection: A Cross-Sectional Pilot Study

Lisa Goudman [1,2,3,4,5,*,†], Ann De Smedt [1,3,6,†], Stijn Roggeman [6], César Fernández-de-las-Peñas [7,8], Samar M. Hatem [1,6], Marc Schiltz [1,6], Maxime Billot [9], Manuel Roulaud [9], Philippe Rigoard [9,10,11] and Maarten Moens [1,2,3,4,12]

1. STIMULUS Research Group, Vrije Universiteit Brussel, Laarbeeklaan 103, 1090 Brussels, Belgium
2. Department of Neurosurgery, Universitair Ziekenhuis Brussel, Laarbeeklaan 101, 1090 Brussels, Belgium
3. Center for Neurosciences (C4N), Vrije Universiteit Brussel, Laarbeeklaan 103, 1090 Brussels, Belgium
4. Pain in Motion (PAIN) Research Group, Department of Physiotherapy, Human Physiology and Anatomy, Faculty of Physical Education and Physiotherapy, Vrije Universiteit Brussel, Laarbeeklaan 103, 1090 Brussels, Belgium
5. Research Foundation Flanders (FWO), Egmontstraat 5, 1000 Brussels, Belgium
6. Department of Physical Medicine and Rehabilitation, Universitair Ziekenhuis Brussel, Laarbeeklaan 101, 1090 Brussels, Belgium
7. Department of Physical Therapy, Occupational Therapy, Rehabilitation and Physical Medicine, Universidad Rey Juan Carlos, 28922 Alcorcón, Spain
8. Center for Neuroplasticity and Pain (CNAP), SMI, Department of Health Science and Technology, Faculty of Medicine, Aalborg University, 9220 Aalborg, Denmark
9. PRISMATICS Lab (Predictive Research in Spine/Neuromodulation Management and Thoracic Innovation/Cardiac Surgery), Poitiers University Hospital, 86021 Poitiers, France
10. Department of Spine Surgery & Neuromodulation, Poitiers University Hospital, 86021 Poitiers, France
11. Pprime Institute UPR 3346, CNRS, ISAE-ENSMA, University of Poitiers, 86360 Chasseneuil-du-Poitou, France
12. Department of Radiology, Universitair Ziekenhuis Brussel, Laarbeeklaan 101, 1090 Brussels, Belgium
* Correspondence: lisa.goudman@vub.be; Tel.: +32-24775514
† These authors contributed equally to this work.

Abstract: Fatigue, pain, headache, brain fog, anosmia, ageusia, mood symptoms, and sleep disorders are symptoms commonly experienced by people with post-COVID-19 condition. These symptoms could be considered as manifestations of central sensitization. The aim of this study is to evaluate whether there are indicators of central sensitization by using experimental pain measurements and to determine their association with patient-reported outcome measures (PROMs). A cross-sectional study including 42 patients after COVID-19 infection was conducted. The central sensitization inventory (CSI) was administered as a PROM to evaluate central-sensitization-associated symptoms. Pressure pain thresholds (PPT), temporal summation, and descending nociceptive pain inhibition (CPM) were assessed as experimental pain measurements. The median score on the CSI was 46.5 (Q1–Q3: 33–54). The presence of central-sensitization-associated symptoms was seen in 64.3% of patients based on the CSI ($\geq$40/100 points). A deficient CPM was seen in 12% and 14% of patients when measured at the trapezius and rectus femoris, respectively. A negative correlation between pressure sensitivity on the rectus femoris and the CSI score (r = -0.36, 95%CI -0.13 to -0.65, $p = 0.007$) was observed. Central-sensitization-associated symptoms were present in up to 64.3% of patients post-COVID-19 infection, based on a PROM, i.e., the CSI. A more objective evaluation of nociceptive processing through experimental pain measurements was less suggestive of indicators of central sensitization. Only a small negative correlation between pressure sensitivity and the CSI was observed, thereby pointing towards the discrepancy between the CSI and experimental pain measurements and presumably the complementary need for both to evaluate potential indicators of central sensitization in this population.

Keywords: post-COVID-19 condition; persisting symptoms; sensitivity; central sensitization

1. Introduction

The coronavirus disease 2019 (COVID-19) pandemic, caused by severe acute respiratory syndrome coronavirus 2 (SARS-CoV-2) infection, has resulted in worldwide strict lockdowns, physical distancing, and home isolation to slow down the spread of the pandemic and to avoid fatalities [1,2]. Due to the lack of a definitive treatment option for COVID-19, more than 230 vaccine candidates have been proposed, with 49 approved vaccines up until now [3]. A network meta-analysis revealed that COVID-19 vaccines provided a significant reduction in the risk of contracting symptomatic SARS-CoV-2 and a significant reduction in the risk of developing severe COVID-19 in comparison to a placebo [2]. Nevertheless, despite the efficacy of COVID-19 vaccines, the prevalence of persons infected and confronted with persisting symptoms for months or years after SARS-CoV-2 infection is estimated to be up to 31% [4,5]. Fatigue, pain, headache, brain fog, anosmia, ageusia, and emotional or sleep disorders are among the most common persistent post-COVID manifestations [4,6–8]. A meta-analysis reported that fatigue is the most prevalent post-COVID symptom with a prevalence rate of up to 45% [9]. Patients with these persistent debilitating symptoms are classified as suffering from post-COVID-19 condition, defined as "a condition that occurs in people who have a history of probable or confirmed SARS-CoV-2 infection; usually within three months from the onset of COVID-19, with symptoms and effects that last for at least two months" [10,11]. It is specifically denoted by the WHO that the symptoms of post-COVID-19 condition cannot be explained by an alternative medical diagnosis [10,11].

Fatigue is one of the core symptoms in central-sensitization-associated disorders [12,13], leading to the hypothesis that central sensitization might be an underlying common etiology in chronic pain patients and in patients with post-COVID-19 condition [14]. Post-COVID-19 condition has previously been described as having considerable overlapping symptoms with myalgic encephalomyelitis/chronic fatigue syndrome [15,16], a condition associated with central sensitization [17]. Emerging evidence suggests the presence of central sensitization in a subgroup of patients with post-COVID-19 condition. By using the self-rated questionnaire, the central sensitization inventory (CSI), a Belgian study showed that 70% of individuals with post-COVID-19 condition exhibited sensitization-associated symptomatology [18] whereas a Spanish study reported a prevalence of only 34% in a group of patients exhibiting post-COVID pain [19]. Another rational supporting the presence of central sensitization is the fact that individuals with post-COVID-19 condition exhibit several central nervous-system-derived symptoms, e.g., fatigue, sleep problems, memory loss, concentration problems, or psychological disturbances [4].

The exclusive use of a screening questionnaire such as the CSI for inferring sensitization in people with post-COVID-19 condition is not recommended because a self-reported tool cannot capture the complexity of a nervous system impairment such as central sensitization [20]. Accordingly, besides patient-reported outcome measure (PROMs), i.e., CSI, to identify the presence of central-sensitization-associated symptoms, quantitative sensory testing could be used to quantify sensory dysfunctions by evaluating pain thresholds, nociceptive pain facilitation, and endogenous pain inhibition [21,22]. A less efficacious descending nociceptive inhibitory system, combined with increased nociceptive facilitation and decreased pain thresholds, is commonly related to an increased excitability of the central nervous system, namely central sensitization [23,24]. To the best of our knowledge, no study has previously investigated the presence of altered nociceptive processing by conducting experimental pain measurements in individuals post-COVID-19 infection. Therefore, the aims of this study were to further evaluate whether there are indicators of central sensitization in patients with post-COVID-19 infection by using experimental pain measurements and to determine their association with PROMs such as the CSI.

2. Materials and Methods

2.1. Study Participants

This is a cross-sectional study investigating the symptoms of central sensitization and impaired nociceptive processing in individuals post-COVID-19 infection. Both male and female patients who had been previously infected with SARS-CoV-2 were eligible to participate. The patients were only eligible if they had had a positive COVID-19 test at least 3 months before inclusion. The patients were recruited through various ways. Firstly, the patients were invited to participate by physicians in cases where they were consulted after a SARS-CoV-2 infection at the Department of Physical Medicine and Rehabilitation of UZ Brussel. Secondly, advertisements and announcements from patient support groups were used as an additional recruitment strategy. Finally, social media was used to recruit patients. The study protocol was approved by the central ethics committee of Universitair Ziekenhuis Brussels (B.U.N. 1432020000348) on 16 December 2020. The study was registered on clinicaltrials.gov (NCT04703452) and was conducted according to the revised Declaration of Helsinki (1998).

2.2. Study Protocol

The patients included had one study visit to UZ Brussel, which was scheduled according to patient preferences. During the study visit, the patients first filled out the following three PROMs in a randomized order: the central sensitization inventory, the post-COVID-19 functional status scale, and the London chest activity of daily living. After filling out the questionnaires, the following experimental pain measurements were performed: pressure pain thresholds (PPT), temporal summation, and descending nociceptive inhibition. The complete testing protocol lasted for maximally 1 h. All of the participants were asked to refrain from consuming caffeine, alcohol, or nicotine 24 h before the study.

2.3. Self-Reported Questionnaires

The primary outcome was the presence of central-sensitization-associated symptoms, as assessed by the central sensitization inventory (CSI). The CSI consists of 25 symptom-related items that the patient has to score on a five-point Likert scale [25]. A total score of $\geq 40/100$ is indicative of the presence of central sensitization symptomatology (sensitivity: 81% and specificity: 75%) [25]. The participants were categorized based on central-sensitization-related severity into three subgroups: (i) low level, (ii) medium level, or (iii) high level of central-sensitization-related symptom severity using an accessible calculator (https://www.pridedallas.com/questionnaires, accessed on 19 November 2021) [26]. The CSI has good psychometric properties for assessing symptoms of central sensitization [21] and it is validated in Dutch and French [27,28].

Post-COVID-19 functional status was evaluated by the post-COVID-19 functional status scale (PCFS). This scale is ordinal, has six steps ranging from 0 (no symptoms) to 5 (death) and covers the entire range of functional outcomes by focusing on limitations in usual activities either at home or at work/study, as well as lifestyle changes. More specifically, the following scale grades are included: 0 (no functional limitations), 1 (negligible functional limitation), 2 (slight functional limitation), 3 (moderate functional limitation), 4 (severe functional limitation), and death. The PCFS was assessed twice, once by the interviewers during a short-structured interview, as well as with self-reporting by the patient [29,30].

The London chest activity of daily living (LCADL) scale was assessed to evaluate the level of dyspnea during activities of daily living (0–75 points). This questionnaire consists of 15 items and contains the following answer options: 0 (I do not perform this activity because I've never had to do it or it is irrelevant), 1 (I do not feel any breathless when performing this activity), 2 (I feel moderate breathless when performing this activity), 3 (I feel a lot of breathless in performing this activity), 4 (I cannot perform this activity due to breathless and I have no one who can perform the activity for me) or 5 (I cannot perform this activity anymore and I need someone to perform it for me or help me because of breathless). Greater dyspnea-related limitation in activities of daily living translates into higher scores on the LCADL. It has four domains: self-care (0–20 points), domestic activities (0–30 points), physical activities (0–8 points), and leisure time (0–12 points) [31,32].

2.4. Experimental Pain Measurements

Pressure pain sensitivity was measured at the middle of the trapezius muscle (i.e., midway between the spinous process of the seventh cervical vertebra and the lateral edge of the acromion) [33] and at the center of the rectus femoris muscle (i.e., the middle of the distance between the anterior inferior iliac spine and the upper edge of the patella) [34] on the dominant side with a hand-held manual algometer (Wagner FPX™ Algometer, Wagner Instruments, Greenwich, CT, USA). On each location, two measurements (interval 30 s) were obtained, generating a mean pressure pain threshold (PPT) per area that was used in subsequent analyses. To determine the PPT, pressure was increased at a rate of approximately 1 kg/s until the participants indicated that the sensation became painful. Consequently, the pressure was immediately released. The pressure established at that moment was used as PPT, measured in kg/cm^2. Pressure algometry has been found to be an efficient and reliable technique for PPT determination and examination of sensitivity to pressure pain [35].

Temporal summation (TS) was evaluated with 10 consecutive pressure pulses at the intensity of the PPT (previously determined) on the same areas. For each pulse of the TS procedure, the pressure was increased at a rate of 2 kg/s until the previously determined PPT, where it was maintained for one second before being released. An inter-stimulus interval of one second was used. The participants were instructed to rate the pain intensity of the first, fifth, and tenth pressure pulse according to a verbal numeric pain rating scale (vNPRS). The TS score was obtained by subtracting the first vNPRS score from the last vNPRS [36]. The higher the TS score, the more efficient the nociceptive signaling to the brain. The TS procedure is found to be reliable and valid and is supported for use in chronic pain patients [37].

To assess the efficacy of endogenous pain inhibition, the conditioned pain modulation (CPM) paradigm was used [38–40]. An occlusion cuff was used as a conditioning stimulus and pressure stimuli were used as the test stimulus on the trapezius and quadriceps locations. The conditioning stimulus was applied to the non-dominant side [34] for 2 min. In order to apply the conditioning stimulus, an occlusion cuff was inflated to a painful intensity and maintained at that level as a heterotopic noxious conditioning stimulus. The cuff was inflated at approximately 20 mmHg/s until the point that the sensation first became painful. Next, patients adapted for 30 s to the stimulus and subsequently rated their pain intensity on the vNPRS. Cuff inflation was then increased or decreased until the participant indicated that the pain level was equal to a score of 3/10 on the vNPRS. Thirty seconds after application of the conditioning stimulus, the first test stimulus (via PPT) was measured on the trapezius. After 60 s, the second test stimulus on the trapezius was assessed. Again, 30 s later (at 1′30″ after application of the conditioning stimulus), the first test stimulus on the quadriceps muscle was applied (via PPT) and the last test stimulus on the quadriceps was applied again 30 s later (at 2′) [34]. The CPM effect is calculated as PPT after conditioning stimulation—PPT before conditioning stimulation [41]. Negative scores (decreased PPTs) indicate no CPM effect and positive scores (increased PPTs) indicate effective CPM.

2.5. Statistical Analysis

All of the analyses were performed in R Studio version 1.4.1106 (R version 4.0.5, R Foundation). *p*-values of 0.05 or less were considered statistically significant. Statistics for quantitative variables included median and 1st and 3rd quartiles, the number of observations, and number of missing values. For categorical variables, the absolute counts (n) and percentages (%) of patients were presented.

The primary outcome of this study is to identify whether patients post-COVID-19 infection suffer from central-sensitization-associated symptoms, based on the total CSI score. Therefore, the percentages of patients with central sensitization were reported based on the cut-off value of 40/100 on the CSI and the central-sensitization-related symptom severity categories. Furthermore, correlation analyses were performed between total CSI scores and experimental pain measurements (i.e., PPT, TS, and CPM) and the total LCADL score using Spearman rank correlations. A Bonferroni correction was applied to correct for multiple testing (seven comparisons for each variable). Agreement between the PCFS scores rated by the patient and the physician was evaluated using a weighted kappa with linear weights. Kruskal–Wallis tests were used to explore the effect of the presence of symptoms of central sensitization on experimental pain measurements, total LCADL scores, and PCFS scores.

Finally, K-means clustering was performed to classify patients according to shared features of self-reported data and experimental measurements. For the clustering, the centroids of hierarchical clustering (squared Euclidean distances with the method of Ward) were used as starting points. All of the variables were standardized before clustering and only patients with complete data were incorporated into the cluster analysis. All of the analyses were performed on the data as observed. This means that no data imputation strategies, nor observation carried forward techniques, were performed.

3. Results

3.1. Demographic Statistics

In total, 42 patients were included in this study (12 males and 30 females) with a mean age of 48 (SD: 12) years. All of the visits took place between 19 January 2021 and 20 December 2021, whereby only one patient was hospitalized for COVID-19 infection at the time of the study visit. The median time between confirmation of SARS-CoV-2 infection and the study visit was 190.5 (Q1–Q3: 117–360) days. Four patients were on non-steroidal anti-inflammatory drugs, four patients were on paracetamol, five patients were on antidepressants, one patient was on opioids, two patients were on benzodiazepines, and one patient received a combination product. For female patients, oral anticonceptives were taken by two patients and two patients took hormone replacement therapy.

3.2. Symptoms of Central Sensitization, Functionality, and Disability

The median score on the CSI was 46.5 points (Q1–Q3: 33–54), whereby 15 patients (35.7%) had a score < 40/100 on the CSI and 27 patients (64.3%) had a score ≥ 40/100. In terms of severity, 5 patients (11.9%) could be classified as low level of central-sensitization-related symptom severity (CSI median score: 18 points, Q1–Q3: 8–21), 12 (28.6%) as medium-level (CSI median score: 33 points, Q1–Q3: 29.75–36.25), and 25 (59.5%) as high-level of central-sensitization-related symptom severity (CSI median score 53 points, Q1–Q3: 48–60). The median CSI score in males (CSI median score: 33.5 points, Q1–Q3: 26.25–46.5) was significantly lower compared to females (CSI median score: 49.5 points, Q1–Q3: 37.75–58) (sample difference -13 (95% CI -2 to -24), $p = 0.02$).

Concerning the PCFS, 4 persons (9.5%) had no functional limitations (grade 0), 7 (16.7%) had negligible functional limitations (grade 1), 15 (35.7%) reported slight functional limitations (grade 2), 14 (33.3%) indicated moderate functional limitations (grade 3), and 2 (4.8%) scored severe functional limitations (grade 4) according to the patient ratings. For the interviews conducted by the physician, 2 persons (4.8%) had no functional limitations (grade 0), 6 (14.3%) had negligible functional limitations (grade 1), 14 (33.3%) reported slight functional limitations (grade 2), 18 (42.8%) indicated moderate functional limitations (grade 3), and 1 (2.4%) scored severe functional limitations (grade 4). There was missing data for one patient (2.4%). The median time to conduct this interview entailed 1245 (Q1–Q3: 738–2218) seconds, corresponding to 20.75 min. There was a statistically significant agreement between both ratings, kw = 0.546 (95% CI 0.345 to 0.748, $p < 0.001$). The strength of agreement was classified as moderate [42]. No statistically significant differences were revealed for PCFS scores between the males and females, based on patient ratings (W = 136.5, p = 0.21) and interviews (W = 160.5, p = 0.90). Table 1 provides an overview of the classifications based on self-reports and interviews.

Table 1. Agreement and disagreement in PCFS scores between patient self-reporting and physician interviews. Green boxes indicate agreement between both ratings; blue boxes indicate a lower self-reporting score compared to the physician interview; and yellow boxes indicate a higher self-reporting score compared to the physician interview. Abbreviations. PFCS: post-COVID-19 functional status scale.

		Physician PCFS Score					
		0	1	2	3	4	5
Patient PCFS score	0	2	1	0	0	0	0
	1	0	4	2	1	0	0
	2	0	1	7	7	0	0
	3	0	0	5	9	0	0
	4	0	0	0	1	1	0
	5	0	0	0	0	0	0

Concerning the LCADL, median scores of 22/75 (Q1–Q3: 17.25–27.50) were revealed, whereby higher scores indicate higher dyspnea-related limitation in activities of daily living. For self-care, a median value of 4.5/20 (Q1–Q3: 4–6) was revealed. For domestic activities, physical activities and leisure time median values of 8.5/30 (Q1–Q3: 6–11.75), 4/8 (Q1–Q3: 3–4) and 4/12 (Q1–Q3: 3–5) were reported, respectively. The median LCADL score in males (LCADL median score: 16 points, Q1–Q3: 15–22.75) was significantly lower compared to females (LCADL median score: 23.5 points, Q1–Q3: 20–30.25) (sample difference −6 (95% CI −1 to −10), p = 0.02).

3.3. Experimental Pain Measurements

The median PPT on the trapezius muscle was 4.4 (Q1–Q3: 3.1–5.6) kg/cm^2 and 4.4 (Q1–Q3: 3.4–6.5) kg/cm^2 on the quadriceps muscle. For temporal summation, the first score was subtracted from the final score, leading to a median value of 3 (Q1–Q3: 1.25–4) for the trapezius and 4 (Q1–Q3: 2–5) for the quadriceps point.

For functioning of the descending inhibitory pathways, 35 patients demonstrated an efficient CPM (median CPM effect: 1.28, Q1–Q3: 0.73 to 1.79) and 5 patients did not (median CPM effect: −0.50, Q1–Q3: −0.82 to −0.22) when measured on the trapezius muscle. On the quadriceps muscle, 6 patients did not demonstrate an efficient CPM (median CPM effect: −0.01, Q1–Q3: −0.04 to 0.0), while 34 patients demonstrated an efficient CPM (median CPM effect: 1.53, Q1–Q3: 0.85 to 2.32). In two patients, no CPM effect was measured.

3.4. Associations between Self-Reported and Experimental Measurements

Table 2 presents outcome measurements by severity of central-sensitization-associated symptoms.

A significant positive correlation between PPTs on the trapezius and quadriceps (r = 0.65, 95% CI 0.54 to 0.85, p < 0.001) and between TS on the trapezius and quadriceps (r = 0.65, 95% CI 0.44 to 0.8, p < 0.001) was observed. The total scores on the LCADL and CSI were also positively correlated (r = 0.8, 95% CI 0.54 to 0.85, p < 0.001). A negative correlation between PPTs on the quadriceps and the CSI score (r = −0.36, 95% CI −0.13 to −0.65, p = 0.0067) was also identified (Figure 1).

Table 2. Total scores on LCADL and PCFS, and results from experimental pain measurements from the complete sample, as well as those separated by the presence or absence (CSI < 40) of symptoms of central sensitization (CSI ≥ 40). Abbreviations: CPM: conditioned pain modulation, CSI: central sensitization inventory, LCADL: London chest activity of daily living, PFCS: post-COVID-19 functional status scale, PPT: pressure pain threshold, and TS: temporal summation.

Variable	Level	Total Sample (*n* = 42)	CSI Score < 40/100 (*n* = 15)	CSI Score ≥ 40/100 (*n* = 27)
Sex	Male/Female	28.6%/71.4%	46.7%/53.3%	18.5%/81.5%
Age (years)		48 (SD: 12)	49 (SD: 15)	48 (SD: 11)
Time since COVID-19 (days)		190.5 (Q1–Q3: 117–360)	184 (Q1–Q3: 96–200)	212 (Q1–Q3: 127–387)
PPT Trapezius		4.37 (Q1–Q3: 3.12–5.60)	5.21 (Q1–Q3: 3.89–7.22)	3.96 (Q1–Q3: 2.82–5.05)
PPT Quadriceps		4.43 (Q1–Q3: 3.40–6.49)	6.21 (Q1–Q3: 3.82–9.13)	4.33 (Q1–Q3: 3.28–5.88)
TS Trapezius		3 (Q1–Q3: 1.25–4)	3 (Q1–Q3: 1.5–3)	4 (Q1–Q3: 1.5–5)
TS Quadriceps		4 (Q1–Q3: 2–5)	3 (Q1–Q3: 2.5–4)	4 (Q1–Q3: 2–5.5)
CPM Trapezius		1.17 (Q1–Q3: 0.53–1.75)	1.36 (Q1–Q3: 0.90–1.75)	0.94 (Q1–Q3: 0.50–1.57)
CPM Quadriceps		1.30 (Q1–Q3: 0.58–2.24)	0.89 (Q1–Q3: 0.47–1.87)	1.52 (Q1–Q3: 0.77–2.31)
LCADL		22/75 (Q1–Q3: 17.25–27.50)	15 (Q1–Q3: 15–17.5)	25 (Q1–Q3: 22.5–32.5)
PCFS patient	Grade 0	9.5%	26.7%	0.0%
	Grade 1	16.7%	33.3%	7.4%
	Grade 2	35.7%	26.7%	40.7%
	Grade 3	33.3%	13.3%	44.4%
	Grade 4	4.8%	0.0%	7.4%
PCFS physician	Grade 0	4.8%	13.3%	0.0%
	Grade 1	14.3%	33.3%	3.7%
	Grade 2	33.3%	26.7%	37.0%
	Grade 3	42.8%	20.0%	55.5%
	Grade 4	2.4%	0.0%	3.7%
	Unknown	2.4%	6.7%	0.0%

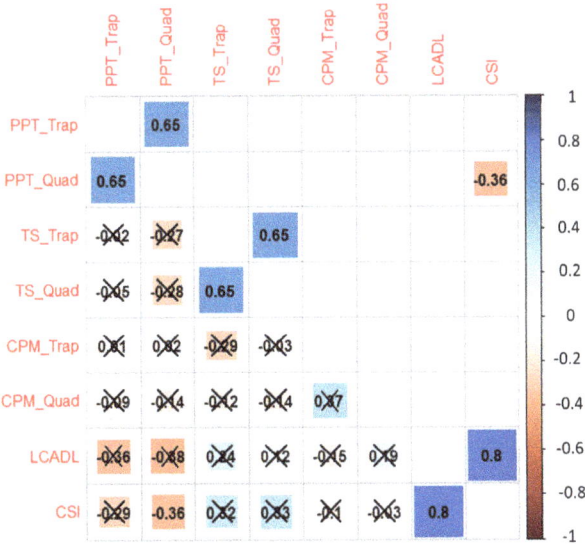

Figure 1. Correlation plot. The correlation coefficients range from −1 (red) to +1 (blue) and are presented with their actual values on the plot. In the lower triangle, correlations that are not statistically significant are marked with a cross. On the upper triangle, only statistically significant correlations are presented. Abbreviations: CPM: conditioned pain modulation, CSI: central sensitization inventory, LCADL: London chest activity of daily living, PFCS: post-COVID-19 functional status scale, PPT: pressure pain threshold, Quad: quadriceps, Trap: trapezius, and TS: temporal summation.

Based on Kruskal–Wallis tests, there was a significant effect of central sensitization-associated symptoms on PPT on the trapezius at the 5% level (χ^2 (df = 1) = 4.46, p = 0.03) (Figure S1). The effect of the presence of symptoms of central sensitization did not result in statistically significant differences for the other experimental pain measurements.

For the LCADL, the median score in patients with the presence of symptoms of central sensitization was higher compared to patients with the absence of these symptoms (χ^2 (df = 1) = 27.18, p < 0.001). There was a significant effect of central sensitization-associated symptoms on the PCFS with higher median values in patients with sensitization symptomatology, both for the PCFS scores derived from the self-reporting of patients (χ^2 (df = 1) = 12.67, p < 0.001) as well as from the interviews (χ^2 (df = 1) = 9.91, p = 0.002, Figure S2).

The K-means clustering resulted in five clusters, whereby 5, 8, 10, 13, and 3 patients were classified (n = 39). A visual presentation of the clusters is graphically presented in Figure 2.

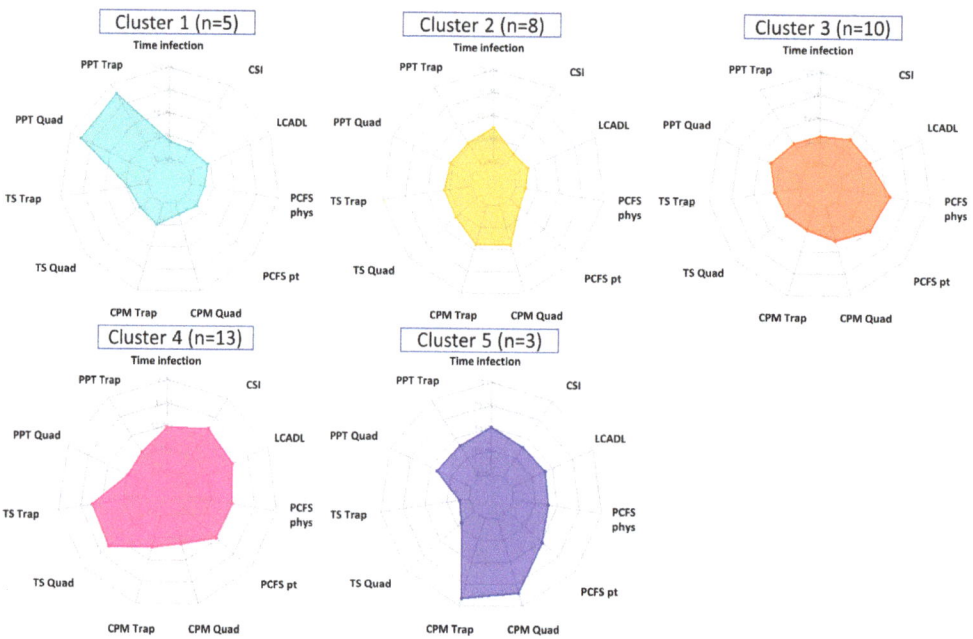

Figure 2. K-means clustering algorithm with five distinct clusters. CPM was coded negatively in case there was a malfunctioning of the descending nociceptive inhibitory pathways and positive in case of functioning of these pathways. For temporal summation, higher scores indicate more nociceptive facilitation. Abbreviations. CPM: conditioned pain modulation, CSI: central sensitization inventory, LCADL: London chest activity of daily living, PFCS: post-COVID-19 functional status scale, phys: physician, PPT: pressure pain threshold, pt: patient, Quad: quadriceps, Trap: trapezius, and TS: temporal summation.

Cluster 4 represented 33.3% of the patients and could be interpreted as a typical chronic pain patient showing a relatively high CSI score, nociceptive facilitation, malfunctioning of the nociceptive inhibitory pathways, and lower PPTs as compared to the remaining clusters. Cluster 1 (12.8%) is characterized by high PPTs on the trapezius and rectus femoris, while cluster 5 (7.7%) is characterized by high values of descending nociceptive inhibitory control. Cluster 3 (25.6%) predominantly reveals a high contribution of limitations in usual activities based on the PCFS. Finally, 20.5% of patients are attributed to cluster 2 in which rather low

PPTs, lower contribution of PROMs, high values of descending inhibitory control and a limited contribution of nociceptive facilitation are present.

4. Discussion

The current study observed the presence of central-sensitization-associated symptomatology in up to 64.3% of patients post-COVID-19 infection, based on self-reporting through the CSI. Most patients (69%) reported slight to moderate functional limitations. Physical activities were responsible for most of the dyspnea-related limitations in activities of daily life. For patients with central-sensitization-associated symptoms, greater dyspnea-related limitations and higher limitations in functional status were observed. A small negative correlation between pressure pain sensitivity on the rectus femoris and the CSI score was observed. No other correlations between experimental pain measurements and CSI were observed. Clustering analysis identified that 33% of patients in this sample demonstrated a profile featuring a high CSI score, nociceptive pain facilitation, and malfunctioning of the nociceptive inhibitory pathways.

Based on the WHO definition, individuals with a history of probable or confirmed SARS-CoV-2 infection, usually 3 months from the onset of COVID-19 with symptoms that last for at least 2 months, could be classified as suffering from post-COVID-19 condition [10]. The patients included in this study had a positive COVID-19 test at least 3 months before study inclusion, nevertheless the exact duration of symptomatology was not asked. Only 9.5% of patients did not report any symptoms of functional limitations, therefore it is assumed that more than 90% of patients suffered from post-COVID-19 condition. We identified the presence of central-sensitization-associated symptomatology in up to 64.3% of our patients post-COVID-19 infection based on PROMs. This result is similar to our previous study [18], but much higher than the prevalence rate of 34% observed in individuals with just post-COVID pain [19]. This discrepancy may be related to the fact that the sample of patients included by Fernández-de-las-Peñas et al. mainly suffered from solely post-COVID pain [19] whereas the Belgian sample [18] reported more heterogeneous post-COVID symptoms such as fatigue or memory loss, which are also evaluated in the CSI [25]. In fact, the presence of psychological and physical post-COVID symptoms are related to the CSI score. Interestingly, higher CSI scores were associated with greater dyspnea-related limitations and higher functional limitations in the current study, thus supporting the previous assumption.

Since the use of PROMs such as the CSI is not able to further ascertain the presence of altered nociceptive pain processing, we included, for the first time, experimental pain measurements in people post-COVID-19 infection. The presence of pressure pain hyperalgesia increased temporal summation and impaired descending inhibition are manifestations of central nervous system sensitization [43]. We were unable to determine the presence of pressure hyperalgesia in our sample of individuals post-COVID-19 infection since we did not include a control group without post-COVID symptoms; however, it would be expected for lower PPTs in individuals with persistent symptoms to be found. Historical data are available for pain-free populations with testing on the trapezius whereby mean values ranging from 4.96 (SD: 3.33) [44] to 5.32 (SD: 3.28) [44], and 5.75 (SD: 2.88) [45] were revealed. Mean PPT values of 4.02 (SD: 1.60) [45] have been observed in patients with whiplash-associated disorders and 2.90 (SD: 2.49) [44] in patients with fibromyalgia. The currently obtained values in patients post-COVID-19 infection seem to be in line with the findings observed in patients with whiplash-associated disorders, suggesting that patients post-COVID-19 infection could also demonstrate pressure pain hyperalgesia.

Nevertheless, our main objective was to further identify the association of experimental pain measurements with the self-reported CSI. We identified a small correlation between sensitivity to pressure pain and the CSI score suggesting that both outcomes represent different aspects of the sensitization spectrum. This weak correlation is in line with previous data in chronic spinal pain patients where a weak correlation was found between the CSI and PPT [46], as was the case in patients with knee osteoarthritis [47].

Statistically, non-significant results were revealed between the CSI and PPT in patients with shoulder pain [48] and patients with chronic whiplash-associated disorders [49]. No other association between the CSI with temporal summation or CPM was identified in the present study, as was the case in patients with chronic whiplash-associated disorders [49]. These results further support the belief that the CSI assessed a broad spectrum of sensitization symptomatology and not just altered nociceptive pain processing. As such, the CSI only marginally reflects direct alterations in central nociceptive processing and is better at identifying psychosocial factors that patients experience than identifying central nervous system adaptations due to central sensitization [49]. It is also possible that the small percentage of patients showing an impaired CPM explains the lack of association.

Concerning the PROMs, a positive correlation was revealed between the LCADL and the CSI ($r = 0.8$, 95% CI 0.54 to 0.85, $p < 0.001$), meaning that patients with higher symptomatology of central sensitization present more dyspnea during activities of daily living. Furthermore, patients with high central sensitization symptomatology also revealed more limitations in functional outcomes. Previous studies have already demonstrated correlations between CSI and functionality, work ability, depression, and social support scales in patients with spinal pain [50–52]. These findings further support the previous hypothesis that the CSI captures a broad spectrum of symptomatology and not only evaluates central nervous system processing in response to nociception. The currently obtained values on the LCADL (median 22/75, Q1–Q3: 17.25–27.50) for dyspnea-related limitation in activities of daily living are in line with the mean value of 17 (SD: 5.7) that was revealed in a population of post-COVID-19 patients in Turkey [53]. Despite the fact that most patients in this study were female (71.4%), females had more dyspnea-related limitations in activities of daily living and more central-sensitization-associated symptoms compared to males. A previous study explored phenotypes based on clinical data obtained in a post-COVID-19 care clinic and revealed that the fatigue-predominant phenotype was more common in females, while the dyspnea-predominant phenotype was more common in males [54]. Since fatigue is one of the core symptoms in central-sensitization-associated disorders, the results of higher CSI scores in females compared to males is not surprising. Further research is needed to further evaluate the dominance of dyspnea-related limitations in patients post-COVID-19 infection.

Although preliminary due to the low number of participants and no external validation, clustering analysis identified that 33% of patients demonstrated a central sensitization profile featuring a high CSI score, nociceptive pain facilitation, and malfunctioning of the nociceptive inhibitory pathways. This subgroup of patients fulfills all of the criteria for a nociplastic condition [55] as has been proposed recently [56] and this could need particular attention in their management. For instance, early treatment of these subgroups of patients could be applied to avoid the further development of central sensitization. Similarly, more multidisciplinary interventions targeting the nervous system, e.g., acceptance and commitment therapy and pain neuroscience education [57], should be applied to this subgroup of patients. These hypotheses should be confirmed or refuted in future clinical trials. Additionally, further exploration and validation of the clustering analysis should still be performed, incorporating the clinical features of pain.

Despite the innovative aspect of conducting experimental pain measurements in patients post-COVID-19 infection, certain limitations should be taken into account when considering the results of this study. The patients included in this study were recruited through convenience sampling, which could limit the generalizability of the results. Nevertheless, the results obtained in this study seem to be comparable to findings in other chronic pain populations. Additionally, no control group was included; therefore, experimental pain measurements could only be compared to data from historical studies. In terms of experimental pain measurements, only one modality (i.e., pressure stimuli) was used, whereas the available guidelines recommend the use of different modalities [39]. This choice was made not to further increase the burden on the study participants, since this was a pilot study exploring indicators of central sensitization in this population. Additionally, standardized sites of stimulation (i.e., trapezius muscle and quadriceps muscle) were used to enable interpretation of the results at the cohort level, regardless of the location of symptomatology of individual patients. Moreover, this study only explored indicators of central sensitization post-COVID-19 infection, without evaluating previous existing comorbidities. Finally, no information was collected on the duration of sick leave or work status after COVID-19 infection.

5. Conclusions

In patients post-COVID-19 infection, symptoms of central sensitization were present in 64.3% of the sample based on a self-reported questionnaire. A more objective evaluation of nociceptive pain processing was less suggestive for indicators of central sensitization, thereby pointing towards a discrepancy between the CSI and experimental pain measurements in patients post-COVID-19 infection.

Supplementary Materials: The following supporting information can be downloaded at: https://www.mdpi.com/article/10.3390/jcm12020661/s1, Figure S1: Boxplots of the different experimental pain measurements by the presence of symptoms of central sensitization. Figure S2: Boxplots of the LCADL and PCFS scores, separated by the presence of symptoms of central sensitization.

Author Contributions: Conceptualization, L.G., A.D.S., S.M.H., M.S. and M.M.; data curation, A.D.S., S.R. and M.S.; formal analysis, A.D.S., S.M.H. and L.G.; methodology, L.G., A.D.S., S.M.H., M.S. and M.M.; writing—original draft, L.G., C.F.-d.-l.-P. and M.M.; writing—review and editing, all authors. All authors have read and agreed to the published version of the manuscript.

Funding: This research received no external funding.

Institutional Review Board Statement: The study protocol was approved by the central ethics committee of Universitair Ziekenhuis Brussel (B.U.N. 1432020000348) on 16 December 2020.

Informed Consent Statement: Informed consent was obtained from all subjects involved in the study.

Data Availability Statement: The data presented in this study are available on motivated request from the corresponding author.

Acknowledgments: The authors are grateful to Levi Wauman for his help with the data collection.

Conflicts of Interest: L.G. is a postdoctoral research fellow funded by the Research Foundation Flanders (FWO), Belgium (project number 12ZF622N). P.R. reports grants from Medtronic, Abbott and Boston Scientific and consultant fees and payments for lectures from Medtronic and Boston Scientific, outside the submitted work. M.M. has received speaker fees from Medtronic and Nevro. STIMULUS received independent research grants from Medtronic. There are no other conflicts of interest to declare.

References

1. Kim, D.Y.; Shinde, S.K.; Lone, S.; Palem, R.R.; Ghodake, G.S. COVID-19 Pandemic: Public Health Risk Assessment and Risk Mitigation Strategies. *J. Pers. Med.* **2021**, *11*, 1243. [CrossRef] [PubMed]
2. Kumar, S.; Saikia, D.; Bankar, M.; Saurabh, M.K.; Singh, H.; Varikasuvu, S.R.; Maharshi, V. Efficacy of COVID-19 vaccines: A systematic review and network meta-analysis of phase 3 randomized controlled trials. *Pharmacol. Rep.* **2022**, *10*, 321. [CrossRef] [PubMed]
3. VIPER Group COVID19 Vaccine Tracker Team. COVID19 Vaccine Tracker. Available online: https://covid19.trackvaccines.org/ (accessed on 10 November 2022).
4. Lopez-Leon, S.; Wegman-Ostrosky, T.; Del Valle, N.C.A.; Perelman, C.; Sepulveda, R.; Rebolledo, P.A.; Cuapio, A.; Villapol, S. Long-COVID in children and adolescents: A systematic review and meta-analyses. *Sci. Rep.* **2022**, *12*, 9950. [CrossRef] [PubMed]
5. Han, Q.; Zheng, B.; Daines, L.; Sheikh, A. Long-Term Sequelae of COVID-19: A Systematic Review and Meta-Analysis of One-Year Follow-Up Studies on Post-COVID Symptoms. *Pathogens* **2022**, *11*, 269. [CrossRef]
6. Logue, J.K.; Franko, N.M.; McCulloch, D.J.; McDonald, D.; Magedson, A.; Wolf, C.R.; Chu, H.Y. Sequelae in Adults at 6 Months after COVID-19 Infection. *JAMA Netw. Open* **2021**, *4*, e210830. [CrossRef]
7. Carfi, A.; Bernabei, R.; Landi, F. Persistent Symptoms in Patients after Acute COVID-19. *JAMA* **2020**, *324*, 603–605. [CrossRef]
8. Moens, M.; Duarte, R.V.; De Smedt, A.; Putman, K.; Callens, J.; Billot, M.; Roulaud, M.; Rigoard, P.; Goudman, L. Health-related quality of life in persons post-COVID-19 infection in comparison to normative controls and chronic pain patients. *Front. Public Health* **2022**, *10*, 991572. [CrossRef]

9. Salari, N.; Khodayari, Y.; Hosseinian-Far, A.; Zarei, H.; Rasoulpoor, S.; Akbari, H.; Mohammadi, M. Global prevalence of chronic fatigue syndrome among long COVID-19 patients: A systematic review and meta-analysis. *BioPsychoSoc. Med.* **2022**, *16*, 21. [CrossRef]
10. World Health Organization. Coronavirus Disease (COVID-19): Post COVID-19 Condition. Available online: https://www.who.int/news-room/questions-and-answers/item/coronavirus-disease-(covid-19)-post-covid-19-condition?gclid=Cj0KCQiA37KbBhDgARIsAIzce14fsUS4hL4RdKOXZ6qNRx_LD6BH9EvsFQq2MFLBNx7MFF1HLGhCAkUaAgPBEALw_wcB (accessed on 10 November 2022).
11. Soriano, J.B.; Murthy, S.; Marshall, J.C.; Relan, P.; Diaz, J.V. A clinical case definition of post-COVID-19 condition by a Delphi consensus. *Lancet Infect. Dis.* **2022**, *22*, e102–e107. [CrossRef]
12. Aaron, L.A.; Buchwald, D. A review of the evidence for overlap among unexplained clinical conditions. *Ann. Intern. Med.* **2001**, *134*, 868–881. [CrossRef]
13. Yunus, M.B. Editorial review: An update on central sensitivity syndromes and the issues of nosology and psychobiology. *Curr. Rheumatol. Rev.* **2015**, *11*, 70–85. [CrossRef]
14. Bierle, D.M.; Aakre, C.A.; Grach, S.L.; Salonen, B.R.; Croghan, I.T.; Hurt, R.T.; Ganesh, R. Central Sensitization Phenotypes in Post Acute Sequelae of SARS-CoV-2 Infection (PASC): Defining the Post COVID Syndrome. *J. Prim. Care Community Health* **2021**, *12*, 21501327211030826. [CrossRef] [PubMed]
15. Sukocheva, O.A.; Maksoud, R.; Beeraka, N.M.; Madhunapantula, S.V.; Sinelnikov, M.; Nikolenko, V.N.; Neganova, M.E.; Klochkov, S.G.; Kamal, M.A.; Staines, D.R.; et al. Analysis of post COVID-19 condition and its overlap with myalgic encephalomyelitis/chronic fatigue syndrome. *J. Adv. Res.* **2022**, *40*, 179–196. [CrossRef] [PubMed]
16. Komaroff, A.L.; Bateman, L. Will COVID-19 Lead to Myalgic Encephalomyelitis/Chronic Fatigue Syndrome? *Front. Med.* **2020**, *7*, 606824. [CrossRef]
17. Bourke, J.H.; Wodehouse, T.; Clark, L.V.; Constantinou, E.; Kidd, B.L.; Langford, R.; Mehta, V.; White, P.D. Central sensitisation in chronic fatigue syndrome and fibromyalgia; a case control study. *J. Psychosom. Res.* **2021**, *150*, 110624. [CrossRef] [PubMed]
18. Goudman, L.; De Smedt, A.; Noppen, M.; Moens, M. Is Central Sensitisation the Missing Link of Persisting Symptoms after COVID-19 Infection? *J. Clin. Med.* **2021**, *10*, 5594. [CrossRef]
19. Fernández-de-las-Peñas, C.; Parás-Bravo, P.; Ferrer-Pargada, D.; Cancela-Cilleruelo, I.; Rodríguez-Jiménez, J.; Nijs, J.; Arendt-Nielsen, L.; Herrero-Montes, M. Sensitization symptoms are associated with psychological and cognitive variables in COVID-19 survivors exhibiting post-COVID pain. *Pain Pract.* **2022**, *23*, 23–31. [CrossRef]
20. Nijs, J.; Huysmans, E. Clinimetrics: The Central Sensitisation Inventory: A useful screening tool for clinicians, but not the gold standard. *J. Physiother.* **2022**, *68*, 207. [CrossRef]
21. Mayer, T.G.; Neblett, R.; Cohen, H.; Howard, K.J.; Choi, Y.H.; Williams, M.J.; Perez, Y.; Gatchel, R.J. The development and psychometric validation of the central sensitization inventory. *Pain Pract.* **2012**, *12*, 276–285. [CrossRef]
22. Treede, R.D. The role of quantitative sensory testing in the prediction of chronic pain. *Pain* **2019**, *160* (Suppl. S1), S66–S69 [CrossRef]
23. Curatolo, M.; Arendt-Nielsen, L.; Petersen-Felix, S. Central hypersensitivity in chronic pain: Mechanisms and clinical implications. *Phys. Med. Rehabil. Clin. N. Am.* **2006**, *17*, 287–302. [CrossRef] [PubMed]
24. Weaver, K.R.; Griffioen, M.A.; Klinedinst, N.J.; Galik, E.; Duarte, A.C.; Colloca, L.; Resnick, B.; Dorsey, S.G.; Renn, C.L. Quantitative Sensory Testing across Chronic Pain Conditions and Use in Special Populations. *Front. Pain Res.* **2021**, *2*, 779068. [CrossRef] [PubMed]
25. Neblett, R.; Cohen, H.; Choi, Y.; Hartzell, M.M.; Williams, M.; Mayer, T.G.; Gatchel, R.J. The Central Sensitization Inventory (CSI): Establishing clinically significant values for identifying central sensitivity syndromes in an outpatient chronic pain sample. *J. Pain Off. J. Am. Pain Soc.* **2013**, *14*, 438–445. [CrossRef]
26. Cuesta-Vargas, A.I.; Neblett, R.; Nijs, J.; Chiarotto, A.; Kregel, J.; van Wilgen, C.P.; Pitance, L.; Knezevic, A.; Gatchel, R.J.; Mayer, T.G.; et al. Establishing Central Sensitization-Related Symptom Severity Subgroups: A Multicountry Study Using the Central Sensitization Inventory. *Pain Med.* **2020**, *21*, 2430–2440. [CrossRef] [PubMed]
27. Kregel, J.; Vuijk, P.J.; Descheemaeker, F.; Keizer, D.; van der Noord, R.; Nijs, J.; Cagnie, B.; Meeus, M.; van Wilgen, P. The Dutch Central Sensitization Inventory (CSI): Factor Analysis, Discriminative Power, and Test-Retest Reliability. *Clin. J. Pain* **2016**, *32*, 624–630. [CrossRef]
28. Pitance, L.; Piraux, E.; Lannoy, B.; Meeus, M.; Berquin, A.; Eeckhout, C.; Dethier, V.; Robertson, J.; Roussel, N. Cross cultural adaptation, reliability and validity of the French version of the central sensitization inventory. *Man. Ther.* **2016**, *25*, e83–e84. [CrossRef]
29. Corsi, G.; Nava, S.; Barco, S. A novel tool to monitor the individual functional status after COVID-19: The Post-COVID-19 Functional Status (PCFS) scale. *G. Ital. Cardiol.* **2020**, *21*, 757. [CrossRef]
30. Klok, F.A.; Boon, G.; Barco, S.; Endres, M.; Geelhoed, J.J.M.; Knauss, S.; Rezek, S.A.; Spruit, M.A.; Vehreschild, J.; Siegerink, B. The Post-COVID-19 Functional Status scale: A tool to measure functional status over time after COVID-19. *Eur. Respir. J.* **2020**, *56*, 2001494. [CrossRef]
31. Muller, J.P.; Goncalves, P.A.; Fontoura, F.F.; Mattiello, R.; Florian, J. Applicability of the London Chest Activity of Daily Living scale in patients on the waiting list for lung transplantation. *J. Bras. Pneumol.* **2013**, *39*, 92–97. [CrossRef]

32. Garrod, R.; Bestall, J.C.; Paul, E.A.; Wedzicha, J.A.; Jones, P.W. Development and validation of a standardized measure of activity of daily living in patients with severe COPD: The London Chest Activity of Daily Living scale (LCADL). *Respir. Med.* **2000**, *94*, 589–596. [CrossRef]
33. Coppieters, I.; Ickmans, K.; Cagnie, B.; Nijs, J.; De Pauw, R.; Noten, S.; Meeus, M. Cognitive Performance Is Related to Central Sensitization and Health-related Quality of Life in Patients with Chronic Whiplash-Associated Disorders and Fibromyalgia. *Pain Physician* **2015**, *18*, E389–E401. [PubMed]
34. Mertens, M.G.; Hermans, L.; Crombez, G.; Goudman, L.; Calders, P.; Van Oosterwijck, J.; Meeus, M. Comparison of five conditioned pain modulation paradigms and influencing personal factors in healthy adults. *Eur. J. Pain* **2021**, *25*, 243–256. [CrossRef] [PubMed]
35. Kosek, E.; Ekholm, J.; Hansson, P. Pressure pain thresholds in different tissues in one body region. The influence of skin sensitivity in pressure algometry. *Scand. J. Rehabil. Med.* **1999**, *31*, 89–93. [CrossRef] [PubMed]
36. Malfliet, A.; Pas, R.; Brouns, R.; De Win, J.; Hatem, S.M.; Meeus, M.; Ickmans, K.; van Hooff, R.J.; Nijs, J. Cerebral Blood Flow and Heart Rate Variability in Chronic Fatigue Syndrome: A Randomized Cross-Over Study. *Pain Physician* **2018**, *21*, E13–E24. [CrossRef]
37. Cathcart, S.; Winefield, A.H.; Rolan, P.; Lushington, K. Reliability of temporal summation and diffuse noxious inhibitory control. *Pain Res. Manag.* **2009**, *14*, 433–438. [CrossRef]
38. Moont, R.; Pud, D.; Sprecher, E.; Sharvit, G.; Yarnitsky, D. 'Pain inhibits pain' mechanisms: Is pain modulation simply due to distraction? *Pain* **2010**, *150*, 113–120. [CrossRef]
39. Yarnitsky, D.; Bouhassira, D.; Drewes, A.M.; Fillingim, R.B.; Granot, M.; Hansson, P.; Landau, R.; Marchand, S.; Matre, D.; Nilsen, K.B.; et al. Recommendations on practice of conditioned pain modulation (CPM) testing. *Eur. J. Pain* **2015**, *19*, 805–806. [CrossRef]
40. Staud, R.; Craggs, J.G.; Robinson, M.E.; Perlstein, W.M.; Price, D.D. Brain activity related to temporal summation of C-fiber evoked pain. *Pain* **2007**, *129*, 130–142. [CrossRef]
41. Coppieters, I.; De Pauw, R.; Kregel, J.; Malfliet, A.; Goubert, D.; Lenoir, D.; Cagnie, B.; Meeus, M. Differences Between Women with Traumatic and Idiopathic Chronic Neck Pain and Women without Neck Pain: Interrelationships among Disability, Cognitive Deficits, and Central Sensitization. *Phys. Ther.* **2017**, *97*, 338–353. [CrossRef]
42. Sim, J.; Wright, C.C. The kappa statistic in reliability studies: Use, interpretation, and sample size requirements. *Phys. Ther.* **2005**, *85*, 257–268. [CrossRef]
43. Uddin, Z.; MacDermid, J.C. Quantitative Sensory Testing in Chronic Musculoskeletal Pain. *Pain Med.* **2016**, *17*, 1694–1703. [CrossRef] [PubMed]
44. Coppieters, I.; Cagnie, B.; Nijs, J.; van Oosterwijck, J.; Danneels, L.; De Pauw, R.; Meeus, M. Effects of Stress and Relaxation on Central Pain Modulation in Chronic Whiplash and Fibromyalgia Patients Compared to Healthy Controls. *Pain Physician* **2016**, *19*, 119–130. [PubMed]
45. Meeus, M.; Van Oosterwijck, J.; Ickmans, K.; Baert, I.; Coppieters, I.; Roussel, N.; Struyf, F.; Pattyn, N.; Nijs, J. Interrelationships between pain processing, cortisol and cognitive performance in chronic whiplash-associated disorders. *Clin. Rheumatol.* **2015**, *34*, 545–553. [CrossRef] [PubMed]
46. Kregel, J.; Schumacher, C.; Dolphens, M.; Malfliet, A.; Goubert, D.; Lenoir, D.; Cagnie, B.; Meeus, M.; Coppieters, I. Convergent Validity of the Dutch Central Sensitization Inventory: Associations with Psychophysical Pain Measures, Quality of Life, Disability, and Pain Cognitions in Patients with Chronic Spinal Pain. *Pain Pract.* **2018**, *18*, 777–787. [CrossRef]
47. Gervais-Hupé, J.; Pollice, J.; Sadi, J.; Carlesso, L.C. Validity of the central sensitization inventory with measures of sensitization in people with knee osteoarthritis. *Clin. Rheumatol.* **2018**, *37*, 3125–3132. [CrossRef]
48. Coronado, R.A.; George, S.Z. The Central Sensitization Inventory and Pain Sensitivity Questionnaire: An exploration of construct validity and associations with widespread pain sensitivity among individuals with shoulder pain. *Musculoskelet. Sci. Pract.* **2018**, *36*, 61–67. [CrossRef]
49. Hendriks, E.; Voogt, L.; Lenoir, D.; Coppieters, I.; Ickmans, K. Convergent Validity of the Central Sensitization Inventory in Chronic Whiplash-Associated Disorders; Associations with Quantitative Sensory Testing, Pain Intensity, Fatigue, and Psychosocial Factors. *Pain Med.* **2020**, *21*, 3401–3412. [CrossRef]
50. Kosińska, B.; Tarnacka, B.; Turczyn, P.; Gromadzka, G.; Malec-Milewska, M.; Janikowska-Hołowenko, D.; Neblett, R. Psychometric validation of the Polish version of the Central Sensitization Inventory in subjects with chronic spinal pain. *BMC Neurol.* **2021**, *21*, 483. [CrossRef]
51. Akeda, K.; Yamada, J.; Takegami, N.; Fujiwara, T.; Murata, K.; Kono, T.; Sudo, T.; Imanishi, T.; Asanuma, Y.; Kurata, T.; et al. Evaluation of Central Sensitization Inventory in Patients Undergoing Elective Spine Surgery in a Multicenter Study. *Glob. Spine J.* **2021**, 21925682211047473. [CrossRef]
52. Holm, L.A.; Nim, C.G.; Lauridsen, H.H.; Filtenborg, J.B.; O'Neill, S.F. Convergent validity of the central sensitization inventory and experimental testing of pain sensitivity. *Scand. J. Pain* **2022**, *22*, 597–613. [CrossRef]
53. Çalik Kütükcü, E.; Çakmak, A.; Kinaci, E.; Uyaroğlu, O.A.; Yağli, N.V.; Güven, G.S.; Sağlam, M.; Özişik, L.; Başaran, N.Ç.; Ince, D.I. Reliability and validity of the Turkish version of Post-COVID-19 Functional Status Scale. *Turk. J. Med. Sci.* **2021**, *51*, 2304–2310. [CrossRef]

54. Ganesh, R.; Grach, S.L.; Ghosh, A.K.; Bierle, D.M.; Salonen, B.R.; Collins, N.M.; Joshi, A.Y.; Boeder, N.D., Jr.; Anstine, C.V.; Mueller, M.R.; et al. The Female-Predominant Persistent Immune Dysregulation of the Post-COVID Syndrome. *Mayo Clin. Proc.* **2022**, *97*, 454–464. [CrossRef] [PubMed]
55. Kosek, E.; Cohen, M.; Baron, R.; Gebhart, G.F.; Mico, J.A.; Rice, A.S.C.; Rief, W.; Sluka, A.K. Do we need a third mechanistic descriptor for chronic pain states? *Pain* **2016**, *157*, 1382–1386. [CrossRef] [PubMed]
56. Fernández-de-Las-Peñas, C.; Nijs, J.; Neblett, R.; Polli, A.; Moens, M.; Goudman, L.; Patil, M.S.; Knaggs, R.D.; Pickering, G.; Arendt-Nielsen, L. Phenotyping Post-COVID Pain as a Nociceptive, Neuropathic, or Nociplastic Pain Condition. *Biomedicines* **2022**, *10*, 2562. [CrossRef] [PubMed]
57. Moens, M.; Jansen, J.; De Smedt, A.; Roulaud, M.; Billot, M.; Laton, J.; Rigoard, P.; Goudman, L. Acceptance and Commitment Therapy to Increase Resilience in Chronic Pain Patients: A Clinical Guideline. *Medicina* **2022**, *58*, 499. [CrossRef] [PubMed]

Disclaimer/Publisher's Note: The statements, opinions and data contained in all publications are solely those of the individual author(s) and contributor(s) and not of MDPI and/or the editor(s). MDPI and/or the editor(s) disclaim responsibility for any injury to people or property resulting from any ideas, methods, instructions or products referred to in the content.

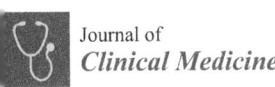

Article

The Very Long COVID: Persistence of Symptoms after 12–18 Months from the Onset of Infection and Hospitalization

Marco Ranucci [1,*], Ekaterina Baryshnikova [1], Martina Anguissola [1], Sara Pugliese [1], Luca Ranucci [1], Mara Falco [2] and Lorenzo Menicanti [3]

1. Department of Cardiovascular Anesthesia and Intensive Care, IRCCS Policlinico San Donato, 20097 Milan, Italy
2. Department of Radiology, Koelliker Hospital, 10134 Turin, Italy
3. Scientific Directorate, IRCCS Policlinico San Donato, 20097 Milan, Italy
* Correspondence: marco.ranucci@grupposandonato.it; Tel.: +39-(02)-5277-4754

Abstract: According to the World Health Organization's definition, long COVID is the persistence or development of new symptoms 3 months after the initial infection. Various conditions have been explored in studies with up to one-year follow-up but very few looked further. This prospective cohort study addresses the presence of a wide spectrum of symptoms in 121 patients hospitalized during the acute phase of COVID-19 infection, and the association between factors related to the acute phase of the disease and the presence of residual symptoms after one year or longer from hospitalization. The main results are as follows: (i) post-COVID symptoms persist in up to 60% of the patient population at a mean follow-up of 17 months; (ii) the most frequent symptoms are fatigue and dyspnea, but neuropsychological disturbances persist in about 30% of the patients (iii) when corrected for the duration of follow-up with a freedom-from-event analysis; only complete (2 doses) vaccination at the time of hospital admission remained independently associated with persistence of the major physical symptoms, while vaccination and previous neuropsychological symptoms remained independently associated with persistence of major neuropsychological symptoms.

Keywords: COVID-19; long COVID; post-acute; long follow-up; persistent symptoms; major physical symptoms; major neurological symptoms

1. Introduction

The World Health Organization's definition of long COVID is the continuation or development of new symptoms 3 months after the initial SARS-CoV-2 infection, with these symptoms lasting for at least 2 months with no other explanation [1]. Common symptoms of long COVID can include fatigue, shortness of breath, and cognitive dysfunction. Over 200 different symptoms have been reported that can have an impact on everyday functioning [1]. A post-acute COVID-19 study from the USA [2] included patients hospitalized due to COVID-19 and re-evaluated after 60 days from discharge. Within this period of time, 6.7% of the patients died, 15.1% required re-admission, and 32.6% reported persistent symptoms. The most common symptoms were dyspnea while walking up the stairs, cough, and loss of taste and/or smell. Other studies extended the observation period up to 3–4 months after hospital admission and found similar results [3–8], with approximately 30% of the patient population reporting fatigue, dyspnea, psychological distress, anxiety, depression, concentration, and sleep abnormalities.

There are studies addressing mortality [9], cardiovascular risk [10], pulmonary function [11], and neuropsychological changes [12] at one year or longer after COVID-19 infection.

However, few studies extended the window of observation longer than 12 months. The present study addresses the persistence of a wide spectrum of symptoms after hospital discharge of COVID-19 patients, and the association between factors related to the acute

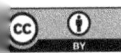

phase of the disease and the presence of residual symptoms after one year or longer from hospitalization.

2. Materials and Methods

This is a single-center prospective cohort study conducted at the IRCCS San Donato, a Clinical Research Hospital partially funded by the Italian Ministry of Health. The Local Ethics Committee (San Raffaele Hospital) approved the experimental design on 3 March 2022, registry number 28/INT/2022. All the patients gave written informed consent. The study has been financed by a grant from the Italian Ministry of Health for the research projects of the Cardiac Network of the Italian IRCCS (Clinical Research Hospitals). The eligible patient population was represented by subjects hospitalized at our institution with a diagnosis of COVID-19 infection between January 2021 and July 2022. The planned patient population was 100 patients. The primary endpoint was the persistence of major physical and neuropsychological symptoms from 3 up to 12–18 months from the hospital discharge, and the assessment of factors associated with the time-related freedom from residual symptomatology.

2.1. Patient Population and Study Procedures

The patients were recruited through an initial telephone contact; those who were reachable and agreed to participate received a date for the study procedure at our hospital. The telephone calls started in April 2022 and ended on 15 November 2022. The first patient hospital admission date was 8 January 2021, and the last hospital admission date was 4 July 2022. The first follow-up visit date was 12 April 2022, and the last follow-up visit was 21 November 2022. The recruitment flow is shown in Figure 1. The final patient population comprised 121 subjects. The study has three work packages. Work package 1 is a clinical assessment of the patient, comprehensive of the parameters at the time of hospital admission in the acute phase, main laboratory data, and investigation of the presence of residual symptomatology linked to COVID-19. Work package 2 is an evaluation of the coagulation profile of the patient, and work package 3 includes a proteomic assessment of the patient. The present report deals with the results of work package 1.

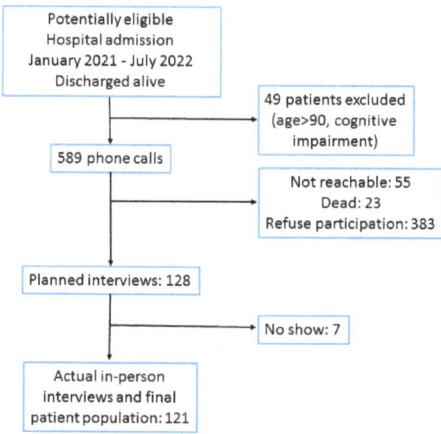

Figure 1. Patient screening and selection.

2.2. Data Collection and Definitions

Data collection was based on (i) the retrieval of the relevant data from the original patient's files and (ii) a personal interview conducted in a hospital office by dedicated biologists and a medical doctor.

The following items regarding the acute phase hospitalization were collected: demographics (with age classes ≤50 years, 51–60 years, 61–70 years, 71–80 years, and >80 years);

disease severity (mild: no oxygen therapy; moderate: nasal oxygen or oxygen mask; and severe: non-invasive or invasive ventilation), hospital stay, the unit of admission, and vaccination (2 doses) at the time of hospital admission; co-morbidities: obesity, hypertension, diabetes, history of coronary disease, heart failure, atrial fibrillation, chronic obstructive pulmonary disease, asthma, active cancer, chronic kidney failure, chronic liver failure, previous cerebrovascular accident, anxiety, or depression; therapy at the time of hospitalization; laboratory exams: peak fibrinogen levels, peak D-Dimer, peak platelet count, nadir platelet count, or nadir antithrombin.

A specific COVID-19 treatment was applied to all the patients, following the indications of the Italian Drug Agency: a prophylactic dose of low molecular weight heparin; low-dose steroids; and remdesivir in selected patients (within 7 days from the onset of COVID-19 symptoms; a moderate degree of severity and at least one risk factor for progression to a severe form).

Follow-up items included follow-up duration; any symptom after discharge; work capacity reduced; fatigue, fever, cough, or dyspnea (these last four items combined as "Major physical symptoms"—MPS—adjudicated in the presence of one or more symptoms); and chest pain, palpitations, headache, sleep disturbances, anxiety, depression (new symptoms starting or worsening during hospitalization), memory dysfunction, brain fog, (these last four items combined as "Major neuropsychological symptoms"—MNS—adjudicated in presence of one or more symptoms), paresthesias, muscle pain, joint pain, and sensorial deficit. For each symptom or combination of symptoms, there was a distinction between resolved and ongoing status. Data were collected in an electronic platform (Research Electronic Data Capture—RedCAP).

2.3. Statistical Analysis

Data are shown as number (percentage), mean (standard deviation) or median (interquartile range) as appropriate. Differences between categorical variables were assessed using Pearson's chi-square, while differences in continuous variables were explored with Student's t-test (normally distributed variables) or a non-parametric test (non-normally distributed variables). Survival curves were applied in univariate (Kaplan–Meier with log-rank test) and multivariable (Cox regression with hazard ratios and 95% confidence intervals) analyses. For the statistical calculations and graphical support data were exported from RedCAP into statistical packages (SPSS 20.0, IBM, Chicago, IL, USA, and MedCalc, MedCalc Software, Ostend, Belgium). For all tests, a $p < 0.05$ was considered significant.

3. Results

The general characteristics of the patient population are shown in Table 1, according to the severity of the disease in its acute phase. The body mass index (BMI) was significantly higher for increasing degrees of severity as well as the length of hospital stay. A previous smoking habit was significantly less frequent in those with a mild degree of severity, and patients with a severe pattern of disease had significantly higher peak fibrinogen values during the acute phase.

The data collected at follow-up are reported in Table 2 for the whole patient population and separately for the different degrees of severity of the disease during the acute phase. The follow-up period significantly differed, with a shorter follow-up for patients with a mild severity. Overall, 96% of the patients reported one or more symptoms from the hospital discharge to follow-up; however, this rate was significantly lower (79%) in patients with a mild pattern of the disease. MPS were reported as still present at the time of follow-up by 61% of the patient population, again with a significant lower rate (37%) in patients who experienced a mild pattern of disease. It is of notice that this patient population reported a significantly higher rate of fever; however, it was resolved at the time of follow-up. Among symptoms still present at the time of follow-up, fatigue was reported by 50% of the patients and dyspnea by 42%, followed by joint pain (35%), memory dysfunction (34%), sleep disturbances, muscle pain (27%), anxiety, brain fog and paresthesias (20%), and depression (18%). MPS were significantly more frequent for an increasing severity of the disease during the acute phase, and this particularly applied to ongoing dyspnea, whereas the other component of the MPS (fatigue and cough) did not differ for different degrees of the severity of the disease. The MNS rate was not significantly different for different degrees of the severity of the disease.

Table 1. Patient population (N = 121) details at hospital admission and during the acute phase of the disease, according to the severity of the disease.

Item	Mild N = 19	Moderate N = 68	Severe N = 34	p
Age at hospital admission (years)	59.5 (15.3)	66.3 (11.6)	63.6 (14.6)	0.129
Gender male	12 (63.2)	46 (67.6)	22 (64.7)	0.916
Body mass index (kg/m^2)	25.3 (4.1)	27.5 (6.0)	29.4 (6.0)	0.047
Hospital stay (days)	8 (6–18)	14 (10–20)	23 (16–32)	0.001
Unit of admission				
Ward	19 (100)	67 (98.5)	30 (91.2)	0.205
ICU	0 (0)	1 (1.5)	3 (8.8)	
Vaccination (at least 2 doses)	7 (36.8)	14 (19.1)	4 (11.8)	0.096
Obesity	3 (15.8)	14 (20.6)	11 (32.4)	0.294
Arterial hypertension	5 (26.3)	32 (47.1)	18 (52.9)	0.34
Diabetes	3 (15.8)	11 (16.2)	6 (17.6)	0.978
Coronaropathy	2 (10.5)	15 (22.1)	3 (8.8)	0.177
Heart failure	0 (0)	7 (10.3)	2 (5.9)	0.293
Smoking habit				0.008
No	11 (58)	33 (48.5)	15 (44.1)	
Previous	4 (21.1)	32 (47)	19 (56)	
Ongoing	4 (21.1)	3 (4.4)	0 (0)	
Atrial fibrillation	0 (0)	7 (10.3)	4 (11.8)	0.315
Active cancer previous 5 years	5 (26.3)	5 (7.4)	1 (2.9)	0.013
COPD	2 (10.5)	3 (4.4)	1 (2.9)	0.452
Chronic kidney failure	0 (0)	6 (8.8)	2 (5.9)	0.384
Previous CVA	2 (10.5)	1 (1.5)	3 (8.8)	0.13
Anxiety	3 (15.8)	9 (13.2)	7 (20.6)	0.629
Depression	3 (15.8)	6 (8.8)	5 (14.7)	0.56
Chronic liver failure	1 (5.3)	3 (4.4)	0 (0)	0.438

Data are mean (standard deviation), median (interquartile range), or number (%). CVA: cerebrovascular accident; COPD: chronic obstructive pulmonary disease; ICU: intensive care unit.

Table 2. Residual symptomatology after discharge from the hospital according to the severity of the acute phase.

Item	All	Mild N = 121	Moderate N = 19	Severe N = 68	p N = 34
Follow-up time (months)	17 (12–18)	12 (8–17)	17 (12–18)	17 (14–19)	0.011
Symptoms after discharge	112 (95.6)	15 (78.9)	75 (95.6)	32 (94.1)	0.046
Major physical symptoms					
Resolved	38 (31.4)	12 (63.2)	26 (38.2)	9 (26.5)	
Ongoing	74 (61.2)	7 (36.8)	42 (61.8)	25 (73.5)	0.031
Work capacity reduced	39 (32.2)	4 (21.1)	21 (30.9)	14 (41.2)	0.303
Fever	5 (4.1)	3 (15.8)	2 (2.9)	0 (0)	0.016
Resolved	4 (3.3)	2 (10.5)	2 (2.9)	0 (0)	
Ongoing	1 (0.8)	1 (5.3)	0 (0)	0 (0)	0.348
Fatigue	86 (71.1)	11 (57.9)	50 (73.5)	25 (73.5)	0.386
Resolved	26 (21.5)	4 (21.1)	15 (22.1)	7 (20.6)	
Ongoing	60 (49.6)	7 (36.8)	35 (51.5)	17 (50)	0.596

Table 2. Cont.

Item	All	Mild N = 121	Moderate N = 19	Severe N = 68	p N = 34
Cough	29 (24)	4 (21.1)	16 (23.5)	9 (26.5)	0.911
Resolved	9 (7.4)	1 (5.3)	6 (8.8)	2 (5.9)	
Ongoing	20 (16.5)	3 (15.8)	10 (14.7)	7 (20.6)	0.919
Dyspnea	59 (48.8)	1 (5.3)	37 (54.4)	21 (61.8)	0.001
Resolved	8 (6.6)	0 (0)	4 (5.9)	4 (11.8)	
Ongoing	51 (42.1)	1 (5.3)	33 (48.5)	17 (50)	0.001
Chest pain	12 (9.9)	1 (5.3)	7 (10.3)	4 (11.8)	0.845
Resolved	3 (2.5)	1 (5.3)	1 (1.5)	1 (2.9)	
Ongoing	9 (7.4)	0 (0)	6 (8.8)	3 (8.8)	0.62
Palpitations	13 (10.7)	1 (5.3)	8 (11.8)	4 (11.8)	0.215
Resolved	2 (1.7)	0 (0)	0 (0)	2 (5.9)	
Ongoing	11 (9.0)	1 (5.3)	8 (11.8)	2 (5.9)	0.17
Headache	14 (11.6)	2 (10.5)	7 (10.3)	5 (14.7)	0.211
Resolved	2 (1.7)	0 (0)	2 (2.9)	0 (0)	
Ongoing	12 (9.9)	2 (10.5)	5 (7.4)	5 (14.7)	0.582
Major neuropsychological symptoms	58 (47.9)	7 (36.8)	35 (51.5)	16 (47.1)	0.525
Resolved	0 (0)		2 (5.3)	2 (2.9)	
Ongoing	54 (44.6)	7 (36.8)	33 (48.5)	14 (41.2)	0.592
Anxiety	26 (21.5)	3 (15.8)	16 (23.5)	7 (20.6)	0.76
Resolved	2 (1.7)	0 (0)	0 (0)	2 (5.9)	
Ongoing	24 (19.8)	3 (15.8)	16 (23.5)	5 (14.7)	0.177
Depression	24 (19.8)	2 (10.5)	14 (20.6)	8 (23.5)	0.509
Resolved	2 (1.7)	0 (0)	0 (0)	2 (0)	
Ongoing	22 (18.1)	2 (10.5)	14 (20.6)	6 (17.6)	0.183
Sleep disturbances	36 (29.8)	3 (15.8)	22 (32.4)	11 (32.4)	0.35
Resolved	3 (2.5)	1 (5.3)	1 (1.5)	1 (2.9)	
Ongoing	33 (27.3)	2 (10.5)	21 (30.9)	10 (29.4)	0.425
Memory dysfunction	46 (38)	6 (31.6)	26 (38.2)	14 (41.2)	0.787
Resolved	4 (3.3)	1 (5.3)	2 (2.9)	1 (2.9)	
Ongoing	42 (34.7)	5 (26.3)	24 (35.3)	13 (38.2)	0.916
Brain fog	29 (24)	4 (21.1)	17 (25)	8 (23.5)	0.936
Resolved	4 (3.3)	1 (5.3)	2 (2.9)	1 (2.9)	
Ongoing	25 (20.6)	3 (15.8)	15 (22.1)	7 (20.6)	0.966
Paresthesia	31 (25.6)	1 (5.3)	21 (30.9)	9 (25.5)	0.077
Resolved	6 (5.0)	0 (0)	3 (4.4)	3 (8.8)	
Ongoing	26 (20.6)	1 (5.3)	18 (26.5)	5 (14.7)	0.13
Muscle pain	39 (32.2)	6 (31.6)	22 (32.4)	11 (32.4)	0.998
Resolved	7 (5.8)	1 (5.3)	5 (7.4)	1 (2.9)	
Ongoing	32 (26.5)	5 (26.3)	17 (25)	10 (29.4)	0.919
Joint pain	45 (37.2)	5 (26.3)	27 (39.7)	13 (38.2)	0.559
Resolved	3 (2.5)	1 (5.3)	2 (2.9)	0 (0)	
Ongoing	42 (34.7)	4 (21.1)	25 (36.8)	13 (38.2)	0.533
Residual sensory deficit	48 (39.6)	3 (15.8)	30 (44.1)	15 (44.1)	0.068
Sight	19 (15.7)	1 (5.3)	8 (11.8)1	0 (29.4)	0.037
Smell	5 (4.1)	1 (5.3)	2 (2.9)	2 (5.9)	0.786
Hearing	12 (9.9)	1 (5.3)	10 (14.7)	1 (2.9)	0.543
Taste	12 (9.9)	0 (0)	10 (14.7)	2 (5.9)	0.653

Data are median (interquartile range) or number (%).

The analysis of the determinants of ongoing MPS and MNS was based on survival curves, given the different follow-up times between groups. Figure 2 reports the persistence of MPS in the general patient population. Starting with 95% of persistence after 3 months from hospital discharge, MPS remained present in 82% of the patients after 1 year, and 45% of the patients after 18 months, reaching about 10% only after 20 months. With a Kaplan–Meier analysis with log-rank test, factors associated with the freedom from MPS at a level of $p < 0.1$ were age class (with a faster resolution of symptoms for patients ≥ 70 years, $p = 0.098$) and vaccination, with vaccinated patients having a hazard ratio for the persistence of symptoms of 0.305 (95% confidence interval 0.164–0.568, $p = 0.001$) with respect to non-vaccinated patients. No other factor demonstrated an association with the persistence of MPS (Supplementary Table S1). Figure 3 reports the freedom from the persistence of MPS in vaccinated vs. non-vaccinated patients. After 1 year, 92% of the non-vaccinated patients still reported MPS vs. 50% of the vaccinated patients. After 18 months the percentages decreased to 50% and 22%, respectively.

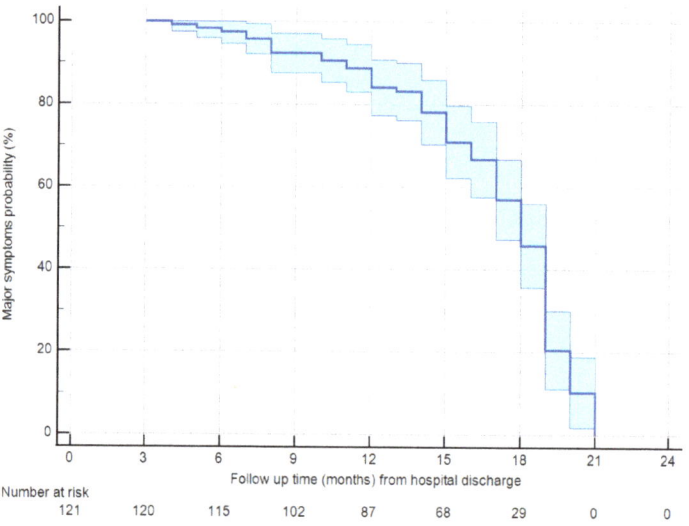

Figure 2. Freedom from major physical symptoms in the overall population.

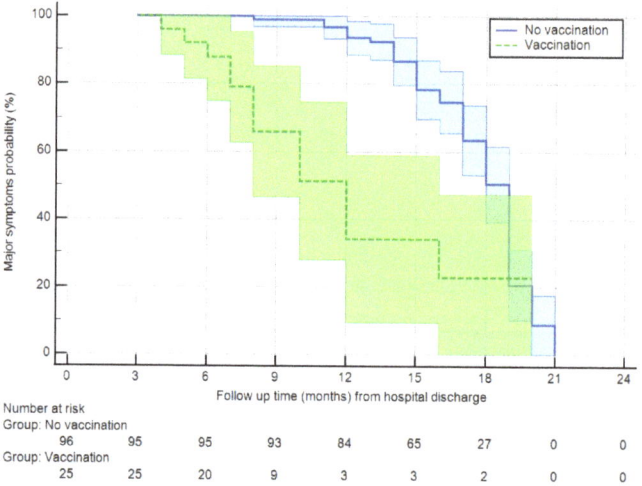

Figure 3. Freedom from major physical symptoms in vaccinated vs. non-vaccinated patients (Log-rank test, $p = 0.001$). Light blue and light green areas are 95% confidence intervals.

A Cox regression analysis was applied to the persistence of MPS with vaccination, severity of disease, and age class as covariates. In this model, vaccination remained independently associated with the persistence of MPS (hazard ratio 0.309, 95% confidence interval 0.160–0.6, $p = 0.001$), whereas age class (hazard ratio 1.01, 95% confidence interval

0.843–1.212, $p = 0.910$) and severity of the disease (hazard ratio 0.970, 95% confidence interval 0.651–1.446, $p = 0.880$) lost significant association.

To investigate the intercorrelation between age class and vaccination, a sensitivity analysis was conducted (Table 3). Although without reaching statistical significance ($p = 0.338$); patients aged >80 years had a higher (40%) vaccination rate than patients ≤ 80 years (14 to 23%).

Table 3. Vaccination rate according to age class.

Age class	<50	50–60	61–70	70–80	>80	p
	N = 17	N = 26	N = 28	N = 35	N = 15	
Vaccination	4 (23.5)	5 (19.2)	5 (17.9)	5 (14.3)	6 (40)	0.338

Data are number (%).

The persistence of MNS was significantly associated with vaccination (hazard ratio 0.206, 95% confidence interval 0.108–0.394, $p = 0.001$), ICU admission (hazard ratio 0.340, 95% confidence interval 0.184–0.628, $p = 0.001$), and presence of neurological symptoms (anxiety or depression) at the time of the acute phase (hazard ratio 2.87, 95% confidence interval 1.56–5.27, $p = 0.001$). The other factors showed no association with persistence of MNS (Supplementary Table S2). Once tested in a Cox regression multivariable analysis, the factors that remained associated with the persistence of MNS were vaccination (hazard ratio 0.205, 95% confidence interval 0.099–0.426, $p = 0.001$) and previous neurological symptoms (hazard ratio 3.42, 95% confidence interval 1.83–6.39, $p = 0.001$), while admission to the ICU lost significance (hazard ratio 0.59, 95% confidence interval 0.30–1.16, $p = 0.126$). Figure 4 shows the freedom from persistence of MNS in vaccinated and non-vaccinated patients, adjusted for previous neurological symptoms. At 1-year follow-up, vaccinated patients had MNS in 24% of the cases vs. 94% in non-vaccinated patients. At 18 months follow-up these rates remained stable for vaccinated patients and decreased to 32% in non-vaccinated patients.

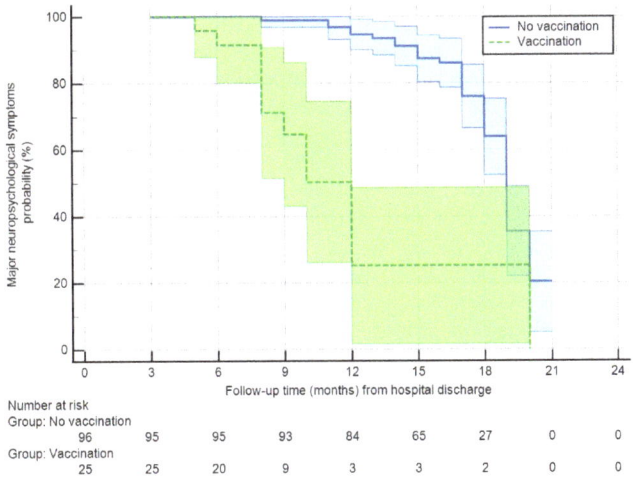

Figure 4. Freedom from major neuropsychological symptoms in vaccinated vs. non-vaccinated patients (Log-rank test, $p = 0.001$). Light blue and light green areas are 95% confidence intervals. Adjusted for previous neurological symptoms.

Overall, at the time of the acute phase, 25 (20.7%) patients were vaccinated with two doses. After discharge, at the time of follow-up, 113 (93.4%) received a vaccination, with 9 patients (7.4%) receiving a total of one dose, 62 (51.2%) two doses, and 40 (33.1%) three doses. The type of vaccine was Pfizer in 77 (63.6%) patients, Moderna in 21 (17.4%) patients, Astra Zeneca in 7 (5.8%) patients, Janssen in 2 (1.7%) patients, and unknown in 6 patients.

4. Discussion

The main results of our study are that (i) post-COVID symptoms persist in up to 60% of the patient population at a mean follow-up of 17 months; (ii) the most frequent symptoms are fatigue and dyspnea, but neuropsychological disturbances persist in about 30% of the patients (iii) when corrected for the duration of follow-up with a freedom-from-event analysis; only complete (2 doses) vaccination at the time of hospital admission remained independently associated with persistence of MPS, while vaccination and previous neuropsychological symptoms remained independently associated with persistence of MNS. Immediately after discharge, all the patients (vaccinated and non-vaccinated) showed residual symptoms, but they were compatible with the hospital discharge. The survival curves between vaccinated and non-vaccinated patients start diverging only after 3 months of follow-up.

Other studies investigated, with different experimental designs, the long-term persistence of symptoms after the hospital discharge of COVID-19 patients. Kalak and associates [13], in a series of 166 patients, 135 of whom had been admitted to a hospital during the acute phase, found residual weakness (21%), dyspnea (16%), and brain fog (7%) after 18 months from hospital discharge. These results are in line with our observation. The only predictors of dyspnea at 18 months follow-up were dyspnea during the acute phase and dexamethasone therapy, likely markers of the severity of the disease. Gutierrez-Canales and associates [14] addressed post-COVID symptoms in a series of patients (non-vaccinated) who did not require hospitalization during the acute phase. As expected, in these low-severity disease patients, those who were followed for 5 months or longer showed a lower rate of persistent symptoms (22%) with respect to our series. However, the frequency of each symptom followed our pattern, with fatigue, dyspnea, and neuropsychological disturbances being the most represented. A study performed in India [15] included 371 patients followed 6 months after the infection, with 22% of patients being admitted to a hospital during the acute phase. Again, the frequency of long COVID symptoms was lower (9%) than in our series. Of notice, patients who received two doses of vaccine before the infection had a higher probability of developing long COVID symptoms. The authors explained their findings as the result of a better survival. Our results show the opposite, with a time-adjusted probability of developing long COVID symptoms in vaccinated patients that is one-third for MPS and one-fifth for MNS with respect to non-vaccinated patients. In this regard, our study confirms what was reported by the United Kingdom Health Security Agency [16] that people vaccinated before COVID-19 infection are 50% less likely to develop long COVID symptoms 1 to 6 months after the infection. Our data show that this effect is prolonged and even more pronounced from 3 up to 18 months after the infection. The positive effects of vaccination in limiting the probability of developing long COVID symptoms were reported in a Spanish study on 681 patients (23% hospitalized during the acute phase) [17]. This study included only patients who developed long COVID symptoms after an unspecified period of time from the infection. Major symptoms like fatigue were significantly less frequent in vaccinated patients (odds ratio 0.19, 95% confidence interval 0.04–0.79).

A comprehensive and multidisciplinary evaluation of patients hospitalized for COVID-19 infection was undertaken by Bellan and associates [18] one year after hospital discharge. Three hundred twenty-four patients received clinical investigation with lung function test, and a subgroup was tested for circulating cytokines. Patients admitted during the first wave had a persistence of symptoms of 41.1% vs. 31.2% in patients admitted during the third wave ($p = 0.09$) and showed a significantly ($p = 0.02$) lower diffusion lung for carbon monoxide. Although the authors did not address this point, no patient was vaccinated during the first wave in Italy, whereas many were during the third wave. Risk factors for the development of long COVID symptoms were gender female and previous neuropsychological symptoms (anxiety and depression), with no association with the severity of the disease. This finding is in agreement with our results. A Norwegian study [19] directly addressed the effects of vaccination on the presence of long COVID symptoms, in a population of 360 vaccinated and 1060 non-vaccinated patients. No significant differences were noticed with respect to permanent symptoms at 3–15 months. However, it was unspecified whether or not these patients were hospitalized during the acute phase.

Overall, the majority of the studies agree that long COVID symptoms are a frequent pattern, even if the window of observation is variable within and between studies. There is no consensus on the potential factors that may predict the onset of a long COVID pattern, and, namely, the severity of the disease in the acute phase, the age, and the role of vaccination. Conversely, the authors agree on the most common type of symptoms, which are fatigue, dyspnea, anxiety, and depression.

Our study differs from the existing ones and offers a different point of view. First of all, our patient population has been observed for a quite long period of time, up to 20 months after the hospital discharge, whereas the majority of the studies limit the follow-up to 6–12 months. Secondly, our patient population is homogeneous (only hospitalized patients) and single-center. This allowed us to review the patients' files and retrieve objective information on a number of items, including vaccination state and laboratory exams. Third, and most important, our data have been retrieved through a direct interview of the patients rather than through telephone interviews or web-based questionnaires. This allowed a sounder and less subjective identification of the various symptoms. Finally, and differently from the existing studies, we could assess the freedom from long COVID symptoms using adequate statistical tools like actuarial curves with univariate and multivariable estimates of the role of various factors as determinants of MPS and MNS. This allowed us to discriminate the weight of each variable, and, in particular, we could demonstrate that, in our series, the apparent impact of the severity of the disease was blunted when analyzed in a model based on the follow-up time. The same happened for the age of the patients: the apparent paradox of a lower rate of residual symptoms in the elderly patients is explained by the higher rate of vaccinated patients in the age class >80 years. This is easily explainable considering that in Italy the first vaccinations were reserved for elderly people. Another possible explanation for the higher rate of long COVID pattern in young (<50 years) patients could be related to the fact that young and active subjects are probably more sensitive to a decrease in work capacity and endurance than elderly people. As a matter of fact, neuropsychological symptoms behave differently, with a trend toward a higher rate of persistence in elderly people.

The main result of our study pertains to the role of vaccination. In our series, patients vaccinated at the time of the acute phase had a one-third probability of developing major physical long COVID symptoms than non-vaccinated patients, and a one-fifth probability of developing major neuropsychological symptoms, independently from the severity of the disease. Therefore, the protective role of vaccination is not due to a lower severity of the acute phase, but to some alternative unknown mechanism that involves the immune system.

Limitations

There are limitations to our study. The first one is that physical symptoms and diseases present at the time of hospitalization were retrieved from the patient's files and are therefore reliable information; conversely, the pre-existence of symptoms comprising the MNS was explored in part from the patient's files (anxiety and depression) and in part at the time of the follow-up interview, and it is possible that this last piece of information could be biased by the subjective interpretation and memory of the patient.

Even the severity of the symptoms is assessed based on subjective judgment and not on objective measures. The window of observation includes only 29 patients after 15 months of follow-up and therefore data at 18 months could be less reliable (full resolution of symptoms after 21 months is an extrapolation and cannot be proven). Finally, our patient population comprised only patients who, at the time of the acute phase, had symptoms requiring hospitalization. Hence, our results cannot be generalized to the general patient population and namely to those suffering an acute infection not requiring hospitalization.

Even the single-center design limits the generalizability of our results, and a selection bias cannot be excluded.

In conclusion, long COVID represents an important sequela of the COVID-19 infection both in terms of physical and mental state. The wide diffusion of vaccination should however guarantee a significant containment of this pattern.

Supplementary Materials: The following supporting information can be downloaded at: https://www.mdpi.com/article/10.3390/jcm12051915/s1, Table S1: Therapies and laboratory exams at the time of hospitalization; Table S2: Patient population (N = 121) data and association with major physical symptoms persistence; Table S3: Patient population (N = 121) data and association with major neurological symptoms persistence.

Author Contributions: Conceptualization, M.R., M.F. and L.M.; methodology, E.B.; formal analysis, M.R.; investigation, E.B., M.A., S.P. and L.R.; data curation, E.B., M.A. and S.P.; writing—original draft preparation, M.R. and M.F.; writing—review and editing, M.R. and E.B.; project administration, E.B., M.A. and S.P.; funding acquisition, M.R. All authors have read and agreed to the published version of the manuscript.

Funding: The study has been financed by a grant from the Italian Ministry of Health for the research projects of the Cardiac Network of the Italian IRCCS (Clinical Research Hospitals).

Institutional Review Board Statement: The study was conducted in accordance with the Declaration of Helsinki and approved by the Local Ethics Committee (San Raffaele Hospital) on 3 March 2022, registry number 28/INT/2022. All the patients gave a written informed consent.

Informed Consent Statement: Informed consent was obtained from all subjects involved in the study.

Data Availability Statement: The original dataset supporting the findings of this study will be deposited in the public repository Zenodo after the publication of the paper and accessible upon a reasonable request to the corresponding author.

Conflicts of Interest: The authors declare no conflict of interest. The funding organization had no role in the design of the study; in the collection, analyses, or interpretation of data; in the writing of the manuscript; or in the decision to publish the results.

References

1. Post COVID-19 Condition (Long COVID). Available online: https://www.who.int/europe/news-room/fact-sheets/item/post-covid-19-condition (accessed on 7 January 2023).
2. Chopra, V.; Flanders, S.A.; O'Malley, M.; Malani, A.N.; Prescott, H.C. Sixty-Day Outcomes Among Patients Hospitalized with COVID-19. *Ann. Intern. Med.* **2021**, *174*, 576–578. [CrossRef]
3. Nalbandian, A.; Sehgal, K.; Gupta, A.; Madhavan, M.V.; McGroder, C.; Stevens, J.S.; Cook, J.R.; Nordvig, A.S.; Shalev, D.; Sehrawat, T.S.; et al. Post-acute COVID-19 syndrome. *Nat. Med.* **2021**, *27*, 601–615. [CrossRef] [PubMed]
4. Arnold, D.T.; Hamilton, F.W.; Milne, A.; Morley, A.J.; Viner, J.; Attwood, M.; Noel, A.; Gunning, S.; Hatrick, J.; Hamilton, S.; et al. Patient outcomes after hospitalisation with COVID-19 and implications for follow-up: Results from a prospective UK cohort. *Thorax* **2021**, *76*, 399–401. [CrossRef] [PubMed]
5. Moreno-Pérez, O.; Merino, E.; Leon-Ramirez, J.M.; Andres, M.; Ramos, J.M.; Arenas-Jiménez, J.; Asensio, S.; Sanchez, R.; Ruiz-Torregrosa, P.; Galan, I.; et al. COVID19-ALC research group. Post-acute COVID-19 syndrome. Incidence and risk factors: A Mediterranean cohort study. *J. Infect.* **2021**, *82*, 378–383. [CrossRef] [PubMed]
6. Halpin, S.J.; McIvor, C.; Whyatt, G.; Adams, A.; Harvey, O.; McLean, L.C.; Kemp, S.; Corrado, J.; Singh, R.; Collins, T.; et al. Postdischarge symptoms and rehabilitation needs in survivors of COVID-19 infection: A cross-sectional evaluation. *J. Med. Virol.* **2021**, *93*, 1013–1022. [CrossRef] [PubMed]
7. Jacobs, L.G.; Gourna Paleoudis, E.; Lesky-Di Bari, D.; Nyirenda, T.; Friedman, T.; Gupta, A.; Rasouli, L.; Zetkulic, M.; Balani, B.; Ogedegbe, C.; et al. Persistence of symptoms and quality of life at 35 days after hospitalization for COVID-19 infection. *PLoS ONE* **2020**, *15*, e0243882. [CrossRef] [PubMed]
8. Garrigues, E.; Janvier, P.; Kherabi, Y.; Le Bot, A.; Hamon, A.; Gouze, H.; Doucet, L.; Berkani, S.; Oliosi, E.; Mallart, E.; et al. Post-discharge persistent symptoms and health-related quality of life after hospitalization for COVID-19. *J. Infect.* **2020**, *81*, e4–e6. [CrossRef]
9. Novelli, L.; Raimondi, F.; Carioli, G.; Carobbio, A.; Pappacena, S.; Biza, R.; Trapasso, R.; Anelli, M.; Amoroso, M.; Allegri, C.; et al. HPG23 Covid19 Study Group. One-year mortality in COVID-19 is associated with patients' comorbidities rather than pneumonia severity. *Respir. Med. Res.* **2022**, *83*, 100976.

10. Ortega-Paz, L.; Arévalos, V.; Fernández-Rodríguez, D.; Jiménez-Díaz, V.; Bañeras, J.; Campo, G.; Rodríguez-Santamarta, M.; Díaz, J.F.; Scardino, C.; Gómez-Álvarez, Z.; et al. CV COVID-19 registry investigators. One-year cardiovascular outcomes after coronavirus disease 2019: The cardiovascular COVID-19 registry. *PLoS ONE* **2022**, *17*, e0279333. [CrossRef]
11. Watanabe, A.; So, M.; Iwagami, M.; Fukunaga, K.; Takagi, H.; Kabata, H.; Kuno, T. One-year follow-up CT findings in COVID-19 patients: A systematic review and meta-analysis. *Respirology* **2022**, *27*, 605–616. [CrossRef] [PubMed]
12. Cavaco, S.; Sousa, G.; Gonçalves, A.; Dias, A.; Andrade, C.; Pereira, D.; Aires, E.A.; Moura, J.; Silva, L.; Varela, R.; et al. Predictors of cognitive dysfunction one-year post COVID-19. *Neuropsychology*, **2023**, *epub ahead of print*. [CrossRef]
13. Kalak, G.; Jarjou'i, A.; Bohadana, A.; Wild, P.; Rokach, A.; Amiad, N.; Abdelrahman, N.; Arish, N.; Chen-Shuali, C.; Izbicki, G. Prevalence and Persistence of Symptoms in Adult COVID-19 Survivors 3 and 18 Months after Discharge from Hospital or Corona Hotels. *J. Clin. Med.* **2022**, *11*, 7413. [CrossRef] [PubMed]
14. Gutiérrez-Canales, L.G.; Muñoz-Corona, C.; Barrera-Chávez, I.; Viloria-Álvarez, C.; Macías, A.E.; Guaní-Guerra, E. Quality of Life and Persistence of Symptoms in Outpatients after Recovery from COVID-19. *Medicina* **2022**, *58*, 1795. [CrossRef] [PubMed]
15. Arjun, M.C.; Singh, A.K.; Pal, D.; Das, K.; Alekhya, G.; Venkateshan, M.; Mishra, B.; Patro, B.K.; Mohapatra, P.R.; Subba, S.H. Characteristics and predictors of Long COVID among diagnosed cases of COVID-19. *PLoS ONE* **2022**, *17*, e0278825. [CrossRef] [PubMed]
16. UKHSA Review Shows Vaccinated Less Likely to Have Long COVID than Unvaccinated. Available online: https://www.gov.uk/government/news/ukhsa-review-shows-vaccinated-less-likely-to-have-long-covid-than-unvaccinated (accessed on 13 January 2022).
17. Romero-Rodríguez, E.; Pérula-de Torres, L.Á.; Castro-Jiménez, R.; González-Lama, J.; Jiménez-García, C.; González-Bernal, J.J.; González-Santos, J.; Vélez-Santamaría, R.; Sánchez-González, E.; Santamaría-Peláez, M. Hospital admission and vaccination as predictive factors of long COVID-19 symptoms. *Front. Med.* **2022**, *9*, 1016013. [CrossRef] [PubMed]
18. Bellan, M.; Apostolo, D.; Albè, A.; Crevola, M.; Errica, N.; Ratano, G.; Tonello, S.; Minisini, R.; D'Onghia, D.; Baricich, A.; et al. Determinants of long COVID among adults hospitalized for SARS-CoV-2 infection: A prospective cohort study. *Front. Immunol.* **2022**, *13*, 1038227. [CrossRef] [PubMed]
19. Brunvoll, S.H.; Nygaard, A.B.; Fagerland, M.W.; Holland, P.; Ellingjord-Dale, M.; Dahl, J.A.; Søraas, A. Post-acute symptoms 3-15 months after COVID-19 among unvaccinated and vaccinated individuals with a breakthrough infection. *Int. J. Infect. Dis.* **2023**, *126*, 10–13. [CrossRef] [PubMed]

Disclaimer/Publisher's Note: The statements, opinions and data contained in all publications are solely those of the individual author(s) and contributor(s) and not of MDPI and/or the editor(s). MDPI and/or the editor(s) disclaim responsibility for any injury to people or property resulting from any ideas, methods, instructions or products referred to in the content.

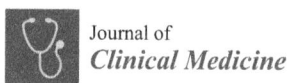 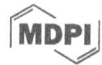

Article

Long-COVID-19 in Asymptomatic, Non-Hospitalized, and Hospitalized Populations: A Cross-Sectional Study

Aysegul Bostanci [1], Umut Gazi [1,*], Ozgur Tosun [2], Kaya Suer [3], Emine Unal Evren [4], Hakan Evren [4] and Tamer Sanlidag [5]

1. Department of Medical Microbiology and Clinical Microbiology, Faculty of Medicine, Near East University, Nicosia 99138, Cyprus
2. Department of Biostatistics, Faculty of Medicine, Near East University, Nicosia 99138, Cyprus
3. Department of Infectious Diseases and Clinical Microbiology, Faculty of Medicine, Near East University, Nicosia 99138, Cyprus
4. Department of Infectious Diseases and Clinical Microbiology, Faculty of Medicine, University of Kyrenia, Kyrenia 99320, Cyprus
5. DESAM Research Institute, Near East University, Nicosia 99138, Cyprus
* Correspondence: umut.gazi@neu.edu.tr

Citation: Bostanci, A.; Gazi, U.; Tosun, O.; Suer, K.; Unal Evren, E.; Evren, H.; Sanlidag, T. Long-COVID-19 in Asymptomatic, Non-Hospitalized, and Hospitalized Populations: A Cross-Sectional Study. *J. Clin. Med.* **2023**, *12*, 2613. https://doi.org/10.3390/jcm12072613

Academic Editors: Domingo Palacios-Ceña and César Fernández De Las Peñas

Received: 6 February 2023
Revised: 15 March 2023
Accepted: 28 March 2023
Published: 30 March 2023

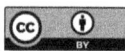

Copyright: © 2023 by the authors. Licensee MDPI, Basel, Switzerland. This article is an open access article distributed under the terms and conditions of the Creative Commons Attribution (CC BY) license (https://creativecommons.org/licenses/by/4.0/).

Abstract: A substantial proportion of coronavirus disease 2019 (COVID-19) survivors continue to suffer from long-COVID-19 (LC) symptoms. Our study aimed to determine the risk factors for LC by using a patient population from Northern Cyprus. Subjects who were diagnosed with severe acute respiratory syndrome-2 (SARS-CoV-2) infection in our university hospital were invited and asked to fill in an online questionnaire. Data from 296 survivors who had recovered from COVID-19 infection at least 28 days prior the study was used in the statistical analysis. For determination of risk factors for "ongoing symptomatic COVID-19 (OSC)" and "Post-COVID-19 (PSC)" syndromes, the patient population was further divided into group 1 (Gr1) and group 2 (Gr2), that included survivors who were diagnosed with COVID-19 within 4–12 weeks and at least three months prior the study, respectively. The number of people with post-vaccination SARS-CoV-2 infection was 266 (89.9%). B.1.617.2 (Delta) (41.9%) was the most common SARS-CoV-2 variant responsible for the infections, followed by BA.1 (Omicron) (34.8%), B.1.1.7 (Alpha) (15.5%), and wild-type SARS-CoV-2 (7.8%). One-hundred-and-nineteen volunteers (40.2%) stated an increased frequency of COVID-19-related symptoms and experienced the symptoms in the week prior to the study. Of those, 81 (38.8%) and 38 (43.7%) were from Gr1 and Gr2 groups, respectively. Female gender, chronic illness, and symptomatic status at PCR testing were identified as risk factors for developing OSC syndrome, while only the latter showed a similar association with PSC symptoms. Our results also suggested that ongoing and persistent COVID-19-related symptoms are not influenced by the initial viral cycle threshold (Ct) values of the SARS-CoV-2, SARS-CoV-2 variant as well as vaccination status and type prior to COVID-19. Therefore, strategies other than vaccination are needed to combat the long-term effect of COVID-19, especially after symptomatic SARS-CoV-2 infection, and their possible economic burden on healthcare settings.

Keywords: long COVID; questionnaire; asymptomatic; symptomatic; risk factors; Post-COVID-19 syndrome; cross-sectional study

1. Introduction

Since its emergence in late 2019, coronavirus disease 2019 (COVID-19) has caused serious health problems worldwide. While the current rates of severe disease and hospitalization are on the decline due to the effective vaccination regimens [1], a substantial proportion of survivors continue to suffer from long-COVID-19 (LC) symptoms for weeks or months after the onset of COVID-19 [2–6]. Today, as the number of people infected with SARS-CoV-2 continues to rise, LC is heralded as the next threat to healthcare systems, which were already overwhelmed during the ongoing COVID-19 pandemic; recently, the Office for National Statistics estimated that almost two million people are experiencing LC symptoms in the United Kingdom [7].

A wide variety of symptoms, such as fatigue, malaise, shortness of breath, cough, and cognitive impairments, can occur in COVID-19 survivors. The prevalence of LC is still not known; due to the differences in study designs including follow-up, the definition of the disease, and region, a broad prevalence range of 22% to 81% was estimated by previous reports [8]. However, a recent review that analyzed more than 190 reports published until January 2022 revealed that at least 45% of COVID-19 survivors experience one and more unresolved symptoms at four months after the onset of SARS-CoV-2 infection [9].

Moreover, the underlying mechanisms responsible for LC are still not well established since LC symptoms may not be specific to COVID-19 and can be associated with post-intensive care syndrome or an exacerbation of pre-existing health conditions. Nevertheless, both the organ damage from the acute infection phase and specific long-lasting inflammatory mechanisms are thought to be involved in the pathophysiology [2]. On the other hand, while the literature on the risk factors is not yet clear on the association of LC with the severity of COVID-19 infection, it consistently reported higher incidence rates in subjects with female gender, old age, and comorbidities [8].

Literature on LC is also difficult to interpret because of variable terms (such as post-acute COVID-19 syndrome or post-COVID conditions) used to define the condition. In an attempt to standardize the terms, the National Institute for Health and Care Excellence (NICE) proposed the use of the term "Long-COVID-19". The term also covered the "ongoing symptomatic COVID-19 (OSC)" and "Post-COVID-19 syndrome (PSC)", which are defined as the persistence of symptoms for periods between 4 and 12 weeks, and beyond 12 weeks from the onset of COVID-19, respectively, without any alternative diagnosis [10,11]. Our study aimed to identify the associated risk factors and prevalence of both OSC and PSC in Northern Cyprus, which is yet to receive attention in the literature. For this purpose, COVID-19 survivors who were tested with reverse-transcriptase polymerase chain reaction (RT-PCR) for SARS-CoV-2 at a university hospital were invited to join our study, and then asked to complete an online questionnaire.

2. Materials and Methods

2.1. Study Design

This retrospective cohort study was conducted with COVID-19 survivors in Northern Cyprus. Subjects who were previously diagnosed with SARS-CoV-2 infection at the Near East University Hospital COVID-19 PCR Diagnosis Laboratory were reached by phone and invited to participate in an online survey developed on Google Forms. Only data from those who were diagnosed with COVID-19 at least 28 days prior to study was included. Duplicate database entries with the same user ID were eliminated before analysis. Data collected from a total of 296 volunteers between September 2021 and February 2022 was used in a statistical analysis to determine the risk factors associated with LC among the population studied. Information on SARS-CoV-2 variants, RT-PCR Ct values, and vaccination status of the participants were obtained from the hospital database.

2.2. Detection of SARS-CoV-2 and its Variants

SARS-CoV-2 infection was diagnosed by RT-PCR performed on nasopharyngeal swab samples, utilizing Uniplex RT-qPCR SARS-CoV-2 RT-qPCR Detection Kit (IKAS Medical, Nicosia, Northern Cyprus) that is based on amplification of viral ORF1ab, N1, and N2 genes and uses human Rnase P as an internal control. SARS-CoV-2 variant analysis was conducted by using Multiplex SARS-CoV-2 VoC RT-qPCR Detection Kit (IKAS Medical, Nicosia, Northern Cyprus) that identifies variants of concern, including B.1.1.7 (Alpha), B.1.351 (Beta), B.1.617.2 (Delta), P.1 (Gamma), and B.1.1.529 (Omicron) variants, by simultaneously detecting mutations (del69/70, N501Y, K417N, T478K, Y144del, and P681R) in the Spike protein gene [12,13].

2.3. Ethics

The study was conducted in line with the guidelines of the Declaration of Helsinki, and was approved by the ethics committee of the Institutional Review Board at Near East University (YDU/2021-92-1359). Written informed consent was obtained from all participants prior to study enrolment.

2.4. Survey

The survey (Supplementary Material) was comprised of three sections. The first section focused on the sociodemographic characteristics, including age, gender, pre-existing medical comorbidities, and the vaccination status of the participants. The second section included questions on acute symptoms, disease severity, hospitalization, and admission to the intensive care unit (ICU). The third part focused on health status after COVID-19 and LC symptoms.

2.5. Statistical Analysis

Descriptive statistics for the qualitative variables were provided as frequencies and percentages, while the arithmetic mean, standard deviation, median, minimum, and maximum values were calculated for the quantitative variables. The factors that might be associated with post-COVID symptoms were tested using the Pearson chi-square test or Fisher's exact test, where appropriate. Odds ratios with a 95% confidence interval were calculated. Binary logistic regression analysis was performed to calculate the odds ratios and significance for ordinal qualitative risk factors with more than 2 categories. The level of significance was accepted as 0.05. All statistical analyses were performed with SPSS (Version 26.0 for Mac) software.

3. Results

3.1. Characteristics of Participants

A total of 296 participants, with an average age of 37.2 ± 14.9 years (range: 12–83 years), were included in the study. The average time interval between the onset of SARS-CoV-2 infection and filling the questionnaire was 3.4 months (range: 1–23 months, ± 3.5).

The numbers of COVID-19 survivors aged ≤ 17, 18–55, and ≥ 56 years were 23 (7.8%), 233 (78.7%), and 40 (13.5%), respectively. Of the participants, 149 (50.3%) were male, and 147 (49.7%) were female. A total of 81 (27.4%) participants have at least one chronic disease (comorbidity). The numbers of smokers and non-smokers were 67 (22.6%) and 227 (76.7%), respectively, while no relevant data on smoking habit was obtained from the two subjects (Table 1).

Two-hundred-and-sixty-six participants (89.9%) were vaccinated before SARS-CoV-2 infection. Of those, while 191 (71.8%) completed vaccination regimens with Coronavac (n = 58; 30.4%), Pfizer (n = 94; 49.2%), Moderna (n = 3; 1.6%), Johnson & Johnson (n = 28; 14.7%), and Oxford-Astra Zeneca (n = 8; 4.2%), the remaining (n = 75, 28.2%) took one dose of the Coronavac (n = 9; 12.0%), Pfizer (n = 65; 86.7%), and Oxford-Astra Zeneca (n = 1; 1.3%) vaccine. For our analysis, data from only those who completed the vaccination regiments were used, and in order to increase the sample size for higher statistical power, the groups were merged according to the type of vaccine received; killed-virus (Coronavac), mRNA (Pfizer +Moderna), and vector-based (Johnson +Astra Zeneca) (Table 1).

Among the COVID-19 survivors, 254 (85.8%) declared that they were symptomatic during the RT-PCR detectable phase. Twenty-nine of the participants (9.8%) were hospitalized and eight (27.6%) required admission to the ICU. According to the variant analysis, the numbers of B.1.617.2 (Delta), BA.1 (Omicron), B.1.1.7 (Alpha) variants, and wild-type cases SARS-CoV-2 were 124 (41.9%), 103 (34.8%), 46 (15.5%), and 23 (7.8%), respectively (Table 1).

Table 1. Demographic characteristics and clinical profile of the participants.

Characteristics		Gr1 n (%)	Gr2 n (%)	Total n (%)
Gender	Female	102 (48.8)	45 (51.7)	147 (100.0)
	Male	107 (51.2)	42 (48.3)	149 (100.0)
Age	12–17 years	18 (8.6)	5 (5.7)	23 (100.0)
	18–55 years	170 (81.3)	63 (72.4)	233 (100.0)
	≥56 years	21 (10.0)	19 (21.8)	40 (100.0)
Smoking status	Smoker	47 (22.5)	20 (23.0)	67 (100.0)
	Non-smoker	147 (70.3)	62 (71.3)	209 (100.0)
	Former-smoker	13 (6.2)	5 (5.7)	18 (100.0)
Chronic disease	Present	55 (26.3)	26 (29.9)	81 (100.0)
	Absent	154 (73.7)	61 (70.1)	215 (100.0)
Vaccination status	Vaccinated	190 (90.9)	79 (90.8)	269 (100.0)
	Unvaccinated	19 (9.1)	8 (9.2)	27 (100.0)
Vaccination time	Before COVID-19	178 (85.2)	35 (40.2)	213 (100.0)
	After COVID-19	11 (5.3)	45 (51.7)	56 (100.0)
Vaccination regimen	Killed-virus	42 (72.4)	16 (27.6)	58 (100.0)
	mRNA	58 (59.8)	39 (40.2)	97 (100.0)
	Vector-based	29 (80.6)	7 (19.4)	36 (100.0)
SARS-CoV-2 variant	B.1.617.2 (Delta)	98 (79.0)	26 (21.0)	124 (100.0)
	BA.1 (Omicron)	101 (98.1)	2 (1.9)	103 (100.0)
	B.1.1.7 (Alpha)	7 (15.2)	39 (87.8)	46 (100.0)
	Wild Type	3 (13)	20 (87.0)	23 (100.0)
COVID-19 symptoms at PCR testing	Present	181 (86.6)	73 (83.9)	254 (100.0)
	Absent	28 (13.4)	14 (16.1)	42 (100.0)
Hospitalization	Yes	15 (7.2)	14 (16.1)	29 (100.0)
	No	194 (92.8)	73 (83.9)	267 (100.0)
ICU admission	Yes	4 (26.7)	4 (28.6)	8 (100.0)
	No	11 (73.3)	10 (71.4)	21 (100.0)

3.2. Risk Factors Associated with OSC and PSC

According to the survey results, 136 volunteers (45.9%) experienced an increased frequency of COVID-19-related symptoms, such as fatigue (n = 56, 41.1%), cough (n = 35, 25.7%), memory problems (n = 28, 20.6%), dyspnea (n = 26, 19.1%), and headache (n = 22, 16.2%), after recovering from SARS-CoV-2 infection. The number of subjects with ongoing LC symptoms (i.e., volunteers who experienced at least one LC symptom in the week prior to the study) was 119 (40.2%) (Table 2).

Table 2. The most commonly reported LC symptoms experienced by volunteers.

LC Symptoms	Gr1 n (%)	Gr2 n (%)	Total n (%)
Fatigue	34 (37.7)	22 (47.8)	56 (41.1)
Cough	27 (30.0)	8 (17.4)	35 (25.7)
Memory problems	22 (24.4)	6 (13.0)	28 (20.6)
Dyspnea	16 (17.8)	10 (21.7)	26 (19.1)
Headache	15 (16.7)	7 (15.2)	22 (16.2)

For determination of risk factors associated with OSC and PSC, the COVID-19 survivors were divided into two groups depending on the time since COVID-19 diagnosis; while group 1 (Gr1) included survivors, who were diagnosed with SARS-CoV-2 infection from 4 to 12 weeks before the study conducted, Gr2 included participants who joined the study at least three months after the onset of infection.

The prevalence of the LC symptoms in the Gr1 and Gr2 groups were 66.2% and 33.8%, respectively. The most common symptoms in Gr1 subjects were fatigue and cough, while they were fatigue and dyspnea in Gr2 members. Of Gr1 subjects, the number of patients with ongoing LC symptoms was 81 (38.8%), while the corresponding number was 38 (43.7%) for Gr2 volunteers. The most common ongoing symptoms reported by Gr1 and Gr2 volunteers were fatigue (n = 34, 37.7% for Gr1; n = 22, 47.8% for Gr2), cough (n = 27, 30.0% for Gr1; n = 8, 17.4% for Gr2), memory problems (n = 22, 24.4% for Gr1; n = 6, 13.0% for Gr2), dyspnea (n = 16, 17.8% for Gr1; n = 10, 21.7% for Gr2), and headache (n = 15, 16.7% for Gr1; n = 7, 15.2% for Gr2) (Table 2).

The associations of OSC and PSC with different risk factors were evaluated by using data provided by subjects with ongoing LC symptoms (81 Gr1 and 38 Gr2 volunteers). Among the different risk factors evaluated, female gender ($p = 0.006$), presence of chronic disease ($p = 0.007$), and symptomatic status at PCR testing ($p = 0.001$) displayed a statically significant association with the incidence of persistent COVID-19 symptoms in Gr1 (Table 3). The incidence rate of OSC was 2.3 higher in female than in male participants, while subjects with chronic disease and COVID-19 symptoms at PCR testing displayed a 2.4- and 14.8-fold higher risk for OSC, respectively, than those without (Table 3). In contrast, among the risk factors associated with OSC, only symptomatic status at PCR testing ($p = 0.015$) showed an association with PSC; volunteers with symptoms exhibited a 9.0 higher incidence rate of persistent symptoms (Table 4). Nevertheless, data on SARS-CoV-2 variants and vaccination regimens could not be used to evaluate their correlation with LC sub-groups due to restrictions imposed by low sample size. However, our statistical analysis revealed that neither of the variables was associated with LC (Table 5).

Table 3. Risk factors associated with OSC syndrome in Gr1. Abbreviations: OR, odds ratio; CI, confidence interval; ref, reference value. Significant p values were indicated with bold to assist the readers.

Risk Factors	OSC Symptoms		χ^2 Test		Logistic Regression	
	Present n/N (%)	Absent n/N (%)	OR (95% CI)	p Value	OR (95% CI)	p Value
Gender						
Male	24/107 (22.4)	83/107 (77.6)	1 (ref)	**0.006**	-	-
Female	41/102 (40.2)	61/102 (59.8)	2.32 (1.27–4.25)			
Age						
12–17 years	2/18 (11.1)	16/18 (88.9)	-	0.143	0.31 (0.05–1.80)	0.192
18–55 years	57/170 (33.5)	113/170 (66.5)			1.26 (0.46–3.42)	0.649
≥56 years	6/21 (28.6)	15/21 (71.4)			1 (ref)	
Smoking Status						
Smoker	12/47 (25.5)	35/47 (74.5)	-	0.441	1.14 (0.27–4.86)	0.856
Non-smoker	50/147 (34.0)	97/147 (66.0)			1.72 (0.45–6.53)	0.427
Former-smoker	3/13 (23.1)	10/13 (76.9)			1 (ref)	
Chronic disease						
Present	25/55 (45.5)	30/55 (54.5)	2.38 (1.25–4.50)	**0.007**	-	-
Absent	40/154 (26.0)	114/154 (74.0)	1 (ref)			
Vaccination status						
Vaccinated	60/190 (31.6)	130/190 (68.4)	1.29 (0.45–3.76)	0.637		
Unvaccinated	5/19 (26.3)	14/19 (73.7)	1 (ref)			
Vaccination Time						
Before COVID-19	57/178 (32.0)	121/178 (68.0)	1.26 (0.32–4.90)	1.000		
After COVID-19	3/11 (27.3)	8/11 (72.7)	1 (ref)			

Table 3. Cont.

Risk Factors	OSC Symptoms		χ² Test		Logistic Regression	
	Present n/N (%)	Absent n/N (%)	OR (95% CI)	p Value	OR (95% CI)	p Value
COVID-19 symptoms at PCR testing						
Present	64/181 (35.4)	117/181 (64.6)	14.77 (1.96–111.23)	**0.001**	-	-
Absent	1/28 (3.6)	27/28 (96.4)	1 (ref)			
Hospitalization						
Present	8/15 (53.3)	7/15 (46.7)	2.75 (0.95–7.94)	0.079		
Absent	57/194 (29.4)	137/194 (70.6)	1 (ref)			

Table 4. Risk factors associated with PSC syndrome in Gr2. Abbreviations: OR, odds ratio; CI, confidence interval; ref, reference value; *, chi square statistics could not be calculated. Significant p values were indicated with bold to assist the readers.

Risk Factors	PSC Symptoms		χ² Test		Logistic Regression	
	Present n/N (%)	Absent n/N (%)	OR (95% CI)	p Value	OR (95% CI)	p Value
Gender						
Male	15/42 (35.7)	27/42 (64.3)	1 (ref)	0.988	-	-
Female	16/45 (35.6)	29/45 (64.4)	0.99 (0.41–2.39)			
Age						
12–17 years	2/5 (40.0)	3/5 (60.0)	-	*	1.87 (0.24–14.65)	0.553
18–55 years	24/63 (38.1)	39/63 (61.9)			1.72 (0.55–5.39)	0.350
≥56 years	5/19 (26.3)	14/19 (73.7)			1 (ref)	
Smoking Status						
Smoker	10/20 (50.0)	10/20 (50.0)	-	*	1.80 (0.57–5.67)	0.389
Non-smoker	21/62 (33.9)	41/62 (66.1)			1.71 (0.50–5.81)	0.315
Former-smoker	0/5 (0.0)	5/5 (100.0)			1 (ref)	
Chronic disease						
Present	9/26 (34.6)	17/26 (65.4)	0.94 (0.36–2.46)	0.897	-	-
Absent	22/61 (36.1)	39/61 (63.9)	1 (ref)			
Vaccination status						
Vaccinated	29/79 (36.7)	50/79 (63.3)	1.74 (0.33–9.17)	0.706		
Unvaccinated	2/8 (25.0)	6/8 (75.0)	1 (ref)			
Vaccination Time						
Before COVID-19	13/35 (37.1)	22/35 (62.9)	1.08 (0.43–2.68)	0.884		
After COVID-19	16/45 (35.6)	29/45 (64.4)	1 (ref)			
COVID-19 symptoms at PCR testing						
Present	30/73 (41.1)	43/73 (58.9)	9.07 (1.13–73.09)	**0.015**	-	-
Absent	1/14 (7.1)	13/14 (92.9)	1 (ref)			
Hospitalization						
Present	6/14 (42.9)	8/14 (57.1)	1.44 (0.45–4.61)	0.555		
Absent	25/73 (34.2)	48/73 (65.8)	1 (ref)			

Table 5. Association of LC symptoms with vaccination regimen and SARS-CoV-2 variants.

		LC Symptoms		p Value
		Present n (%)	Absent n (%)	
Vaccination regimen	Killed-virus	22 (37.9)	36 (62.1)	0.159
	mRNA	33 (34.0)	64 (66.0)	
	Vector-based	7 (19.4)	29 (80.6)	
SARS-CoV-2 variant	B.1.617.2 (Delta)	52 (41.9)	72 (58.1)	0.395
	BA.1 (Omicron)	49 (47.6)	54 (52.4)	
	B.1.1.7 (Alpha)	21 (45.7)	25 (54.3)	
	Wild Type	14 (60.9)	9 (39.1)	

4. Discussion

The SARS-CoV-2 infection is characterized by a wide spectrum of clinical profiles ranging from asymptomatic to severe COVID-19 disease associated with acute respiratory distress syndrome (ARDS), that can lead to morbidity and mortality from alveolar lumen damage. Today, the risk of becoming severely ill from COVID-19 is significantly lower than that seen in prior estimates because of protection provided by vaccination against SARS-CoV-2. Nevertheless, LC, which is defined by the persistence of COVID-19-related symptoms for weeks and months after the onset of infection with SARS-CoV-2, is predicted to be the next global health crisis with the growing burden on healthcare systems [14,15]. Subjects with persistent LC symptoms may have difficulty to perform daily activities and return to work that can negatively impact their quality of life and lead to great social as well as economic consequences [16]. Our study aimed to evaluate the health status of COVID-19 survivors and determine the risk factors associated with OSC and PSC in Northern Cyprus. The results can provide valuable information for policymakers to develop strategies to combat against long-term effects of SARS-CoV-2 infection.

According to our results, the prevalence of LC among COVID-19 survivors in Northern Cyprus is more than 45%, which is within the range (22–81%) obtained from previous studies [8]. When the prevalence was further analyzed for LC subtypes, 66.2% and 33.8% of participants were found to experience OSC and PSC, respectively. In correlation with previous studies, the most prevalent LC symptoms reported in our study were fatigue and cough [4,5,17]. On the other hand, while the most common symptoms in subjects with OSC syndrome were fatigue and cough, they were fatigue and dyspnea in PSC patients, which is in correlation with previous findings [4,18–20].

The statistical analysis revealed that female gender, chronic disease, and symptomatic status at PCR testing are risk factors associated with OSC, while only the latter exhibited a correlation with PSC [5,11,21]. Female gender and the presence of a comorbidity did not have any influence on the rate of PSC syndrome, which was in contrast to previous findings [20]. Moreover, our study reported a lack of association of OSC and PSC with Ct values detected in the acute phase of infection, which contradicts with the data presented by Perez et al. showing a negative correlation between the viral load and the number of the LC symptoms [22]. Additionally, age, which was also inversely correlated with LC symptoms in a recent report [23], was found to be a significant risk factor for neither OSC nor PSC in our study. While the conflict between our results and previous findings can be because of differences in the methodology and populations used by the studies, it can also be due to the underlying bias related to the self-reported nature of our data.

Increasing the COVID-19 vaccination rate is effective in reducing severe disease and hospitalization; however, it does not influence post-COVID-19 recovery since being unvaccinated was not a risk factor for developing either OSC or PSC in our study. Moreover, the type of vaccine received did not have any effect on the development of LC. Accordingly, in a recent systematic review and meta-analysis, the protective effect of COVID-19 vaccines was suggested for some of the LC symptoms, such as cognitive dysfunction/symptoms, kidney diseases/problems, myalgia, and sleeping disorders/problems, while it was not evident for others, including chest/throat pain, fatigue, headache, and respiratory symptoms [24]. Therefore, the potential protective effect of vaccination against specific OSC and PCS symptoms needs further clarification from future studies. On the other hand, this lack of effect highlights the importance of strategies other than promoting vaccination to combat against the long-term effects of SARS-CoV-2 infection. One such strategy could involve the introduction of a remote patient monitoring (RPM) program that enables the patients to transmit health data at home by using phone calls or telemonitoring applications [25].

While the emergence of new SARS-CoV-2 variants was initially thought to influence LC rates, the previous studies have failed to report any association [26,27]. However, to the best of our knowledge, there has not been any relevant study simultaneously comparing the frequencies of LC syndrome between subjects infected with wild-type, B.1.1.7 (Alpha), B.1.617.2 (Delta), and BA.1 (Omicron) variants of SARS-CoV-2. This was addressed by our study, which demonstrated similar percentages of LC between the volunteers exposed to either SARS-CoV-2 variant. However, due to the small sample size, it was not possible to evaluate their association with OSC and PSC separately. Therefore, studies with bigger sample sizes are required to investigate their potential difference in their ability to cause OSC and PSC.

In our analysis, Delta and Omicron were reported to be the two most common SARS-CoV-2 variants; they were responsible for >75% of infections in our study population, most of whom (>95.0%) tested positive for COVID-19 between January 2021 and February 2022. This is in correlation with literature suggesting Delta and Omicron as the two dominant SARS-CoV-2 variants in 2021 [28]. On the other hand, according to our hospital database, none of the volunteers were infected with the Beta variant, which could be due to its low prevalence during the same period [29].

Apart from the self-reported nature of the presented data that may lead to an overestimation of LC prevalence, the other weaknesses of our study are that the participants were not evenly distributed among groups, and the majority (>90%) of the participants were non-hospitalized patients. Moreover, our study did not include a control group; since ongoing/persistent COVID-19-related symptoms are common and can also be caused by other microbial infections, inclusion of a control group would have helped us to discriminate between the symptoms of those with and without SARS-CoV-2 exposure. Therefore, the results presented in this study should be interpreted with caution. Future studies with the inclusion of bigger sample sizes, physiological assessment/clinical examinations, and controlled or baseline comparison groups are of vital importance to confirm our data.

5. Conclusions

Our findings reveal that more than 45% of COVID-19 survivors in Northern Cyprus experience LC symptoms, while the prevalence of OSC and PSC were more than 60% and 30%, respectively. According to our analysis, COVID-19 survivors with female gender, chronic disease, and symptoms at PCR testing are susceptible to suffering from OSC, while only the latter factor was associated with PSC. Furthermore, the results show a lack of association of vaccination status, SARS-CoV-2 variants, and viral load in the acute phase of SARS-CoV-2 infection with ongoing and persistent COVID-19 symptoms. Therefore, strategies other than promoting vaccination are required to combat against the long-term effects of COVID-19, especially after symptomatic SARS-CoV-2 infection.

Supplementary Materials: The following supporting information can be downloaded at: https://www.mdpi.com/article/10.3390/jcm12072613/s1, File S1. Immune response to SARS-CoV-2 and post-COVID-19 in the upper respiratory tract.

Author Contributions: All authors contributed to the study concept and design. A.B. and U.G. conducted the literature review and wrote the manuscript. A.B., U.G., E.U.E., H.E. and K.S. recruited participants and collected data. U.G. and O.T. performed the statistical analysis. All authors revised and edited the manuscript. U.G. and T.S. supervised the study. All authors have read and agreed to the published version of the manuscript.

Funding: This research did not receive any specific grant from funding agencies in the public, commercial, or not-for-profit sectors.

Institutional Review Board Statement: The study was conducted according to the guidelines of the Declaration of Helsinki, and approved by ethics committee of the Institutional Review Board at Near East University (YDU/2021-92-1359).

Informed Consent Statement: Prior to participating in the survey, participants were given a description and the objectives of the study. Written informed consent was obtained from all participants prior to study enrolment.

Data Availability Statement: Data used for this study is available upon request from corresponding author.

Acknowledgments: The authors would like to thank Near East University Hospital COVID-19 PCR Diagnosis Laboratory.

Conflicts of Interest: The authors declare no conflict of interest.

References

1. Uzun, O.; Akpolat, T.; Varol, A.; Turan, S.; Bektas, S.G.; Cetinkaya, P.D.; Dursun, M.; Bakan, N.; Ketencioglu, B.B.; Bayrak, M.; et al. COVID-19: Vaccination vs. hospitalization. *Infection* **2022**, *50*, 747–752. [CrossRef]
2. Castanares-Zapatero, D.; Chalon, P.; Kohn, L.; Dauvrin, M.; Detollenaere, J.; Maertens de Noordhout, C.; Primus-de Jong, C.; Cleemput, I.; Van den Heede, K. Pathophysiology and mechanism of long COVID: A comprehensive review. *Ann. Med.* **2022**, *54*, 1473–1487. [CrossRef]
3. Chen, C.; Haupert, S.R.; Zimmermann, L.; Shi, X.; Fritsche, L.G.; Mukherjee, B. Global Prevalence of Post-Coronavirus Disease 2019 (COVID-2019) Condition or Long COVID: A Meta-Analysis and Systemic Review. *J. Infect. Dis.* **2022**, *226*, 1593–1607. [CrossRef]
4. Crook, H.; Raza, S.; Nowell, J.; Young, M.; Edison, P. Long-covid-mechanisms, risk factors, and management. *BMJ* **2021**, *374*, n1648. [CrossRef]
5. Nittas, V.; Gao, M.; West, E.A.; Ballouz, T.; Menges, D.; Hanson, S.W.; Puhan, M.A. Long COVID Through a Public Health Lens: An Umbrella Review. *Public Health Rev.* **2022**, *43*, 1604501. [CrossRef]
6. Parker, A.M.; Brigham, E.; Connolly, B.; McPeake, J.; Agranovich, A.V.; Kenes, M.T.; Casey, K.; Reynolds, C.; Schmidt, K.F.R.; Kim, S.Y.; et al. Addressing the post-acute sequelae of SARS-CoV-2 infection: A multidisciplinary model of care. *Lancet Respir. Med.* **2021**, *9*, 1328–1341. [CrossRef]
7. Office for National Statistics. Prevalence of Ongoing Symptoms Following Coronavirus (COVID-19) Infection in the UK: 1 September 2022. Available online: https://www.ons.gov.uk/peoplepopulationandcommunity/healthandsocialcare/conditionsanddiseases/bulletins/prevalenceofongoingsymptomsfollowingcoronaviruscovid19infectionintheuk/1september2022 (accessed on 1 October 2022).
8. Lapa, J.; Rosa, D.; Mendes, J.P.L.; Deusdara, R.; Romero, G.A.S. Prevalence and Associated Factors of Post-COVID-19 Syndrome in a Brazilian Cohort after 3 and 6 Months of Hospital Discharge. *Int. J. Environ. Res. Public Health* **2023**, *20*, 848. [CrossRef]
9. O'Mahoney, L.L.; Routen, A.; Gillies, C.; Ekezie, W.; Welford, A.; Zhang, A.; Karamchandani, U.; Simms-Williams, N.; Cassambai, S.; Ardavani, A.; et al. The prevalence and long-term health effects of Long Covid among hospitalised and non-hospitalised populations: A systematic review and meta-analysis. *Lancet eClin. Med.* **2023**, *55*, 101762. [CrossRef]
10. Jones, R.; Davis, A.; Stanley, B.; Julious, S.; Ryan, D.; Jackson, D.J.; Halpin, D.M.G.; Hickman, H.; Quint, J.K.; Khunti, K.; et al. Risk Predictors and Symptom Features of Long COVID Within a Broad Primary Care Patient Population Including Both Tested and Untested Patients. *Pragmat. Obs. Res.* **2021**, *12*, 93–104. [CrossRef]
11. Ziauddeen, N.; Gurdasani, D.; O'Hara, M.E.; Hastie, C.; Roderick, P.; Yao, G.; Alwan, N.A. Characteristics and impact of Long Covid: Findings from an online survey. *PLoS ONE* **2022**, *17*, e0264331.
12. Ergoren, M.C.; Tuncel, G.; Ozverel, C.S.; Sanlidag, T. Designing In-House SARS-CoV-2 RT-qPCR Assay for Variant of Concerns. *Glob. Med. Genet.* **2022**, *9*, 252–257. [CrossRef] [PubMed]
13. Mamurova, B.; Akan, G.; Mogol, E.; Turgay, A.; Tuncel, G.; Evren, E.U.; Evren, H.; Suer, K.; Sanlidag, T.; Ergoren, M.C. Strong Association between Vitamin D Receptor Gene and Severe Acute Respiratory Syndrome coronavirus 2 Infectious Variants. *Glob. Med. Genet.* **2023**, *10*, 27–33. [CrossRef] [PubMed]
14. Faghy, M.A.; Owen, R.; Thomas, C.; Yates, J.; Ferraro, F.V.; Skipper, L.; Barley-McMullen, S.; Brown, D.A.; Arena, R.; Ashton, R.E.M. Is long COVID the next global health crisis? *J. Glob. Health* **2022**, *12*, 03067. [CrossRef] [PubMed]
15. Loreche, A.M.; Pepito, V.C.F.; Dayrit, M.M. Long Covid: A call for global action. *Public Health Chall.* **2023**, *2*, 2–4. [CrossRef]
16. Buonsenso, D.; Gualano, M.R.; Rossi, M.F.; Gris, A.V.; Sisti, L.G.; Borrelli, I.; Santoro, P.E.; Tumminello, A.; Gentili, C.; Malorni, W.; et al. Post-Acute COVID-19 Sequelae in a Working Population at One Year Follow-Up: A wide Range of Impacts from an Italian Sample. *Int. J. Environ. Res. Public Health* **2022**, *19*, 1093. [CrossRef]

7. Zhu, J.; Ji, P.; Pang, J.; Zhong, Z.; Li, H.; He, C.; Zhang, J.; Zhao, C. Clinical characteristics of 3062 COVID-19 patients: A meta-analysis. *J. Med. Virol.* **2020**, *92*, 1902–1914. [CrossRef] [PubMed]
8. Maestre-Muniz, M.M.; Arias, A.; Mata-Vazquez, E.; Martin-Toledano, M.; Lopez-Larramona, G.; Ruiz-Chicote, A.M.; Nieto-Sandoval, B.; Lucendo, A.J. Long-Term Outcomes of Patients with Coronavirus Disease 2019 at One Year after Hospital Discharge. *J. Clin. Med.* **2021**, *10*, 2945. [CrossRef]
9. Fernandez-de-las-Penas, C.; Palacios-Cena, D.; Gomez-Mayordomo, V.; Florencio, L.L.; Cuadrado, M.L.; Plaza-Mazano, G.; Navarro-Santana, M. Prevalence of Post-COVID-19 symptoms in hospitalized and non-hospitalized COVID-19 survivors: A systematic review and meta-analysis. *Eur. J. Intern. Med.* **2021**, *92*, 55–70. [CrossRef]
10. Fernandez-de-las-Penas, C.; Martin-Guerrero, J.D.; Pellicer-Valero, O.; Navarro-Pardo, E.; Gomez-Mayordomo, V.; Cuadrado, M.L.; Arias-Navalon, J.; Cigaran-Mendez, M.; Hernandez-Barrera Arendt-Nielsen, L. Female Sex Is a Risk Factor Associated with Longer-Term Post-COVID Related-Symptoms but Not with COVID-19 Symptoms: The LONG-COVID-EXP-CM Multicenter Study. *J. Clin. Med.* **2022**, *11*, 413. [CrossRef]
11. Daugherty, S.E.; Guo, Y.; Heath, K.; Dasmarinas, M.C.; Jubilo, K.G.; Samranvedhya, J.; Lipsitch, M.; Cohen, K. Risk of clinical sequelae after the acute phase of SARS-CoV-2 infection: Retrospective cohort study. *BMJ* **2021**, *373*, n1098. [CrossRef] [PubMed]
12. Perez, D.A.G.; Fonseca-Aguero, A.; Toledo-Ibarra, G.A.; Gomez-Valdivia, J.D.J.; Diaz-Resendiz, K.J.G.; Benitez-Trinidad, A.B.; Razura-Carmona, F.F.; Navidad-Murrieta, M.S.; Covantes-Rosales, C.E.; Giron-Perez, M.I. Post-COVID-19 Syndrome in Outpatients and Its Association with Viral Load. *Int. J. Environ. Res. Public Health* **2022**, *19*, 2–11.
13. Subramanian, A.; Nirantharakumar, K.; Hughes, S.; Myles, P.; Williams, T.; Gokhale, K.M.; Taverner, T.; Chandan, J.S.; Brown, K.; Simms-Williams, N.; et al. Symptoms and risk factors for long COVID in non-hospitalized adults. *Nat. Med.* **2022**, *28*, 1706–1714. [CrossRef] [PubMed]
14. Gao, P.; Liu, J.; Lie, M. Effect of COVID-19 Vaccines on Reducing the Risk of Long COVID in the Real World: A Systematic Review and Meta-Analysis. *Int J Environ Res and Public Health* **2022**, *19*, 12422.
15. Bouabida, K.; Malas, K.; Talbot, A.; Desrosiers, M.E.; Lavoie, F.; Lebouche, B.; Taguemout, M.; Rafie, E.; Lessard, D.; Pomey, M.P. Remote Patient Monitoring Program for COVID-19 Patients Following Hospital Discharge: A Cross-Sectional Study. *Front. Digit. Health* **2021**, *3*, 721044. [CrossRef]
16. Morioka, S.; Tsuzuki, S.; Suzuki, M.; Terada, M.; Akashi, M.; Osanai, Y.; Kuge, C.; Sanada, M.; Tanaka, K.; Maruki, T.; et al. Post COVID-19 condition of the Omicron variant of SARS-CoV-2. *J. Infect. Chemother.* **2022**, *28*, 1546–1551. [CrossRef]
17. Magnusson, K.; Kristoffersen, D.T.; Dell'Isola, A.; Kiadaliri, A.; Turkiewicz, A.; Runhaar, J.; Bierma-Zeinstra, S.; Englund, M.; Magnus, P.M.; Kinge, J.M. Post-covid medical complaints after SARS-COV-2 Omicron vs Delta variants—A propective cohort study. *Nat. Commun.* **2022**, *13*, 7363.
18. Duong, B.V.; Larpruenrudee, P.; Fang, T.; Hossain, S.I.; Saha, S.C.; Gu, Y.; Islam, M.S. Is the SARS CoV-2 Omicron Variant Deadlier and More Transmissible Than Delta Variant? *Int. J. Environ. Res. Public Health* **2022**, *19*, 4586.
19. Chen, Z.; Azman, A.S.; Chen, X.; Zou, J.; Tian, Y.; Sun, R.; Xu, X.; Wu, Y.; Lu, W.; Ge, S.; et al. Global landscape of SARS-CoV-2 genomic surveillance and data sharing. *Nat. Genet.* **2022**, *54*, 499–507. [CrossRef]

Disclaimer/Publisher's Note: The statements, opinions and data contained in all publications are solely those of the individual author(s) and contributor(s) and not of MDPI and/or the editor(s). MDPI and/or the editor(s) disclaim responsibility for any injury to people or property resulting from any ideas, methods, instructions or products referred to in the content.

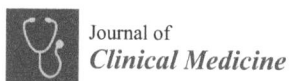

Article

Minimal Clinically Important Differences in Inspiratory Muscle Function Variables after a Respiratory Muscle Training Programme in Individuals with Long-Term Post-COVID-19 Symptoms

Tamara del Corral [1,2], Raúl Fabero-Garrido [1], Gustavo Plaza-Manzano [1,2,*], César Fernández-de-las-Peñas [3,4], Marcos José Navarro-Santana [1] and Ibai López-de-Uralde-Villanueva [1,2]

1. Department of Radiology, Rehabilitation and Physiotherapy, Faculty of Nursing, Physiotherapy and Podiatry, Universidad Complutense de Madrid (UCM), 28040 Madrid, Spain; tamaradelcorral@gmail.com (T.d.C.); rfabero@ucm.es (R.F.-G.); marconav@ucm.es (M.J.N.-S.); ibai.uralde@gmail.com (I.L.-d.-U.-V.)
2. Instituto de Investigación Sanitaria del Hospital Clínico San Carlos (IdISSC), 28040 Madrid, Spain
3. Department of Physical Therapy, Occupational Therapy, Rehabilitation and Physical Medicine, Universidad Rey Juan Carlos, 28922 Alcorcón, Spain; cesar.fernandez@urjc.es
4. Cátedra Institucional en Docencia, Clínica e Investigación en Fisioterapia, Terapia Manual, Punción Seca y Ejercicio Terapéutico, Universidad Rey Juan Carlos, 28922 Alcorcón, Spain
* Correspondence: gusplaza@ucm.es; Tel.: +34-91-394-15-17

Abstract: Objective: To establish the minimal clinically important difference (MCID) for inspiratory muscle strength (MIP) and endurance (IME) in individuals with long-term post-COVID-19 symptoms, as well as to ascertain which of the variables has a greater discriminatory capacity and to compare changes between individuals classified by the MCID. Design: Secondary analysis of randomised controlled trial of data from 42 individuals who performed an 8-week intervention of respiratory muscle training programme. Results: A change of at least 18 cmH$_2$O and 22.1% of that predicted for MIP and 328.5 s for IME represented the MCID. All variables showed acceptable discrimination between individuals who classified as "improved" and those classified as "stable/not improved" (area under the curve ≥0.73). MIP was the variable with the best discriminative ability when expressed as a percentage of prediction (Youden index, 0.67; sensitivity, 76.9%; specificity, 89.7%). Participants classified as "improved" had significantly greater improvements in quality of life and lung function compared with the participants classified as "stable/not improved". Conclusion: In individuals with long-term post-COVID-19 symptoms, the inspiratory muscle function variables had an acceptable discriminative ability to assess the efficacy of a respiratory muscle training programme. MIP was the variable with the best discriminative ability, showing better overall performance when expressed as a percentage of prediction.

Keywords: SARS-CoV-2; minimal clinically important difference; inspiratory muscle training; responsiveness

Citation: del Corral, T.; Fabero-Garrido, R.; Plaza-Manzano, G.; Fernández-de-las-Peñas, C.; Navarro-Santana, M.J.; López-de-Uralde-Villanueva, I. Minimal Clinically Important Differences in Inspiratory Muscle Function Variables after a Respiratory Muscle Training Programme in Individuals with Long-Term Post-COVID-19 Symptoms. *J. Clin. Med.* 2023, 12, 2720. https://doi.org/10.3390/jcm12072720

Academic Editor: Denise Battaglini

Received: 14 March 2023
Revised: 31 March 2023
Accepted: 3 April 2023
Published: 5 April 2023

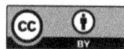

Copyright: © 2023 by the authors. Licensee MDPI, Basel, Switzerland. This article is an open access article distributed under the terms and conditions of the Creative Commons Attribution (CC BY) license (https://creativecommons.org/licenses/by/4.0/).

1. Introduction

Infection with severe acute respiratory syndrome coronavirus 2 (SARS-CoV-2) is responsible for the coronavirus disease 2019 (COVID-19) pandemic, which has resulted in millions of deaths and has put a major strain on health systems worldwide. Although most patients recover spontaneously or after acute-phase management, clinicians are now faced with treating long-term post-COVID-19 symptoms [1]. The most commonly reported persistent symptoms include fatigue, dyspnoea, sleep disorder, and myalgia in up to 41%, 31%, 30%, and 22% of cases, respectively, after more than 1 year of follow-up [2], all of which encourage sedentary lifestyles, induce limited exercise tolerance, and cause considerable deterioration of health-related quality of life (HRQoL) [1]. As recently reported, individuals with long-term post-COVID-19 symptoms can experience respiratory muscle dysfunction [3]. Individuals who have recovered from COVID-19 also exhibit depressed exercise tolerance and an exaggerated hyperventilatory response during exercise [1,4]. These symptoms might be associated with diaphragm fatigue and an increase in the concentration of metabolites that activate the so-called "metaboreflex", causing a peripheral limit to exercise tolerance, characterised by a diffusion defect in oxygen delivery [4,5].

Clinical studies have often reported treatment effects as a change in the outcome measure supported by a measure of variability; however, a statistically significant change might not indicate a clinically meaningful change. There is growing acceptance of the importance of assessing the clinical benefit from the patient's perspective, as well as establishing the outcome measure's ability to detect clinical change and to determine ways to interpret the magnitude of the observed change [6]. The minimal clinically important difference (MCID) was therefore developed to add clinical relevance or patient experience to the reporting of an outcome measure. The MCID is defined as "the smallest difference in score which patients perceive as beneficial and which would mandate a change in the patient's management" [7] and is useful because it links the magnitude of change with treatment decisions in clinical practice and emphasises the primacy of the patient's perception [8]. The MCID of relevant outcomes of respiratory muscle training programs has been established, including the maximal inspiratory pressure (MIP) [9,10], inspiratory muscle endurance (IME) [10], and functional exercise tolerance measured by field tests [11–14] in patients with chronic obstructive pulmonary disease (COPD). Unfortunately, the MCID has not been determined for inspiratory muscle function variables in individuals with long-term post-COVID-19 symptoms. Therefore, the improvements in inspiratory muscle function as a primary outcome in clinical trials for this population remain difficult to interpret. The MCID could help clinicians not only assess whether improvements in inspiratory muscle function are clinically meaningful but also interpret the contribution of changes in muscle strength and endurance to improvement in relevant outcomes (e.g., HRQoL, exercise tolerance, peripheral muscle strength, and lung function) after a respiratory muscle training programme in individuals with long-term post-COVID-19 symptoms.

Thus, the primary aim of this study was to establish the MCIDs for the inspiratory muscle function variables (muscle strength and endurance) in individuals with long-term post-COVID-19 symptoms. The secondary objectives were to ascertain which of the inspiratory muscle function variables has a greater discriminatory capacity and to compare changes in HRQoL, exercise tolerance, peripheral muscle strength, and lung function between individuals who exceed the MCID and those who do not.

2. Materials and Methods

2.1. Study Design

The study consisted of a secondary analysis of data from a previously conducted randomised controlled trial (registered in the United States Clinical Trials Registry: NCT04734561) [15]. This randomised controlled trial was a parallel 4-arm, double-blinded study, and it followed the Consolidated Standards of Reporting Trials guidelines. Participants were randomised into one of the four interventions: (1) inspiratory muscle training; (2) respiratory muscle training (inspiratory and expiratory); (3) sham inspiratory muscle training; or (4) sham respiratory muscle training. The training was 40 min/day, split into two 20 min sessions (morning and afternoon), 6 times per week, over 8 weeks. Clinical assessments were performed at baseline and at 4 and 8 weeks.

For this secondary analysis, data from the 2 real training groups were pooled. In addition, participant data were only included if they had completed their baseline and 8-week assessments. Thus, a total of 42 individuals with long-term post-COVID-19 symptoms were analysed. For a paired 2-tailed t-test with an α of 0.05, a power of 0.80, and an expected effect size of at least 0.5 (a criterion considered by Cohen as the minimum effect size to detect clinically relevant differences) [16], the estimated sample size was 34 individuals. The effect size for respiratory muscle function outcomes could be even larger according to previous studies conducted on other respiratory disease [10], which would imply a slightly smaller sample. Consequently, the analysis of 42 individuals could be considered acceptable if the study were designed with the intention of establishing the MCID for respiratory muscle function outcomes.

2.2. Participants

COVID-19 survivors 18 years of age and older were included in the trial if they presented persistent post-COVID-19 symptoms of fatigue and dyspnoea for at least 3 months after the COVID-19 diagnosis had been confirmed. Candidates were excluded if they (1) presented a diagnosis of progressive respiratory, neuromuscular, or neurological disorders and/or psychiatric or cognitive conditions that hindered their ability to cooperate; (2) presented any contraindication for respiratory muscle training treatment; (3) lacked Internet access; or (4) had been previously included in a rehabilitation programme for their post-COVID-19 symptoms.

2.3. Outcome Measures

- Inspiratory muscle function: Inspiratory muscle strength was assessed by the MIP using a digital mouth pressure meter (MicroRPM; Carefusion, San Diego, CA, USA), according to the American Thoracic Society/European Respiratory Society (ATS/ERS) guidelines [17]. Three trials were performed with a difference of less than 10% between them; the highest value was recorded. The estimated inspiratory muscle strength values were established following the reference equation for the adult population [18]. Inspiratory muscle endurance was measured during a constant load breathing test using the POWERbreathe KH1 device (POWERbreathe International Ltd., Southam, UK), following the instructions established in a previously published protocol [19]. Participants breathed against a submaximal inspiratory load (55% MIP at baseline) until reaching an endpoint limited by their symptoms or their inability to breathe successfully against the load. The length of time for which participants were able to breathe against this load was recorded.
- Health-related quality of life: To measure HRQoL, we employed the EuroQol-5D questionnaire (EQ-5D-5L) [20], which consists of 5 dimensions with 5 response options based on severity level, ranging from 1 to 5. An index score was provided, ranging from 0 (death) to 1 (full health). Participants rated their current overall health on a visual analogue scale, ranging from 0 (poorest imaginable health) to 100 (best imaginable health).
- Exercise tolerance: Cardiorespiratory fitness was assessed by the Ruffier test [21], consisting of 30 squats in 45 s, with a tempo set by a metronome (80 beats per min). Heart rate (HR) was measured after 1 min of resting (HR_0), immediately after completing the 30 squats (HR_1), and after a 1 min recovery (HR_2). Cardiorespiratory fitness was calculated using the following index: $((HR_0 + HR_1 + HR_2) - 200)/10$. Cardiorespiratory fitness correlates with HR due to HR at rest is a general indicator of wellness, while a decline in the HR response to submaximal exercise represents an enhancement in endurance. The linearity of the HR and oxygen consumption relation has been used to predict maximal oxygen uptake in submaximal tasks [22].
- Peripheral muscle strength: Lower-limb muscle strength was determined using the 1 min sit-to-stand (1-min STS) test according to a standardised protocol [23]. The number of times the participant gently touched the chair with their buttocks in 1 min, without using hands or arms to assist the movement, was recorded. Upper limb muscle strength (handgrip force) was assessed using a hand-held dynamometer (Jamar, Patterson Medical, IL, USA) [24]. Three measurements were performed for each hand, alternating sides, and the highest value was recorded.
- Lung function: Pulmonary function testing was assessed using a portable spirometer (Spirobank II USB, MIR, Rome, Italy), according to ATS/ERS guidelines [25]. Measurements included forced vital capacity (FVC), forced expiratory volume in the first second (FEV_1), and their ratio (FEV_1/FVC).

2.4. Anchor Outcome

After the respiratory muscle training, the participants (blinded to the results of their post-training assessments) completed the Global Rating of Change (GROC) scale [7], which was employed as an anchor variable for determining MCID. The GROC consists of a 15-point ordinal scale ranging from −7 ("a great deal worse") to 7 ("a great deal better"). The participants were asked to rate the perceived change in their overall health since the start of the training by answering the following question using the GROC: "Compared with the first assessment/visit, how much change do you perceive in your overall health status after respiratory muscle training (including performance of activities of daily living, efforts/fatigue, and/or dyspnoea)?"

2.5. Data Analysis

The data analysis was performed using SPSS version 27.0 (SPSS Inc., Chicago, IL, USA). For all analyses, the statistical significance was set at 5% ($p < 0.05$).

The change in inspiratory muscle function in the whole sample was assessed using parametric tests, given that a normal distribution of the variables was assumed based on the results of the assumption tests and the central limit theorem (due to the large sample size; N > 30) [26]. Thus, a dependent samples *t*-test was used to determine the differences between pre- and post-training outcomes. Effect sizes were calculated according to Cohen's method: small (0.20–0.49), medium (0.50–0.79), or large (≥ 0.8) [27].

The MCID for improvement perceived by the individual was determined by using an anchor-based method. Concretely, the anchor-based approach was performed using a receiver operating characteristic (ROC) curve analysis. This approach used the anchor variable (external criterion; GROC scale) to determine the optimal cut-off for the respiratory muscle function variables that corresponded to the least misclassification for discriminating between individuals who had improved and those who were unchanged or deteriorated. To calculate the MCID, participants were dichotomised into 2 groups according to GROC scores: (1) stable/not improved (no change or minimal improvement): those who scored +3 or less and (2) improved: those who scored +4 or more. A cut-off of +4 has classically been considered to determine the MCID [7,28].

Group comparisons between individuals with and without a change greater than MCID in inspiratory muscle function outcomes were performed using non-parametric tests due to the sample size (sample size $\leq$ 16 individuals in the groups without exceeding the MCID). In addition, the Shapiro–Wilk test showed a non-normality distribution for almost half of the data. The Mann–Whitney U test was used to detect between-group differences in quality of life, exercise tolerance, peripheral muscle strength, lung function at baseline, post-training, and difference between pre- and post-values (Δpre-post). The Wilcoxon test was used to compare pre- and post-training results within each group. The magnitude of the differences was calculated using an r effect size: small (r < 0.3), medium (0.30–0.5), or large (>0.5) [29].

3. Results

The study sample consisted of 42 individuals with long-term post-COVID-19 symptoms (12 men and 30 women) with a mean age of 47.93 ± 8.84 years (height, 165.9 ± 7.7 cm; weight, 74.69 ± 16.51 kg; and body mass index, 27.13 ± 5.81 kg/m^2). All participants completed more than 95% of the training sessions, and no adverse effects were reported during the respiratory muscle training programme. The mean symptom duration since diagnosis was 354.21 ± 77.56 days, and 13 (31%) participants required hospital admission of whom three required invasive mechanical ventilation. Most participants showed inspiratory and/or expiratory muscle weakness at baseline (n = 32 (76%); MIP and/or maximal expiratory pressure <80% of predicted). This loss of muscle strength could be associated to deconditioning as a result of prolonged inactivity due to hospitalized or quarantined at home. More than half of the participants had smoked at some time in their lives (smokers,

11 (26%); ex-smokers, 12 (29%)). However, only one (2%) participant had impaired lung function (FVC <80% of predicted).

3.1. Findings Related with Minimal Clinically Important Difference

The distribution of participant responses according to their GROC scores was "improved" in 69% and "stable/not improved" in 31% (no change (12%) or minimal improvement (19%)). After 8 weeks of a respiratory muscle training programme, a large and statistically significant increase in both inspiratory muscle strength (ΔMIP in cmH$_2$O, 33.05 $\pm$ 18.99 (95% CI 27.13 to 38.97; $p < 0.001$; $d = 1.43$); ΔMIP in % of predicted, 31.72 $\pm$ 17.60 (95% CI 26.23 to 37.20; $p < 0.001$; $d = 1.75$)) and inspiratory muscle endurance (ΔIME in cmH$_2$O, 272.64 $\pm$ 158.17 (95% CI 223.35 to 321.93; $p < 0.001$; $d = 2.05$)) was observed in the entire sample. Table 1 shows the descriptive statistics for the change in inspiratory muscle function variables for the group classified as "improved" and the group classified as "stable/not improved", as well as the multiple comparisons between them.

Table 1. Descriptive statistics and multiple comparisons between groups for change in inspiratory muscle function.

Outcome	Group	Mean $\pm$ SD; Median (IQR)			Within-Group Differences p-Value; r Effect Size
		Baseline	Post-Training	ΔPre-Post	
MIP (cmH$_2$O)	Improved	78.45 $\pm$ 19.24 75 (64–94)	117.41 $\pm$ 26.3 117 (100.5–130)	38.97 $\pm$ 17.37 36 (28–50)	$p < 0.001$; $r = 0.87$
	Stable/not improved	97.92 $\pm$ 22 93 (82.5–113)	117.77 $\pm$ 20.47 114 (104.5–139)	19.85 $\pm$ 15.97 17 (11–26)	$p < 0.001$; $r = 0.83$
	Between-group differences for ΔPre-Post training p-value; r effect size			$p < 0.001$; $r = 0.50$	
MIP (% pred)	Improved	74.95 $\pm$ 15.57 73.75 (66.63–87.09)	112.19 $\pm$ 20.87 114.10 (100.62–130.55)	37.23 $\pm$ 15.21 365.75 (24.34–52.54)	$p < 0.001$; $r = 0.87$
	Stable/not improved	91.4 $\pm$ 13.86 95.91 (80.24–100.77)	110.82 $\pm$ 16.21 111.61 (99.46–120.88)	19.42 $\pm$ 16.76 18.14 (9.74–21.76)	$p < 0.001$; $r = 0.83$
	Between-group differences for ΔPre-Post training p-value; r effect size			$p < 0.001$; $r = 0.50$	
IME (s)	Improved	200.17 $\pm$ 104.89 173 (117–286.5)	511.48 $\pm$ 151 494 (412–638)	311.31 $\pm$ 149.21 347 (225–428)	$p < 0.001$; $r = 0.87$
	Stable/not improved	166.23 $\pm$ 79.98 145 (113–182.5)	352.62 $\pm$ 128.23 343 (263.5–420.5)	186.38 $\pm$ 147.83 174 (85–291)	$p < 0.001$; $r = 0.83$
	Between-group differences for ΔPre-Post training p-value; r effect size			$p = 0.02$; $r = 0.36$	

Abbreviations: IME, inspiratory muscle endurance; IQR, interquartile range; MIP, maximal inspiratory pressure; SD, standard deviation.

The ROC analysis results for the inspiratory muscle function variables are presented in Table 2. According to the ROC analysis, all variables showed acceptable discrimination between individuals who classified themselves as "improved" and those who classified themselves as "stable/not improved", obtaining an AUC ≥ 0.73 (Figure 1). MIP was the variable with the best discriminative ability, showing better performance when expressed as a percentage of prediction (Youden index, 0.67) rather than in cmH$_2$O (Youden index, 0.58). The ROC curve analysis established that a change of 18 cmH$_2$O (sensitivity, 61.5%; specificity, 96.6%) or of 22.1% of that predicted (sensitivity, 76.9%; specificity, 89.7%) represents a meaningful clinical improvement in MIP. Thus, assuming 18 cmH$_2$O or 22.1% of that predicted as MCID for MIP, 38.5% or 23.1% of the participants who classified themselves as "improved" were misclassified as "stable/not improved", respectively.

Table 2. Receiver operating characteristic (ROC) analysis results for the inspiratory muscle function variables.

Outcome	MCID	AUC (95% CI)	Sensitivity	Specificity	Youden Index	LR+	LR−
MIP (cmH$_2$O)	18	0.82 (0.65 to 0.98)	61.5	96.6	0.581	18.1	0.4
MIP (% pred)	22.1	0.81 (0.65 to 0.98)	76.9	89.7	0.666	7.5	0.3
IME (s)	328.5	0.73 (0.56 to 0.90)	92.3	51.7	0.44	1.9	0.1

Abbreviations: AUC, area under the curve; CI, confidence interval; IME, inspiratory muscle endurance; MCID, minimal clinically important difference; MIP, maximal inspiratory pressure; LR, likelihood ratio.

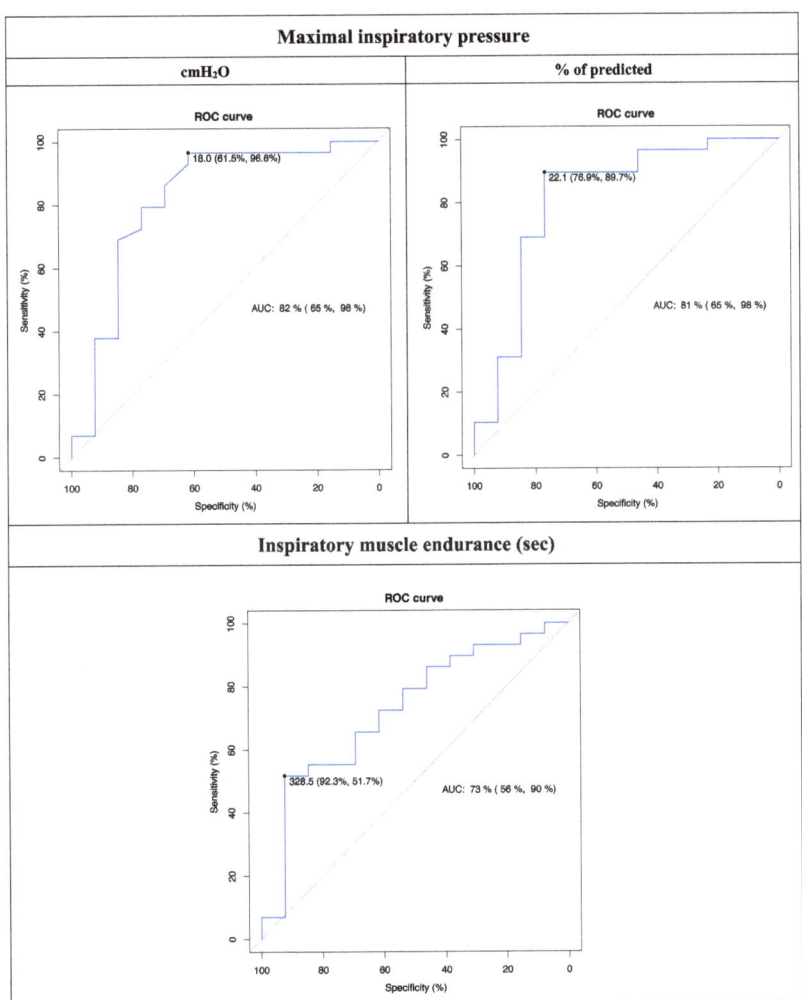

Figure 1. Receiver operating characteristic (ROC) curves for the inspiratory muscle function variables. Values expressed as: AUC (95% CI), area under the curve (95% confidence interval); MCID (Sen, Spe), minimal clinically important difference (sensitivity, specificity).

3.2. Comparison between Individuals with and without a Change Greater than MCID

Table 3 lists the descriptive statistics and multiple comparisons for the change in the assessed variables. The participants with a greater than MCID change in MIP, regardless of measurement unit, showed a medium/large and statistically significant increase in inspiratory muscle strength compared with those with a less than MCID change ($r = 0.45$–0.52). Similarly, the participants who exceeded MCID in IME showed a large and statistically significant increase in MIP compared with those with a change below MCID (MIP in cmH$_2$O, $r = 0.58$; MIP in % of prediction, $r = 0.62$).

The participants with a change greater than the MCID set for the inspiratory muscle function variables (MIP and IME) showed a medium/large and statistically significant increase in HRQoL ($r = 0.31$–0.54) and FVC ($r = 0.35$–0.49) compared with those who did not exceed the MCID, except for the EQ-5D-5L index when the MCID for MIP was set at cmH$_2$O ($p = 0.182$; $r = 0.21$). In addition, only the participants with a change above the MCID in MIP expressed as a percentage of prediction showed a medium and statistically significant increase in the FEV$_1$/FVC ratio ($r = 0.31$) compared with those who did not exceed the MCID. There was no difference in exercise tolerance, peripheral muscle strength, or FEV$_1$ between the participants who exceeded MCID in the inspiratory muscle function variables and those who did not. However, only the participants who exceeded MCID for MIP and IME showed a statistically significant improvement in exercise tolerance compared with their pre-training assessment.

Table 3. Descriptive statistics and multiple comparisons for the change in variables assessed. Values are expressed as mean ± SD and median (IQR).

Outcome	Maximal Inspiratory Pressure (MCID = 18 cmH₂O)			Maximal Inspiratory Pressure (MCID = 22.1% of pred.)			Inspiratory Muscle Endurance (MCID = 328.5 s)			Between-Group Differences p-Value; r Effect Size (a) MCID for MIP in cmH₂O (b) MCID for MIP in % of pred. (c) MCID for IME in sec
	Did not Exceed MCID	Exceeded MCID		Did not Exceed MCID	Exceeded MCID		Did not Exceed MCID	Exceeded MCID		
Inspiratory muscle function										
MIP (cmH₂O)	— —	— —		— —	— —		26.31 ± 19.83 22.5 (14–34) [a]	44 ± 11.15 49 (33.5–51) [a]		(a) — (b) — (c) $p < 0.001$; $r = 0.58$
MIP (% pred)	— —	— —		— —	— —		23.23 ± 14.71 22.78 (14.53–28.67) [a]	45.52 ± 12.57 51.36 (36.4–52.94) [a]		(a) — (b) — (c) $p < 0.001$; $r = 0.62$
IME (s)	116.56 ± 111.07 121 (60–174) [b]	315.21 ± 142.3 310 (229–428) [a]		168.23 ± 125.32 174 (85–250) [a]	319.45 ± 150.24 347 (229–457) [a]		— —	— —		(a) $p < 0.001$; $r = 0.52$ (b) $p = 0.003$; $r = 0.45$ (c) —
HRQoL										
EQ-5D-5L, index	0.145 ± 0.136 0.11 (0.049–0.214) [a]	0.205 ± 0.172 0.22 (0.09–0.302) [a]		0.12 ± 0.155 0.11 (0.023–0.214) [a]	0.225 ± 0.162 0.23 (0.133–0.322) [a]		0.152 ± 0.146 0.167 (0.023–0.253) [a]	0.258 ± 0.178 0.254 (0.166–0.380) [a]		(a) $p = 0.182$; $r = 0.21$ (b) $p = 0.046$; $r = 0.31$ (c) $p = 0.039$; $r = 0.32$
EQ-5D-5L, VAS	6.67 ± 7.5 5 (5–10) [b]	20.67 ± 12.23 20 (14–28) [a]		8.08 ± 11.46 5 (5–15) [b]	21.97 ± 10.88 20 (15–28) [a]		12.46 ± 9.82 14.5 (5–20) [a]	26.12 ± 12.55 24 (17.5–35) [a]		(a) $p < 0.001$; $r = 0.51$ (b) $p < 0.001$; $r = 0.54$ (c) $p < 0.001$; $r = 0.50$
Exercise tolerance										
Ruffier index	−0.62 ± 2.38 −1.2 (−2.2—0.3)	−1.39 ± 2.72 −1.9 (−2.7–0.1) [a]		−0.19 ± 2.34 −0.3 (−1.2–1.3)	−1.69 ± 2.67 −2.2 (−3–0) [a]		−0.87 ± 2.12 −1.2 (−2.3–0.1) [b]	−1.82 ± 3.32 −2.35 (−3.55–0.35) [b]		(a) $p = 0.154$; $r = 0.22$ (b) $p = 0.094$; $r = 0.26$ (c) $p = 0.200$; $r = 0.20$

Table 3. Cont.

Outcome	Maximal Inspiratory Pressure (MCID = 18 cmH$_2$O)		Maximal Inspiratory Pressure (MCID = 22.1% of pred.)		Inspiratory Muscle Endurance (MCID = 328.5 s)		Between-Group Differences p-Value; r Effect Size (a) MCID for MIP in cmH$_2$O (b) MCID for MIP in % of pred. (c) MCID for IME in sec
	Did not exceed MCID	Exceeded MCID	Did not Exceed MCID	Exceeded MCID	Did not Exceed MCID	Exceeded MCID	
Peripheral muscle strength							
1 min STS (n of squats)	10.67 ± 9.57 11 (4–18) [b]	12.52 ± 10.34 13 (7–17) [a]	7.23 ± 11.4 6 (4–13) [b]	14.31 ± 8.8 14 (9–17) [a]	10 ± 10.19 10 (4–16) [a]	15.56 ± 9.23 15.5 (11–20) [a]	(a) $p = 0.085$; $r = 0.27$ (b) $p = 0.058$; $r = 0.29$ (c) $p = 0.102$; $r = 0.25$
Handgrip (Kg)	−1 ± 3.85 −1 (−4–−0.5)	1.21 ± 4.82 2 (−2.5–3)	−0.77 ± 3.53 −1 (−3.5–−0.5)	1.41 ± 5.02 2 (−2.5–3)	0.98 ± 5.43 −0.5 (−2.5–4)	0.34 ± 3.23 1.5 (−2.75–2.5)	(a) $p = 0.262$; $r = 0.17$ (b) $p = 0.236$; $r = 0.18$ (c) $p = 0.876$; $r = 0.02$
Lung function							
FVC (% pred)	−3.78 ± 10.32 −2 (−9–3)	5.27 ± 11.13 3 (0–9) [a]	−0.77 ± 12.36 −2 (−6–3)	5.17 ± 10.77 3 (1–9) [a]	0.5 ± 12.43 0 (−3–3)	7.94 ± 8.12 6 (2–10.5) [a]	(a) $p = 0.034$; $r = 0.33$ (b) $p = 0.025$; $r = 0.35$ (c) $p < 0.001$; $r = 0.49$
FEV$_1$ (% pred)	−1.33 ± 8.63 2 (−4–3)	2.76 ± 10.59 2 (−3–6)	1.92 ± 11.76 2 (−3–3)	1.86 ± 9.71 2 (−3–5)	0.88 ± 11.27 2 (−3–5)	3.5 ± 8.39 2.5 (−1–7.5)	(a) $p = 0.282$; $r = 0.17$ (b) $p = 0.653$; $r = 0.07$ (c) $p = 0.364$; $r = 0.14$
FEV$_1$/FVC (%)	−0.67 ± 2.45 0 (−1–0)	−1.12 ± 3.19 −1 (−2–0) [b]	0.31 ± 3.38 0 (−1–1)	−1.62 ± 2.7 −2 (−3–0) [a]	−0.77 ± 3.3 −0.5 (−2–0)	−1.44 ± 2.56 −1.5 (−3–0) [b]	(a) $p = 0.377$; $r = 0.14$ (b) $p = 0.046$; $r = 0.31$ (c) $p = 0.295$; $r = 0.16$

Abbreviations: EQ-5D-5L, EuroQol-5D questionnaire; FEV$_1$, force expiratory volume at 1st second; FVC, force vital capacity; HRQoL, Health-related quality of life; IQR, interquartile range; IME inspiratory muscle endurance; MCID, minimal clinically important difference; MIP, maximal inspiratory pressure; SD, standard deviation; STS, sit-to-stand; VAS, visual analogue scale; % pred, percentage of predicted value. [a] Statistically significant within-group differences from baseline values, $p < 0.05$, [b] Statistically significant within-group differences from baseline values, $p < 0.01$.

4. Discussion

This study reports the first MCIDs for inspiratory muscle function variables in individuals with long-term post-COVID-19 symptoms after a respiratory muscle training programme. Using an anchor-based approach, our results indicate 18 cmH$_2$O and 22.1% of predicted values as MCID for MIP, and 328.5 s as MCID for IME, suggesting that an increase over these values can be considered clinically relevant in this population. Furthermore, MIP was the variable with the best discriminative ability, showing better overall performance when expressed as a percentage of prediction due to the better metric properties detected. The MCID values presented here provide a way for clinicians to evaluate meaningful change in individual patients and for researchers to evaluate meaningful change between groups.

Both real training groups obtained significant improvements in inspiratory muscle strength and endurance after 8 weeks of a respiratory muscle training programme; these improvements could be considered clinically relevant, given that they were associated with large effect sizes (≥ 0.8). Differences were observed between the group classified as "improved" and the group classified as "stable/not improved", with small to moderate effect sizes. Our results are supported by the study by McNarry et al. [30], who reported that an 8-week inspiratory muscle training programme could strengthen inspiratory muscles in individuals with self-reported COVID-19. Furthermore, participants classified as "improved" had significantly greater improvements in all inspiratory muscle function variables compared with the participants classified as "stable/not improved". This underscores that patient-centred care requires careful and explicit consideration of the patient's perspective to improve patient satisfaction [31].

The AUC ≥ 0.73 from all anchors demonstrated adequate discrimination ability to classify individuals who had undergone important changes from those who had not and therefore rendered this estimate for the MCID clinically useful. To our knowledge, no previous studies have established the MCID for inspiratory muscle function variables in individuals with long-term post-COVID-19 symptoms. We therefore discuss the results considering other respiratory conditions with similar features, while recognising that the differences in the population sample examined would yield larger MCID values. Our determination of the MCID value of 18 cmH$_2$O for MIP is in line with the value of 17.2 cmH$_2$O established for patients with COPD [9] and smaller than the MCID estimate by Gosselink et al. [10] of 13 cmH$_2$O in the same population. With respect to IME, Gosselink et al. [10] reported that a change of at least 261 s was considered clinically significant; in our study, any change greater than 328.5 s was considered clinically important. The discrepancies observed between these studies could lie in the type of population studied in each investigation and by the fact that we used the anchor-based approach—a more conservative and exhaustive method—which is essentially based on the participant's perceived improvement after an intervention and is therefore subjective. This is in contrast to the approach employed in the Gosselink et al. [10] study, which was based on mathematics (summary effect size), with no intervention performed, a better approach to estimate the minimal detectable change (MDC; the smallest change in score that can be detected beyond random error).

Following this argument, the MCID value for MIP reported by the current study could be considered a "real change" because it exceeded the recently redefined MDC of 17 cmH$_2$O in moderate smokers [32]. Given that the MCID is an estimate of how much an outcome measure should change for that change to be considered "important", this value should ideally be similar to or exceed the MDC value, so that the "important" change represented by the MCID also exceeds the value that is estimated to exceed the measurement error in an outcome measure [33]. It is important to note that the MCID value for a particular measure can vary depending on the clinical context and decision at hand, the baseline from which the patient starts, and whether they are improving or deteriorating [34]. Thus, the MCID should be judiciously applied to any particular clinical or research context.

In general terms, MIP expressed as a percentage of prediction was the value with the overall best discriminatory capacity because it assumes the best Youden index (0.67) and an optimal certainty threshold that balances false-negative rates. Specifically, the best balance between the positive and negative likelihood ratio (LR) was detected when the MCID for MIP was set at 22.1% of predicted value (LR+, 7.5; LR−, 0.3; sensitivity, 76.9%; specificity, 89.7%). This is in line with Decramer [35], who reported that MIP had been shown to correlate significantly, albeit weakly, with the response to training in patients with COPD, allowing this outcome to be used to predict the response to the rehabilitation programme and that can be used as a guideline for basing clinical decisions. Reinforcing the relevance of the MIP in detecting the individuals who improved, MIP expressed as cmH_2O showed the highest LR+ (18.1) when a change of ≥ 18 cmH_2O was produced, indicating a large likelihood of determining with greater certainty that the individual would feel clinically better if it exceeded that value. In contrast, the smallest LR− was observed for IME, suggesting that a change lower than 328.5 s assumes a large likelihood that the individual would not perceive clinical improvement. However, the LR+ for IME was trivial; we therefore consider that in clinical practice, it could be more useful to use the MCID established for MIP both in cmH_2O and as a percentage of prediction. MIP expressed as a percentage of prediction is adjusted for anthropometric variables, which affect the results of MIP, thereby possibly explaining the slightly higher diagnostic accuracy over MIP expressed in cmH_2O. This result is supported by the positive correlation of MIP with body composition found in patients with COPD [36] and in healthy individuals [37]. Thus, our results suggest that the use of the MCID for MIP expressed as a percentage of prediction should be the first measure of choice to identify whether a patient has experienced an improvement; also, the probability would increase substantially if we then verify that the change exceeds 18 cmH_2O. Future studies are needed to reinforce or contradict our findings.

We were able to perform group comparisons between the participants with and without a change greater than MCID, which is one of the novelties and strengths of our study, reinforced by the fact that clinical improvements occurred not only in relation to inspiratory muscle function variables but also relative to HRQoL and FVC, making our results more clinically applicable. In fact, only the participants with a change above the MCID in MIP expressed as a percentage of prediction showed a statistically significant decrease in the FEV_1/FVC ratio compared with those who did not exceed the MCID. For reasons beyond our knowledge, participants who did not exceed the MCID of MIP expressed as a percentage of prediction increased FEV_1 without improving FVC. As a result of inspiratory muscle training, FVC is expected to improve due to an increase in inspired volume, so there would be a slight increase in FEV_1 attributed to lung compliance. This trend occurred in all group comparisons of lung function variables between the participants with and without a change greater than MCID, except for MIP expressed as a percentage of prediction. In our opinion, this is the reason why these differences were statistically significant, but not clinically relevant (<2%). In addition, the results showed a non-significant trend towards an increase in exercise capacity and peripheral muscle strength, further reinforcing that this value is slightly higher relative to all reported MCIDs. There is a decompensation between the groups compared, with a higher proportion in the group that exceeded the MCID. Therefore, future studies comparing homogeneous groups are necessary.

This study presents some limitations. The study was derived from a randomised controlled trial that was not primarily designed to estimate the MCID of inspiratory muscle function variables; however, the sample size calculation performed for this new study was adequate for detecting clinically relevant differences. In contrast, the study was not designed to detect differences between individuals with and without a change greater than MCID in inspiratory muscle function variables. Another limitation was the small number of participants without a GROC change, which might have affected the accuracy of estimating the specificity of the cut-off. Lastly, the generalisability of these results is limited to individuals with long-term post-COVID-19 symptoms from a single metropolitan area with characteristics similar to those of this study's sample. Caution should be used in generalising these current findings to patients in other settings with other characteristics, such as acute phase of infection, because the improvements could observed due to the progression of the disease itself.

This study had some clinical implications. The MCIDs reported by the current study may be used to enhance the interpretability and meaningfulness of changes in improvement scores derived from clinical trials that examine the efficacy of interventions designed to improve inspiratory muscle function in individuals with long-term post-COVID-19 symptoms. In addition, researchers could express the results in terms of the proportion of participants in the experimental group who exceeded the MCID values compared with the same proportion of participants in the comparison group, which could provide a more clinically relevant method for examining the differences between intervention strategies. These values can be used to assess the progress of individual patients from a clinical standpoint and to illustrate to patients, caregivers, and third-party payers that "important" change has taken place, which should be a guide for planning patient management.

5. Conclusions

The present study indicated that, in individuals with long-term post-COVID-19 symptoms, the inspiratory muscle function variables (MIP and IME) had an acceptable discriminative ability to assess the efficacy of a respiratory muscle training programme. Specifically, a change of at least 18 cmH$_2$O and 22.1% of the predicted value for MIP and 328.5 s for IME represented the MCID for judging clinical change in inspiratory muscle function. MIP was the variable with the best discriminative ability, showing better overall performance when expressed as a percentage of prediction. Individuals with a change greater than the MCID established for inspiratory muscle function variables showed a statistically significant increase in quality of life and lung function compared with those who did not exceed the MCID.

Author Contributions: T.d.C.: Conceptualization, Data curation, Investigation, Methodology, Resources, Visualization, Project administration, Supervision, Writing—original draft, Writing—review and editing. R.F.-G.: Data curation, Investigation, Resources, Visualization, Project administration, Supervision, Writing—original draft, Writing—review and editing. G.P.-M.: Investigation, Visualization, Writing—original draft, Writing—review and editing. C.F.-d.-l.-P.: Investigation, Visualization, Writing—original draft, Writing—review and editing. M.J.N.-S.: Investigation, Visualization, Writing—original draft, Writing—review and editing. I.L.-d.-U.-V.: Conceptualization, Data curation, Formal analysis, Methodology, Project administration, Resources, Supervision, Validation, Writing—original draft, Writing—review and editing. All authors have read and agreed to the published version of the manuscript.

Funding: Premio "Ayudas a la investigación en fisioterapia y COVID-19" (IP.A.I. Covid-19 2020/03) by the Illustrious Professional Association of Physiotherapists of the Community of Madrid, Spain.

Institutional Review Board Statement: The study consisted of a secondary analysis of data from a previously conducted randomised controlled trial (registered in the United States Clinical Trials Registry: NCT04734561. The study was conducted according to the guidelines of the Declaration of Helsinki and was approved by the Ethics Committee of Hospital Clínico San Carlos (20/715-E_BS).

Informed Consent Statement: Informed consent was obtained from all subjects involved in the study.

Data Availability Statement: Available upon request.

Acknowledgments: The authors thank the participants who took part in this study, the Long Covid ACTS and Covid persistente España (Persistent COVID Spain) for their help.

Conflicts of Interest: The authors declare no conflict of interest.

References

1. Montani, D.; Savale, L.; Noel, N.; Meyrignac, O.; Colle, R.; Gasnier, M.; Corruble, E.; Beurnier, A.; Jutant, E.-M.; Pham, T.; et al. Post-acute COVID-19 syndrome. *Eur. Respir. Rev.* **2022**, *31*, 210185. [CrossRef] [PubMed]
2. Alkodaymi, M.S.; Omrani, O.A.; Fawzy, N.A.; Shaar, B.A.; Almamlouk, R.; Riaz, M.; Obeidat, M.; Obeidat, Y.; Gerberi, D.; Taha, R.M.; et al. Prevalence of post-acute COVID-19 syndrome symptoms at different follow-up periods: A systematic review and meta-analysis. *Clin. Microbiol. Infect.* **2022**, *28*, 657–666. [CrossRef]
3. Hennigs, J.K.; Huwe, M.; Hennigs, A.; Oqueka, T.; Simon, M.; Harbaum, L.; Körbelin, J.; Schmiedel, S.; Wiesch, J.S.Z.; Addo, M.M.; et al. Respiratory muscle dysfunction in long-COVID patients. *Infection* **2022**, *50*, 1391–1397. [CrossRef] [PubMed]
4. Singh, I.; Joseph, P.; Heerdt, P.M.; Cullinan, M.; Lutchmansingh, D.D.; Gulati, M.; Possick, J.D.; Systrom, D.M.; Waxman, A.B. Persistent Exertional Intolerance after COVID-19. *Chest* **2021**, *161*, 54–63. [CrossRef]
5. Sheel, A.W.; Derchak, P.A.; Morgan, B.J.; Pegelow, D.F.; Jacques, A.J.; Dempsey, J.A. Fatiguing inspiratory muscle work causes reflex reduction in resting leg blood flow in humans. *J. Physiol.* **2001**, *537*, 277–289. [CrossRef] [PubMed]
6. Terwee, C.; Dekker, F.; Wiersinga, W.; Prummel, M.; Bossuyt, P. On assessing responsiveness of health-related quality of life instruments: Guidelines for instrument evaluation. *Qual. Life Res.* **2003**, *12*, 349–362. [CrossRef]
7. Jaeschke, R.; Singer, J.; Guyatt, G.H. Measurement of health status: Ascertaining the minimal clinically important difference. *Control. Clin. Trials* **1989**, *10*, 407–415. [CrossRef]
8. Apaza, J.A.S.; Franco, J.V.A.; Meza, N.; Madrid, E.; Loézar, C.; Garegnani, L. Minimal clinically important difference: The basics. *Medwave* **2021**, *21*, e8149. [CrossRef] [PubMed]
9. Iwakura, M.; Okura, K.; Kubota, M.; Sugawara, K.; Kawagoshi, A.; Takahashi, H.; Shioya, T. Estimation of minimal clinically important difference for quadriceps and inspiratory muscle strength in older outpatients with chronic obstructive pulmonary disease: A prospective cohort study. *Phys. Ther. Res.* **2021**, *24*, 35–42. [CrossRef] [PubMed]
10. Gosselink, R.; De Vos, J.; Van Den Heuvel, S.P.; Segers, J.; Decramer, M.; Kwakkel, G. Impact of inspiratory muscle training in patients with COPD: What is the evidence? *Eur. Respir. J.* **2011**, *37*, 416–425. [CrossRef] [PubMed]
11. Zanini, A.; Crisafulli, E.; D'Andria, M.; Gregorini, C.; Cherubino, F.; Zampogna, E.; Azzola, A.; Spanevello, A.; Schiavone, N.; Chetta, A. Minimum Clinically Important Difference in 30-s Sit-to-Stand Test after Pulmonary Rehabilitation in Subjects with COPD. *Respir. Care* **2019**, *64*, 1261–1269. [CrossRef]
12. Vaidya, T.; de Bisschop, C.; Beaumont, M.; Ouksel, H.; Jean, V.; Dessables, F.; Chambellan, A. Is the 1-minute sit-to-stand test a good tool for the evaluation of the impact of pulmonary rehabilitation? Determination of the minimal important difference in COPD. *Int. J. Chronic Obstr. Pulm. Dis.* **2016**, *11*, 2609–2616. [CrossRef]
13. Parreira, V.F.; Janaudis-Ferreira, T.; Evans, R.; Mathur, S.; Goldstein, R.S.; Brooks, D. Measurement Properties of the Incremental Shuttle Walk Test. *Chest* **2014**, *145*, 1357–1369. [CrossRef]
14. Bohannon, R.W.; Crouch, R. Minimal clinically important difference for change in 6-minute walk test distance of adults with pathology: A systematic review. *J. Evaluation Clin. Pract.* **2016**, *23*, 377–381. [CrossRef] [PubMed]
15. Del Corral, T.; Fabero-Garrido, R.; Plaza-Manzano, G.; Fernández-De-Las-Peñas, C.; Navarro-Santana, M.; López-De-Uralde-Villanueva, I. Home-based respiratory muscle training on quality of life and exercise tolerance in long-term post-COVID-19: Randomized controlled trial. *Ann. Phys. Rehabil. Med.* **2023**, *66*, 101709. [CrossRef]
16. Cohen, J. *Statistical Power Analysis for the Behavioral Sciences*; Elsevier Science: Amsterdam, The Netherlands, 2013.
17. American Thoracic Society/European Respiratory Society. ATS/ERS Statement on Respiratory Muscle Testing. *Am. J. Respir. Crit. Care Med.* **2002**, *166*, 518–624. [CrossRef]
18. Morales, P.; Sanchis, J.; Cordero, P.J.; Díez, J.L. Maximum static respiratory pressures in adults. Reference values for a Caucasian Mediterranean population. *Arch. Bronconeumol.* **1997**, *33*, 213–219. [CrossRef]
19. Langer, D.; Charususin, N.; Jácome, C.; Hoffman, M.; McConnell, A.; Decramer, M.; Gosselink, R. Efficacy of a Novel Method for Inspiratory Muscle Training in People with Chronic Obstructive Pulmonary Disease. *Phys. Ther.* **2015**, *95*, 1264–1273. [CrossRef]
20. Herdman, M.; Gudex, C.; Lloyd, A.; Janssen, M.; Kind, P.; Parkin, D.; Bonsel, G.; Badia, X. Development and preliminary testing of the new five-level version of EQ-5D (EQ-5D-5L). *Qual. Life Res.* **2011**, *20*, 1727–1736. [CrossRef] [PubMed]
21. Sartor, F.; Bonato, M.; Papini, G.; Bosio, A.; Mohammed, R.A.; Bonomi, A.G.; Moore, J.P.; Merati, G.; La Torre, A.; Kubis, H.-P. A 45-Second Self-Test for Cardiorespiratory Fitness: Heart Rate-Based Estimation in Healthy Individuals. *PLoS ONE* **2016**, *11*, e0168154. [CrossRef]
22. American College of Sports Medicine. *ACSM's Guidelines for Exercise Testing and Prescription*, 9th ed.; Lippincott Williams & Wilkins: Philadelphia, PA, USA, 2014.
23. Núñez-Cortés, R.; Rivera-Lillo, G.; Arias-Campoverde, M.; Soto-García, D.; García-Palomera, R.; Torres-Castro, R. Use of sit-to-stand test to assess the physical capacity and exertional desaturation in patients post COVID-19. *Chronic Respir. Dis.* **2021**, *18*, 1479973121999205. [CrossRef] [PubMed]
24. Peolsson, R.H.A. Intra- and inter-tester reliability and reference values for hand strength. *J. Rehabil. Med.* **2001**, *33*, 36–41. [CrossRef] [PubMed]
25. Miller, M.R.; Crapo, R.; Hankinson, J.; Brusasco, V.; Burgos, F.; Casaburi, R.; Coates, A.; Enright, P.; van der Grinten, C.P.M.; Gustafsson, P.; et al. General considerations for lung function testing. *Eur. Respir. J.* **2005**, *26*, 153–161. [CrossRef] [PubMed]
26. Nixon, R.; Wonderling, D.; Grieve, R. Non-parametric methods for cost-effectiveness analysis: The central limit theorem and the bootstrap compared. *Health Econ.* **2010**, *19*, 316–333. [CrossRef]

27. Cohen, J. *Statistical Power Analysis for the Behavioral Sciences*; Lawrence Erlbaum Associates Inc.: Hillsdale, NJ, USA, 1988; Volume 18, pp. 131–132.
28. Copay, A.G.; Subach, B.R.; Glassman, S.D.; Polly, D.W., Jr.; Schuler, T.C. Understanding the minimum clinically important difference: A review of concepts and methods. *Spine J.* **2007**, *7*, 541–546. [CrossRef]
29. Pautz, N.; Olivier, B.; Steyn, F. The use of nonparametric effect sizes in single study musculoskeletal physiotherapy research: A practical primer. *Phys. Ther. Sport* **2018**, *33*, 117–124. [CrossRef]
30. McNarry, M.A.; Berg, R.M.; Shelley, J.; Hudson, J.; Saynor, Z.L.; Duckers, J.; Lewis, K.; Davies, G.A.; Mackintosh, K.A. Inspiratory muscle training enhances recovery post-COVID-19: A randomised controlled trial. *Eur. Respir. J.* **2022**, *60*, 2103101. [CrossRef]
31. Joosten, E.; DeFuentes-Merillas, L.; de Weert, G.; Sensky, T.; van der Staak, C.; de Jong, C. Systematic Review of the Effects of Shared Decision-Making on Patient Satisfaction, Treatment Adherence and Health Status. *Psychother. Psychosom.* **2008**, *77*, 219–226. [CrossRef]
32. Balbás-Álvarez, L.; Candelas-Fernández, P.; Del Corral, T.; La Touche, R.; López-De-Uralde-Villanueva, I. Effect of Manual Therapy, Motor Control Exercise, and Inspiratory Muscle Training on Maximum Inspiratory Pressure and Postural Measures in Moderate Smokers: A Randomized Controlled Trial. *J. Manip. Physiol. Ther.* **2018**, *41*, 372–382. [CrossRef]
33. Riddle, D.L.; Stratford, P.W. *Is This Change Real?: Interpreting Patient Outcomes in Physical Therapy*; F.A. Davis Company: Philadelphia, PA, USA, 2013.
34. King, M.T. A point of minimal important difference (MID): A critique of terminology and methods. *Expert Rev. Pharm. Outcomes Res.* **2011**, *11*, 171–184. [CrossRef]
35. Decramer, M. Treatment of chronic respiratory failure: Lung volume reduction surgery versus rehabilitation. *Eur. Respir. J.* **2003**, *22*, 47s–56s. [CrossRef] [PubMed]
36. Souza, R.M.; Cardim, A.B.; Maia, T.O.; Rocha, L.G.; Bezerra, S.D.; Marinho, P.M. Inspiratory muscle strength, diaphragmatic mobility, and body composition in chronic obstructive pulmonary disease. *Physiother. Res. Int.* **2019**, *24*, e1766. [CrossRef] [PubMed]
37. Windisch, W.; Hennings, E.; Sorichter, S.; Hamm, H.; Criée, C. Peak or plateau maximal inspiratory mouth pressure: Which is best? *Eur. Respir. J.* **2004**, *23*, 708–713. [CrossRef] [PubMed]

Disclaimer/Publisher's Note: The statements, opinions and data contained in all publications are solely those of the individual author(s) and contributor(s) and not of MDPI and/or the editor(s). MDPI and/or the editor(s) disclaim responsibility for any injury to people or property resulting from any ideas, methods, instructions or products referred to in the content.

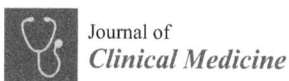

Article

The Association between Dysnatraemia during Hospitalisation and Post-COVID-19 Mental Fatigue

Gerardo Salvato [1,2,3,*], Elvira Inglese [1,4], Teresa Fazia [1], Francesco Crottini [1], Daniele Crotti [1], Federica Valentini [2], Giulio Palmas [2], Alessandra Bollani [2], Stefania Basilico [2,3], Martina Gandola [1,2,3], Giorgio Gelosa [3,5], Davide Gentilini [1,6], Luisa Bernardinelli [1], Andrea Stracciari [7], Francesco Scaglione [4,8], Elio Clemente Agostoni [3,5] and Gabriella Bottini [1,2,3,*]

1 Department of Brain and Behavioral Sciences, University of Pavia, 27100 Pavia, Italy
2 Cognitive Neuropsychology Centre, ASST "Grande Ospedale Metropolitano" Niguarda, 20162 Milan, Italy
3 NeuroMI, Milan Centre for Neuroscience, 20126 Milan, Italy
4 Department of Laboratory Medicine, ASST "Grande Ospedale Metropolitano" Niguarda, 20162 Milan, Italy
5 Neurology Department, ASST "Grande Ospedale Metropolitano" Niguarda, 20162 Milan, Italy
6 Bioinformatics and Statistical Genomic Unit, Istituto Auxologico Italiano IRCCS, 20095 Milan, Italy
7 Department of Psychology, University of Bologna, 40126 Bologna, Italy
8 Department of Oncology and Hemato-Oncology, University of Milan, 20122 Milan, Italy
* Correspondence: gerardo.salvato@unipv.it (G.S.); g.bottini@unipv.it (G.B.)

Abstract: COVID-19 may induce short- and long-term cognitive failures after recovery, but the underlying risk factors are still controversial. Here, we investigated whether (i) the odds of experiencing persistent cognitive failures differ based on the patients' disease course severity and sex at birth; and (ii) the patients' electrolytic profile in the acute stage represents a risk factor for persistent cognitive failures. We analysed data from 204 patients suffering from COVID-19 and hospitalised during the first pandemic wave. According to the 7-point WHO-OS scale, their disease course was classified as severe or mild. We investigated the presence of persistent cognitive failures collected after hospital discharge, while electrolyte profiles were collected during hospitalisation. The results showed that females who suffered from a mild course compared to a severe course of COVID-19 had a higher risk of presenting with persistent mental fatigue after recovery. Furthermore, in females who suffered from a mild course of COVID-19, persistent mental fatigue was related to electrolyte imbalance, in terms of both hypo- and hypernatremia, during hospitalisation in the acute phase. These findings have important implications for the clinical management of hospitalised COVID-19 patients. Attention should be paid to potential electrolyte imbalances, mainly in females suffering from mild COVID-19.

Keywords: mental fatigue; long COVID-19; dysnatraemia; electrolyte imbalance

Citation: Salvato, G.; Inglese, E.; Fazia, T.; Crottini, F.; Crotti, D.; Valentini, F.; Palmas, G.; Bollani, A.; Basilico, S.; Gandola, M.; et al. The Association between Dysnatraemia during Hospitalisation and Post-COVID-19 Mental Fatigue. *J. Clin. Med.* **2023**, *12*, 3702. https://doi.org/10.3390/jcm12113702

Academic Editors: César Fernández De Las Peñas and Domingo Palacios-Ceña

Received: 18 April 2023
Revised: 19 May 2023
Accepted: 24 May 2023
Published: 26 May 2023

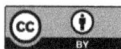

Copyright: © 2023 by the authors. Licensee MDPI, Basel, Switzerland. This article is an open access article distributed under the terms and conditions of the Creative Commons Attribution (CC BY) license (https://creativecommons.org/licenses/by/4.0/).

1. Introduction

Individuals who recovered from Coronavirus disease 2019 (COVID-19) may experience a plethora of persistent symptoms, i.e., 'long COVID' [1]. According to the UK National Institute for Health and Care Excellence (NICE) guidelines, the term long COVID describes signs and symptoms that continue or develop after acute COVID-19. It includes ongoing symptomatic COVID-19 (4 to 12 weeks) and post-COVID-19 syndrome (12 weeks or more). These manifestations may include fatigue, muscle weakness, shortness of breath or cough, as well as joint or chest pain [2], implicating multi-organ alterations following the viral infection. Long COVID also includes persistent cognitive difficulties [3–7], and the most frequently described involves attentional impairments [8]. A systematic review performed on 57 studies with 250,351 survivors of COVID-19 found difficulties in concentration (23.8% of the patient sample) [4]. These failures can be present in the form of (mental) fatigue, one of the most experienced persistent symptoms after hospitalisation [9]. Such persistent symptoms impair an individuals' ability to perform daily activities and affect quality of life [10,11].

Our understanding of the factors underpinning persistent cognitive failures after COVID-19 remains limited. Previous studies have suggested a correlation between persistent cognitive failures and disease severity [6,12,13]. Patients who benefited from invasive ventilation presented with a better cognitive status [13]; however, this topic is a current matter of debate. A growing body of research has also shown that sex at birth may play a role. Females are more likely to suffer from persistent symptoms after recovery, with a higher likelihood of reporting persistent fatigue [14–16]. This evidence sets the state for challenging scientific investigations, as long COVID mainly affects women [15], although vulnerability and mortality from acute COVID-19 infection are higher in men [17]. Studying the different clinical patterns between males and females during the infection could shed new light on this issue. In this perspective, sex at birth determines different pathological profiles in patients affected by COVID-19.

A recent systematic review has shown that electrolytic imbalance is prevalent in COVID-19 patients [18]. Interestingly, studies have also highlighted sex differences in electrolyte imbalances caused by SARS-CoV-2 in the acute phase [19]. Moreover, such electrolyte patterns have been associated with COVID-19 disease in hospitalised patients [20]. In patients with COVID-19, SARS-CoV-2 enters the cells using angiotensin-converting enzyme 2 (ACE2) as a receptor, which is one of the main effectors of the brain renin–angiotensin system (RAS). The virus replicates after entry into the cells, and ACE2 gets downregulated. As a result, there is reduced degradation of angiotensin-II, leading to increased aldosterone secretion and a subsequent electrolyte imbalance. This biochemical condition differs between males and females as sex hormones influence the expression and modulation of the brain RAS pathway responses.

Intriguingly, evidence from other pathologies has shown that dysnatraemia is associated with cognitive failures. For instance, hypernatremia (i.e., sodium levels higher than normal) is associated with cognitive deficits, especially in the elderly [21,22]. Moreover, hyponatremia (i.e., sodium levels lower than normal) may also be associated with adverse cognitive outcomes [23,24]. Specifically, whereas the consequences of acute hyponatremia may be severe, including permanent disability and death, mild and moderate hyponatremia may cause cognitive failures, such as attentional deficits [25,26]. These observations may suggest that the different incidences of persistent cognitive symptoms between males and females who suffered from COVID-19 may be associated with the sex differences in electrolyte imbalances in the acute phase.

Identifying patients at the highest risk is now a research priority to prevent persistent short- and long-term symptoms after recovery. Starting with this clinical and scientific need, the current study aims at exploring whether (i) the probability of experiencing persistent cognitive failures differs on the bases of the disease course severity and the patients' sex at birth; and (ii) the patients' electrolytic profile in the acute stage represents a risk factor for persistent cognitive failures. Based on previous findings showing that disease severity plays a role [13], we expected that the odds of presenting cognitive failures would be higher in patients who did not need ventilation therapy in the acute phase (mild COVID-19). Furthermore, as long COVID symptoms are more likely to occur in females [15], we expected that patients' sex at birth might interact with the disease severity regarding the odds of persistent cognitive difficulties. Lastly, as electrolyte imbalances are one of the recurrent features of COVID-19, which differs between males and females [19], we hypothesised that the odds of cognitive failures could be associated with the electrolyte profile during hospitalisation, particularly in female patients.

2. Materials and Methods

2.1. Patients

Inclusion criteria: We collected data from 275 consecutive patients suffering from COVID-19 admitted to the ASST Grande Ospedale Metropolitano Niguarda in Milan during the first pandemic wave in Italy from February to April 2020 (T0). The diagnosis was based on at least one positive test result with the reverse transcriptase–polymerase chain reaction (PCR) for SARS-CoV-2. After two consecutive negative oropharyngeal swabs (i.e., recovery), patients were discharged and followed up via the outpatient service of the same hospital from May to July 2020 (T1).

Exclusion criteria: As this study focuses on subjective cognitive failures, patients with previous neurological and psychiatric disorders were excluded (n = 41). In addition, patients diagnosed with chronic obstructive pulmonary disease (COPD) and obstructive sleep apnoea syndrome (OSAS) were excluded to ensure that any cognitive outcomes were unrelated to previous chronic respiratory illness (n = 9). Furthermore, those patients who did not complete the questionnaire on cognitive failures (n = 21) were not included, and the final sample comprised 204 patients (see Figure 1).

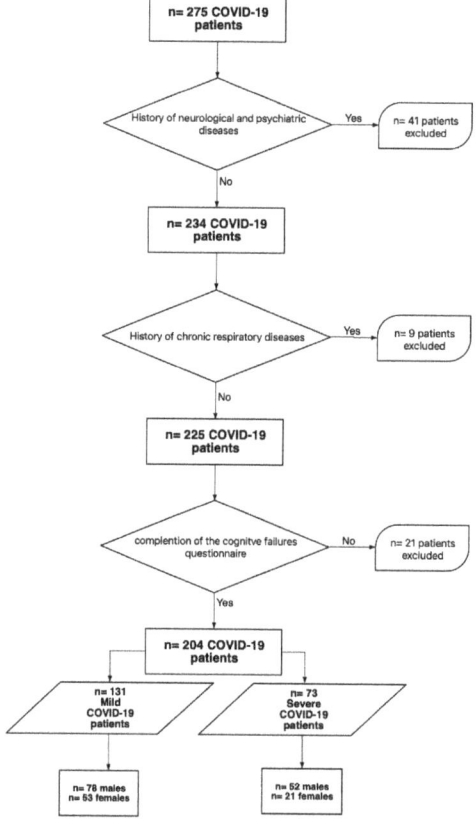

Figure 1. Representation of the patient enrolment workflow of the study.

Based on their medical records, patients were classified into two groups according to whether they received orotracheal intubation or CPAP ventilation (ventilated patients), or oxygen therapy or no oxygen therapy at all (non-ventilated patients), thus creating the covariate severity of the COVID-19 course. According to the 7-point WHO-OS scale, the course of COVID-19 in ventilated patients was classified as severe (severe COVID-19), while in non-ventilated patients, it was classified as mild (mild COVID-19). The Ethical Committee Comitato Etico Area 3 Milano approved the study (N92-15032020 and N408-21072020). The study was conducted following the Declaration of Helsinki. Informed consent was obtained from the patients.

2.2. Clinical Questionnaire on Cognitive Failures

To explore cognitive failures during the health emergency in April 2020, we decided to adopt a clinical tool that could be at the same time effective and quick to administer. Thus, we used a modified version of the Cognitive Failures Questionnaire [27]. We adjusted some of the original questions (such as those involving social interaction) to adapt them to the quarantine situation the patients might have experienced once discharged from the hospital. The questionnaire consisted of 19 statements about possible cognitive failures experienced in everyday life involving several domains, such as attention, memory, gnosis, praxis, orientation in time and space and executive functions (see Table 1 for the complete statements list). Similar questionnaires have also been recently used to test cognitive failures during quarantine/self-isolation for COVID-19 [28]. In our study, patients were asked to indicate the presence or absence of cognitive failures with a "yes/no" response. They could report more than one symptom. At the follow-up visit, the patients came to the Chronicity Service of the ASST "Grande Ospedale Metropolitano" Niguarda, where they underwent a series of assessments throughout the morning. The dedicated healthcare staff administered the Cognitive Failures Questionnaire to all subjects, among other evaluations.

Table 1. Cognitive Failures Questionnaire. The table shows the complete list of statements included in the questionnaire. For each statement, patients provided a yes/no response.

	Self-Administered Cognitive Failures Questionnaire
1	Do you find it difficult to remember things that have recently been said or have recently happened?
2	Are you frequently repetitive, that is, do you often say things more than once because you do not remember saying them the first time?
3	Do you often lose things (e.g., glasses) or fail to remember where you put them?
4	Do you have trouble remembering the names of well-known or familiar people?
5	Do you not remember current social events, such as news heard on television or read in the newspaper?
6	Do you confuse one place with another, for example, are you convinced that you are at home even when you are not?
7	Do you get confused about the date, for example, do you make mistakes with the month or year?
8	Do you struggle to find words?
9	Do you frequently say one word instead of another?
10	Do you sometimes say inconsistent things that make it difficult for others to understand what you are expressing?
11	Do you sometimes feel like you do not understand what is being said?
12	Do you have difficulty recognising commonly used objects?
13	Do you have difficultly using familiar objects, for example, household appliances?
14	Do you use objects incorrectly, for example, using a fork to eat soup?
15	Do you often lose the thread of what someone is saying or struggle to follow a conversation?
16	Are you easily distracted by noise or any external stimuli?
17	Do you have difficulty doing two things at the same time, for example, talking while making coffee?
18	Do you get mentally tired easily?
19	When faced with a problem, do you persist with the same behaviour, even if it has proved ineffective several times?

2.3. Laboratory Test and Data Sources

We retrospectively extracted the electrolytic profile for each patient from a panel of routine clinical laboratory test results. The tested chemical analytes included chloride (Cl^-), potassium (K^+) and sodium (Na^+). All samples were analysed in duplicate, within one hour from blood collection, using the same analyser and the same lot of reagents. Electrolyte parameters were measured by a Roche Cobas 8000 system (ISE modules). Blood samples were processed in a centrifuge at 3000 rpm (revolutions per minute). The number of samples per patient varied according to clinical practice. Each patient was monitored at least once a day, and a pathological value was confirmed by at least two measurements per protocol. To obtain laboratory variables, a query was created to extract anonymised data using the patients' ID (a numeric string) from a SQL-based repository in which all analytical results of the tests performed in the laboratory were stored. The fields extracted were sex, date of birth, day of lab tests execution, test IDs, test results and hospital ward.

2.4. Statistical Analysis Plan

Firstly, we compared the demographic variables reported in Table 1 between the patient groups. We performed a chi-square analysis for categorical variables and the t-test or Wilcoxon for continuous ones. Then, a reliability analysis was carried out on the items included in the Cognitive Failures Questionnaire. As the questionnaire involves dichotomously scored items, we used the Kuder–Richardson formula (KR-20), which is a widely used method to evaluate internal consistency in cognitive and personality tests. To explore whether the COVID-19 course severity impacted the odds of experiencing cognitive failure after recovery differently depending on the patient's sex, a logistic regression model for each item of the questionnaire has been fitted. In each model, disease severity, sex and the interaction between sex and disease severity group were specified as independent variables. We also decided to include the follow-up visit time in the model as it ranged from 3 to 104 days (mean 49.9 ($\pm$16.7) days after recovery). Each item representing a distinct cognitive failure was specified as a dependent variable. If the interaction between the course of disease severity and sex was statistically significant, meaning that the effect of COVID-19 course severity on the investigated endpoint was statistically significantly different in the two sexes, we fitted the logistic regression model as above, stratifying by sex to estimate the effect of COVID-19 course severity in each stratum of the sex variable. If the interaction was not statistically significant, a model was fitted such as that described above but with solely the main effects of disease severity group, sex and follow-up visit.

Lastly, we tested the hypothesis that the odds of presenting specific persistent cognitive failures after recovery could be associated with the electrolyte imbalance observed during hospitalisation. Thus, we fitted logistic regression models considering only the questionnaire items significantly different according to the patient's sex and disease severity. All the laboratory variables were transformed from continuous into binary variables according to their specific cut-off value: if a variable value was out of the normal range, it was labelled "1"; otherwise, the value was labelled "0". Based on the literature indicating, for example, that sodium alterations, defined as hyponatremia and hypernatremia, both lead to a poor clinical outcome in patients with COVID-19 [18] and based on the fact that several patients in our study presented with both hypo- and hyper-alteration (see Supplementary Table S2), we decided to generate three single indices (for Na^+, K^+ and Cl^-) that encapsulated electrolyte alteration in both directions. Thus, for each electrolyte, a score equal to 1 means that the variable values are higher or lower than the normal range. For instance, in the case of Na^+, a score equal to 1 means that patients presented with dysnatraemia (hyponatremia, hypernatremia or both). A normal range for sodium levels in the blood is 135–145 milliequivalents per litre (mEq/L). Levels below 135 mEq/L were considered indicative of hyponatremia, while levels above 145 mEq/L were considered indicative of hypernatremia. For potassium, the normal range is 3.5–5.0 millimoles per liter (mmol/L). Thus, levels below 3.5 mmol/L were considered indicative of hypokalaemia, while levels above 5.5 mmol/L were considered indicative of hyperkalaemia. The normal range of chloride is 98–106 milliequivalents per litre (mEq/L). Thus, levels below 98 mEq/L indicated hypochloraemia, while levels above 106 mEq/L indicated hyperchloremia. Statistical analyses were performed using Jamovi software (version 1.2).

3. Results

The final sample comprised 204 patients with a mean age of 57.1 years (± 11.9), 130 (63%) of whom were males. The patient's sex was defined as sex at birth. Our sample demographics align with those of the Italian National Institute of Health, which reported that participants who tested positive during this period were, on average, 58 years old. Patients were assessed at an average of 49.9 (± 16.7) days after recovery (follow-up time). Following the classification according to the 7-point WHO-OS scale, the sample included 73 patients who received orotracheal intubation or CPAP ventilation (severe COVID-19 patients), and 131 patients who received oxygen therapy or no oxygen therapy at all (mild COVID-19 patients). The clinical characteristics of the sample separated into the two groups of disease severity are reported in Table 2. The pharmacological treatment was in line with the initial recommendations spread during the first wave of the pandemic and was consistent among patients. For example, 92% of enrolled patients were treated with hydroxychloroquine.

Table 2. Demographics and clinical characteristics of the patient samples. The interactions between patient disease severity and sex for the demographic and clinical variables were not statistically significant.

	Mild COVID-19 (N = 131)		Severe COVID-19 (N = 73)		Interaction Disease Severity by Sex
	Males	Females	Males	Females	p-Value
N	78	53	52	21	0.096
Age, mean (SD)	58.3 (14.5)	57.8 (14.3)	55.0 (11.5)	62.4 (11.5)	0.069
Length of hospital stay, mean (SD)	15.5 (9.9)	15.01 (7.6)	22.1 (11.1)	24.7 (13.6)	0.373
Follow-up time, mean (SD)	53.6 (16.6)	49.6 (13.6)	46.8 (17.4)	45.1 (19.6)	0.664

3.1. Persistent Cognitive Failures: The Impact of the Disease Course Severity and Sex

Concerning the socio-demographic and clinical variables, we found no significant difference in terms of the interaction between disease course severity and sex for age ($F_{(1,198)} = 3.3$, $p = 0.069$), sex ($X^2_{(1)} = 2.8$, $p = 0.096$), follow-up time ($F_{(1,188)} = 0.2$, $p = 0.664$) and hospital length stay ($F_{(1,188)} = 0.8$, $p = 0.373$) (see Table 2). Concerning the questionnaire, the reliability analysis of the items showed good internal consistency (KR-20 = 0.851).

Results of the logistic regression analysis aimed at investigating whether the odds of cognitive failures may differ on the bases of the patient's disease severity and sex showed a statistically significant interaction between COVID-19 course severity and sex ($\beta = 0.32$, 95%CI [0.08; 0.55]), $p = 0.009$) for mental fatigue (item 18) only. For this item, we performed a subsequent analysis by stratifying by sex. Results of this latter analysis showed a statistically significant effect of group severity in females ($\beta = 0.29$, 95%CI [0.06; 0.53], $p = 0.01$), meaning that females who suffered from a mild course compared to a severe course of COVID-19 have a higher risk of presenting with persistent mental fatigue after recovery. No effect was observed in males ($\beta = -0.01$, 95%CI [-0.14; 0.11], $p = 0.82$) (see Table 3).

Table 3. Results of the sex-stratified logistic regression model of COVID-19 course severity and cognitive failures, adjusted for the follow-up time.

ITEM 18	Sex = Female			Sex = Male		
	β	95%CI	p-Value	β	95%CI	p-Value
Mild COVID-19	0.29	0.06; 0.53	0.01	−0.01	−0.14; 0.11	0.82
Follow-up time	0.004	−0.003; 0.01	0.27	0.003	−0.0007; 0.006	0.12

A logistic regression model, without interaction terms, was fitted for all the remaining items, in which no statistically significant interaction was observed. As reported in Supplementary Table S1, no statistically significant effect of COVID-19 group severity was observed for any investigated item.

3.2. Association between Persistent Mental Fatigue and the Electrolyte Profile during Hospitalisation

Due to missing data, we retrospectively analysed laboratory test results from 197 patients (out of 204). The sample was composed of n = 125 mild COVID-19 patients (age: $M = 58.08$ (± 14.5) years; sex: 73 males) and n = 72 severe COVID-19 patients (age: $M = 57.21$ (± 11.9) years; sex: 52 males). For an overview of the distribution of the electrolyte imbalance in our patients, see Supplementary Table S2. The results of the logistic regression models performed on item 18, resulting from the previous analysis, showed a statistically significant risk effect of Na^+ alteration ($β = 0.37$, 95%CI [0.09; 0.64], $p = 0.01$) on the odds of presenting with persistent mental fatigue after recovery in females who suffered from a mild course of COVID-19. No statistically significant effects were observed for the remaining electrolytes in females with a mild disease course: K^+ ($β = 0.01$, 95%CI [−0.26; 0.28], $p = 0.94$) and $Cl-$ ($β = -0.04$, 95%CI [−0.33; 0.25], $p = 0.77$).

4. Discussion

In Italy, during the first wave of the COVID-19 outbreak in 2020 (21 February–28 June), there was a total of 240,760 confirmed infections with 34,788 deaths. Depending on the disease severity, many symptoms may persist after recovery, mainly affecting women. Among these symptoms, cognitive failures may also be experienced. Little is known about the risk factors underpinning persistent symptoms after recovery. This study set out the challenge to explore whether cognitive failures after recovery depend upon the disease severity, the patient's sex, and the electrolytic indices during hospitalisation.

We confirm previous evidence by showing that cognitive failures may persist for approximately one month after recovery. Our findings indicated that the disease severity specifically impacted the attentional system by showing that persistent mental fatigue was higher in patients who suffered from a mild course of COVID-19 (i.e., non-ventilated patients). This result is in line with the study by Alemanno and colleagues [13], in which the authors found a better cognitive status in patients who had undergone invasive (orotracheal) ventilation compared to patients who had undergone non-invasive ventilation or no ventilation at all. The authors reported that 12 out of 22 survivors (54.5%) who underwent orotracheal ventilation one month after hospital discharge showed an impaired total score on the MoCA test, a well-known global cognitive screening test. The same applied to 10 out of the 12 survivors who were treated with non-invasive ventilation (83.3%), 17 out of the 20 survivors who needed oxygen therapy (85%), and 2 out of the 2 survivors who did not need oxygen-based treatment (100%). Furthermore, studies exploring cognitive outcomes in COVID-19 survivors reported mental fatigue as one of the most recurrent symptoms [29,30]. Here, we also showed that patient's sex plays a role in developing persistent cognitive failures. Indeed, females who recovered from a mild compared to severe course of COVID-19 were more likely to experience persistent mental fatigue. This result aligns with previous evidence highlighting the role of patient's sex in the presentation of persistent fatigue after recovery. A study on 377 patients has shown that 69% of the sample presented with long COVID. Female sex was independently associated with persistent symptoms, and fatigue was most commonly reported (39.5% of the sample) [16]. Furthermore, another study has shown that females under 50 years reported worse fatigue, with fatigue being more likely in women than in men of the same age [15].

It has been postulated that the aetiology of persistent cognitive failures could be derived from the dual action of the viral infection, which has both direct (immunological and neurological damage) and indirect (hypoxic/respiratory states) consequences [31]. Indeed, two primary routes explain cognition-related deficits in COVID-19 survivors: virus-induced CNS damage (neurotrophic) or non-CNS impairments [32]. Strikingly, we found that in females who suffered from a mild course of COVID-19, persistent mental fatigue was related to an electrolyte imbalance during hospitalisation. The general symptom of fatigue has been previously reported as a consequence of hyponatremia conditions in hospitalised patients [33]. In the case of COVID-19, a possible explanation for the correlation between electrolyte imbalance and mental fatigue in females could be represented by the different sex-dependent expressions of the brain renin–angiotensin system (RAS). In fact, the expression and modulation of the brain RAS pathway responses are influenced by sex hormones. Indeed, with estrogenic stimulation, the ACE2/Ang-(1–7)/MasR system and the ACE2/Ang-(1–8)/AT2 system is increased, while testosterone stimulation mediates the activation of the ACE/Ang-(1–8)/AT1R arm of the RAS. As SARS-CoV-2 enters the cells using ACE2 as a receptor, which is one of the main effectors of the brain RAS, sex differences in the electrolyte imbalance during COVID-19 could be present (see Figure 2).

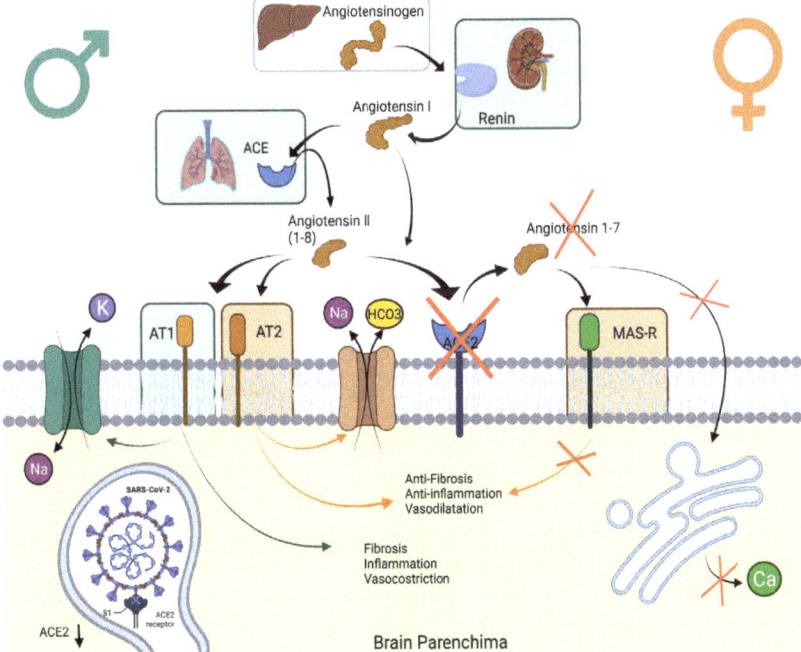

Figure 2. The sex differences in the RAS and response to SARS-CoV-2 injury. Several studies revealed that the AT1 receptor protein is down-regulated by oestrogen, while AT2 receptors are up-regulated. On the other hand, testosterone induced the expression of AT1. AT1 and AT2 receptors have antagonistic actions: Sodium cellular intake is mediated by the AT1 receptor through the increase in Na^+/K^+ ATPase activity, while the AT2 receptor activates phospholipase A2, which contributes to activation of the Na/HCO_3 symporter system (NBC), mediating sodium cell excretion.

5. Conclusions and Clinical Significance

In summary, this study provided new evidence on the aetiological nature of persistent mental fatigue in COVID-19 survivors who required hospitalisation. In particular, females who suffered from a mild course of COVID-19 had a higher frequency of reporting this symptom one month after hospital discharge. On the one hand, epidemiological studies reported a lower frequency of hospitalisation for females during the COVID-19 infection; on the other hand, electrolyte imbalance occurs more frequently in this population, possibly causing such a persistent cognitive failure. These results pave the way for specific electrolyte rebalancing treatment in hospitalised COVID-19 females who do not require ventilation to prevent cognitive failures after recovery. Therefore, adequate laboratory monitoring and subsequent review of appropriate intravenous water balance medications are important management aspects.

6. Limitations

The current study contains some limitations that future investigations may address. Firstly, the nature of the study is retrospective; thus, a prospective case–control study could better define the association between mental fatigue symptoms and the specific direction of sodium imbalance (hypo- or hypernatremia) in hospitalised COVID-19 patients. Moreover, the aetiologies of the changes in sodium concentration could be important contributors to cognitive failures after recovery. Given the association between sodium and fluid balance, sodium may act as a marker for fluid therapies administered during hospitalisation, and future studies may address these issues. Lastly, it would be interesting to correlate the duration of sodium imbalance with the cognitive symptom severity. One of the next challenges could also be to investigate potential factors modulating both the electrolyte and cognitive spheres so that additional confounding factors can be excluded to understand the long-term effects of COVID-19 better.

Supplementary Materials: The following supporting information can be downloaded at: https://www.mdpi.com/article/10.3390/jcm12113702/s1, Table S1: Results; Table S2: Electrolytics imbalance. Figure S1: Cognitive Failures.

Author Contributions: Conceptualisation, G.S., E.I., S.B. and G.B.; Data curation, E.I., T.F., F.C. and D.C.; Formal analysis, G.S., E.I., T.F., F.C., D.C., D.G. and L.B.; Investigation, G.S., E.I., F.C., D.C., F.V., G.P., A.B. and S.B.; Methodology, G.S., E.I. and G.B.; Project administration, G.B.; Supervision, G.B.; Visualisation, T.F.; Writing—original draft, G.S., E.I., F.C., D.C., G.P., A.B. and G.B.; Writing—review and editing, G.S., E.I., T.F., F.V., S.B., M.G., G.G., D.G., L.B., A.S., F.S., E.C.A. and G.B. All authors have read and agreed to the published version of the manuscript.

Funding: This research received no external funding.

Institutional Review Board Statement: The study was conducted according to the guidelines of the Declaration of Helsinki, and was approved by the Ethics Committee Comitato Etico Area 3 Milano (protocol code 92-15032020, date 15 March 2020; and protocol code 408-21072020, date 21 July 2020).

Informed Consent Statement: Informed consent was obtained from all subjects involved in the study.

Data Availability Statement: The data presented in this study are available upon request from the corresponding author.

Conflicts of Interest: The authors declare no conflict of interest.

References

1. Nalbandian, A.; Sehgal, K.; Gupta, A.; Madhavan, M.V.; McGroder, C.; Stevens, J.S.; Cook, J.R.; Nordvig, A.S.; Shalev, D.; Sehrawat, T.S.; et al. Post-acute COVID-19 syndrome. *Nat. Med.* **2021**, *27*, 601–615. Available online: http://www.nature.com/articles/s41591-021-01283-z (accessed on 15 September 2021). [CrossRef] [PubMed]
2. Goërtz, Y.M.; Van Herck, M.; Delbressine, J.M.; Vaes, A.W.; Meys, R.; Machado, F.V.; Houben-Wilke, S.; Burtin, C.; Posthuma, R.; Franssen, F.M.; et al. Persistent symptoms 3 months after a SARS-CoV-2 infection: The post-COVID-19 syndrome? *ERJ Open Res.* **2020**, *6*, 00542–02020. [CrossRef] [PubMed]

8. Manca, R.; De Marco, M.; Ince, P.G.; Venneri, A. Heterogeneity in Regional Damage Detected by Neuroimaging and Neuropathological Studies in Older Adults with COVID-19: A Cognitive-Neuroscience Systematic Review to Inform the Long-Term Impact of the Virus on Neurocognitive Trajectories. *Front. Aging Neurosci.* **2021**, *13*, 646908. [CrossRef] [PubMed]
9. Groff, D.; Sun, A.; Ssentongo, A.E.; Ba, D.M.; Parsons, N.; Poudel, G.R.; Lekoubou, A.; Oh, J.S.; Ericson, J.E.; Ssentongo, P.; et al. Short-term and Long-term Rates of Postacute Sequelae of SARS-CoV-2 Infection: A Systematic Review. *JAMA Netw. Open* **2021**, *4*, e2128568. [CrossRef] [PubMed]
10. On behalf of the "Cognitive and Behavioral Neurology" Study Group of the Italian Neurological Society; Stracciari, A.; Bottini, G.; Guarino, M.; Magni, E.; Pantoni, L. Cognitive and behavioral manifestations in SARS-CoV-2 infection: Not specific or distinctive features? *Neurol. Sci.* **2021**, *42*, 2273–2281. Available online: https://link.springer.com/10.1007/s10072-021-05231-0 (accessed on 15 September 2021). [CrossRef]
11. Almeria, M.; Cejudo, J.C.; Sotoca, J.; Deus, J.; Krupinski, J. Cognitive profile following COVID-19 infection: Clinical predictors leading to neuropsychological impairment. *Brain Behav. Immun.-Health* **2020**, *9*, 100163. Available online: https://linkinghub.elsevier.com/retrieve/pii/S2666354620301289 (accessed on 14 September 2021). [CrossRef]
12. Varatharaj, A.; Thomas, N.; Ellul, M.A.; Davies, N.W.; Pollak, T.A.; Tenorio, E.L.; Sultan, M.; Easton, A.; Breen, G.; Zandi, M.; et al. Neurological and neuropsychiatric complications of COVID-19 in 153 patients: A UK-wide surveillance study. *Lancet Psychiatry* **2020**, *7*, 875–882. Available online: https://linkinghub.elsevier.com/retrieve/pii/S221503662030287X (accessed on 15 September 2021). [CrossRef]
13. Molnar, T.; Varnai, R.; Schranz, D.; Zavori, L.; Peterfi, Z.; Sipos, D.; Tőkés-Füzesi, M.; Illes, Z.; Buki, A.; Csecsei, P. Severe Fatigue and Memory Impairment Are Associated with Lower Serum Level of Anti-SARS-CoV-2 Antibodies in Patients with Post-COVID Symptoms. *J. Clin. Med.* **2021**, *10*, 4337. Available online: https://www.mdpi.com/2077-0383/10/19/4337 (accessed on 15 May 2023). [CrossRef]
14. The Writing Committee for the COMEBAC Study Group; Morin, L.; Savale, L.; Pham, T.; Colle, R.; Figueiredo, S.; Harrois, A.; Gasnier, M.; Lecoq, A.-L.; Meyrignac, O.; et al. Four-Month Clinical Status of a Cohort of Patients After Hospitalization for COVID-19. *JAMA* **2021**, *325*, 1525. Available online: https://jamanetwork.com/journals/jama/fullarticle/2777787 (accessed on 14 April 2022). [CrossRef]
15. Jacobs, L.G.; Paleoudis, E.G.; Bari, D.L.-D.; Nyirenda, T.; Friedman, T.; Gupta, A.; Rasouli, L.; Zetkulic, M.; Balani, B.; Ogedegbe, C.; et al. Persistence of symptoms and quality of life at 35 days after hospitalisation for COVID-19 infection. *PLoS ONE* **2020**, *15*, e0243882. [CrossRef]
16. Poudel, A.N.; Zhu, S.; Cooper, N.; Roderick, P.; Alwan, N.; Tarrant, C.; Ziauddeen, N.; Yao, G.L. Impact of Covid-19 on health-related quality of life of patients: A structured review. *PLoS ONE* **2021**, *16*, e0259164. [CrossRef]
17. Hampshire, A.; Trender, W.; Chamberlain, S.R.; Jolly, A.E.; Grant, J.E.; Patrick, F.; Mazibuko, N.; Williams, S.C.; Barnby, J.M.; Hellyer, P.; et al. Cognitive deficits in people who have recovered from COVID-19. *EClinicalMedicine* **2021**, *39*, 101044. Available online: https://linkinghub.elsevier.com/retrieve/pii/S2589537021003242 (accessed on 14 April 2022). [CrossRef]
18. Alemanno, F.; Houdayer, E.; Parma, A.; Spina, A.; Del Forno, A.; Scatolini, A.; Angelone, S.; Brugliera, L.; Tettamanti, A.; Beretta, L.; et al. COVID-19 cognitive deficits after respiratory assistance in the subacute phase: A COVID-rehabilitation unit experience. *PLoS ONE* **2021**, *16*, e0246590. [CrossRef]
19. Romero-Duarte, Á.; Rivera-Izquierdo, M.; de Alba, I.G.-F.; Pérez-Contreras, M.; Fernández-Martínez, N.F.; Ruiz-Montero, R.; Serrano-Ortiz, Á.; González-Serna, R.O.; Salcedo-Leal, I.; Jiménez-Mejías, E.; et al. Sequelae, persistent symptomatology and outcomes after COVID-19 hospitalisation: The ANCOHVID multicentre 6-month follow-up study. *BMC Med.* **2021**, *19*, 129. [CrossRef]
20. Sigfrid, L.; Drake, T.M.; Pauley, E.; Jesudason, E.C.; Olliaro, P.; Lim, W.S.; Gillesen, A.; Berry, C.; Lowe, D.J.; McPeake, J.; et al. Long Covid in adults discharged from UK hospitals after Covid-19: A prospective, multicentre cohort study using the ISARIC WHO Clinical Characterisation Protocol. *Lancet Reg. Health-Eur.* **2021**, *8*, 100186. Available online: https://linkinghub.elsevier.com/retrieve/pii/S2666776221001630 (accessed on 14 April 2022). [CrossRef]
21. Bai, F.; Tomasoni, D.; Falcinella, C.; Barbanotti, D.; Castoldi, R.; Mulè, G.; Augello, M.; Mondatore, D.; Allegrini, M.; Cona, A.; et al. Female gender is associated with long COVID syndrome: A prospective cohort study. *Clin. Microbiol. Infect.* **2022**, *28*, e9–e611. Available online: https://linkinghub.elsevier.com/retrieve/pii/S1198743X21006297 (accessed on 14 April 2022). [CrossRef]
22. Docherty, A.B.; Harrison, E.M.; Green, C.A.; Hardwick, H.E.; Pius, R.; Norman, L.; Holden, K.A.; Read, J.M.; Dondelinger, F.; Carson, G.; et al. Features of 20133 UK patients in hospital with COVID-19 using the ISARIC WHO Clinical Characterisation Protocol: Prospective observational cohort study. *BMJ* **2020**, *369*, m1985. Available online: https://www.bmj.com/lookup/doi/10.1136/bmj.m1985 (accessed on 14 April 2022). [CrossRef]
23. Song, H.J.J.M.D.; Chia, A.Z.Q.; Tan, B.K.J.; Teo, C.B.; Lim, V.; Chua, H.R.; Samuel, M.; Kee, A. Electrolyte imbalances as poor prognostic markers in COVID-19: A systemic review and meta-analysis. *J. Endocrinol. Investig.* **2022**, *46*, 235–259. Available online: https://link.springer.com/10.1007/s40618-022-01877-5 (accessed on 3 March 2023). [CrossRef]
24. Pani, A.; Inglese, E.; Puoti, M.; Cento, V.; Alteri, C.; Romandini, A.; Di Ruscio, F.; Senatore, M.; Moreno, M.; Tarsia, P.; et al. Sex differences in electrolyte imbalances caused by SARS-CoV-2: A cross-sectional study. *Int. J. Clin. Pract.* **2021**, *75*, e14882. [CrossRef]

20. Zimmer, M.A.; Zink, A.K.; Weißer, C.W.; Vogt, U.; Michelsen, A.; Priebe, H.-J.; Mols, G. Hypernatremia—A Manifestation of COVID-19: A Case Series. *AA Pract.* **2020**, *14*, e01295. Available online: https://journals.lww.com/10.1213/XAA.0000000000001295 (accessed on 2 May 2022). [CrossRef]
21. Adrogué, H.J.; Madias, N.E. Hypernatremia. *N. Engl. J. Med.* **2000**, *342*, 1493–1499. [CrossRef] [PubMed]
22. Tsipotis, E.; Price, L.L.; Jaber, B.L.; Madias, N.E. Hospital-Associated Hypernatremia Spectrum and Clinical Outcomes in an Unselected Cohort. *Am. J. Med.* **2018**, *131*, 72–82.e1. Available online: https://linkinghub.elsevier.com/retrieve/pii/S0002934317308410 (accessed on 2 May 2022). [CrossRef] [PubMed]
23. Nowak, K.L.; Yaffe, K.; Orwoll, E.S.; Ix, J.H.; You, Z.; Barrett-Connor, E.; Hoffman, A.R.; Chonchol, M. Serum Sodium and Cognition in Older Community-Dwelling Men. *Clin. J. Am. Soc. Nephrol.* **2018**, *13*, 366–374. Available online: https://cjasn.asnjournals.org/lookup/doi/10.2215/CJN.07400717 (accessed on 6 April 2022). [CrossRef] [PubMed]
24. Lee, S.; Min, J.-Y.; Kim, B.; Ha, S.-W.; Han, J.H.; Min, K.-B. Serum sodium in relation to various domains of cognitive function in the elderly US population. *BMC Geriatr.* **2021**, *21*, 328. Available online: https://bmcgeriatr.biomedcentral.com/articles/10.1186/s12877-021-02260-4 (accessed on 6 April 2022). [CrossRef]
25. Giuliani, C.; Peri, A. Effects of Hyponatremia on the Brain. *J. Clin. Med.* **2014**, *3*, 1163–1177. Available online: http://www.mdpi.com/2077-0383/3/4/1163 (accessed on 6 April 2022). [CrossRef]
26. Soiza, R.L.; Cumming, K.; Clarke, J.M.; Wood, K.M.; Myint, P.K. Hyponatremia: Special Considerations in Older Patients. *J. Clin. Med.* **2014**, *3*, 944–958. Available online: http://www.mdpi.com/2077-0383/3/3/944 (accessed on 6 April 2022). [CrossRef]
27. Broadbent, D.E.; Cooper, P.F.; FitzGerald, P.; Parkes, K.R. The Cognitive Failures Questionnaire (CFQ) and its correlates. *Br. J. Clin. Psychol.* **1982**, *21*, 1–16. Available online: https://onlinelibrary.wiley.com/doi/10.1111/j.2044-8260.1982.tb01421.x (accessed on 6 April 2022). [CrossRef]
28. Santangelo, G.; Baldassarre, I.; Barbaro, A.; Cavallo, N.D.; Cropano, M.; Maggi, G.; Nappo, R.; Trojano, L.; Raimo, S. Subjective cognitive failures and their psychological correlates in a large Italian sample during quarantine/self-isolation for COVID-19. *Neurol. Sci. Off. J. Ital. Neurol. Soc. Ital. Soc. Clin. Neurophysiol.* **2021**, *42*, 2625–2635. [CrossRef]
29. Fang, X.; Ming, C.; Cen, Y.; Lin, H.; Zhan, K.; Yang, S.; Li, L.; Cao, G.; Li, Q.; Ma, X. Post-sequelae one year after hospital discharge among older COVID-19 patients: A multi-center prospective cohort study. *J. Infect.* **2022**, *84*, 179–186. Available online: https://linkinghub.elsevier.com/retrieve/pii/S016344532100596X (accessed on 14 April 2022). [CrossRef]
30. Iqbal, F.M.; Lam, K.; Sounderajah, V.; Clarke, J.M.; Ashrafian, H.; Darzi, A. Characteristics and predictors of acute and chronic post-COVID syndrome: A systematic review and meta-analysis. *EClinicalMedicine* **2021**, *36*, 100899. Available online: https://linkinghub.elsevier.com/retrieve/pii/S2589537021001796 (accessed on 14 April 2022). [CrossRef]
31. Oliviero, A.; de Castro, F.; Coperchini, F.; Chiovato, L.; Rotondi, M. COVID-19 Pulmonary and Olfactory Dysfunctions: Is the Chemokine CXCL10 the Common Denominator? *Neuroscientist* **2021**, *27*, 214–221. Available online: http://journals.sagepub.com/doi/10.1177/1073858420939033 (accessed on 15 September 2021). [CrossRef]
32. Ritchie, K.; Chan, D.; Watermeyer, T. The cognitive consequences of the COVID-19 epidemic: Collateral damage? *Brain Commun.* **2020**, *2*, fcaa069. Available online: https://academic.oup.com/braincomms/article/doi/10.1093/braincomms/fcaa069/5848404 (accessed on 15 September 2021). [CrossRef]
33. Olsson, K.; Öhlin, B.; Melander, O. Epidemiology and characteristics of hyponatremia in the emergency department. *Eur. J. Intern. Med.* **2013**, *24*, 110–116. Available online: https://linkinghub.elsevier.com/retrieve/pii/S0953620512002877 (accessed on 15 April 2022). [CrossRef]

Disclaimer/Publisher's Note: The statements, opinions and data contained in all publications are solely those of the individual author(s) and contributor(s) and not of MDPI and/or the editor(s). MDPI and/or the editor(s) disclaim responsibility for any injury to people or property resulting from any ideas, methods, instructions or products referred to in the content.

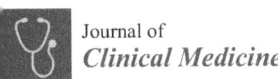

Article

Physical Health-Related Quality of Life Improves over Time in Post-COVID-19 Patients: An Exploratory Prospective Study

Stefan Malesevic [1,2], Noriane A. Sievi [2], Dörthe Schmidt [3], Florence Vallelian [4], Ilijas Jelcic [5], Malcolm Kohler [2] and Christian F. Clarenbach [2,*]

1. Faculty of Medicine, University of Zurich, 8006 Zurich, Switzerland; stefan.malesevic@usz.ch
2. Department of Pulmonology, University Hospital Zurich, 8091 Zurich, Switzerland
3. Department of Cardiology, University Hospital Zurich, 8091 Zurich, Switzerland
4. Department of Internal Medicine, University Hospital Zurich, 8091 Zurich, Switzerland
5. Department of Neurology, University Hospital Zurich, 8091 Zurich, Switzerland
* Correspondence: christian.clarenbach@usz.ch

Abstract: (1) Background: Ongoing symptoms after mild or moderate acute coronavirus disease 19 (COVID-19) substantially affect health-related quality of life (HRQoL). However, follow-up data on HRQoL are scarce. We characterized the change in HRQoL over time in post-COVID-19 patients who initially suffered from mild or moderate acute COVID-19 without hospitalization. (2) Methods: Outpatients who visited an interdisciplinary post-COVID-19 consultation at the University Hospital Zurich and suffered from ongoing symptoms after acute COVID-19 were included in this observational study. HRQoL was assessed using established questionnaires. Six months after baseline, the same questionnaires and a self-constructed questionnaire about the COVID-19 vaccination were distributed. (3) Results: In total, 69 patients completed the follow-up, of whom 55 (80%) were female. The mean (SD) age was 44 (12) years and the median (IQR) time from symptom onset to completing the follow-up was 326 (300, 391) days. The majority of patients significantly improved in EQ-5D-5L health dimensions of mobility, usual activities, pain and anxiety. Furthermore, according to the SF-36, patients showed clinically relevant improvements in physical health, whereas no significant change was found regarding mental health. (4) Conclusions: Physical aspects of HRQoL in post-COVID-19 patients relevantly improved over 6 months. Future studies are needed to focus on potential predictors that allow for establishing individual care and early interventions.

Keywords: post-COVID-19; health-related quality of life; physical health; mental health; follow-up

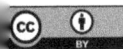

1. Introduction

Long-term health consequences after acute COVID-19 are increasingly recognized and lead to a high individual burden. Multiple organ systems may be affected and lead to variable clinical presentations, including neurocognitive, pulmonary and cardiac symptoms. When symptoms after acute COVID-19 exceed 12 weeks, the National Institute for Health and Care Excellence (NICE) defines the symptom complex as "Post-COVID-19 syndrome" [1]. The most common symptoms reported by patients are fatigue, dyspnea, myalgia and chest pain [2]. However, the puzzle behind the pathophysiological mechanisms remains unsolved. Persistent inflammation, induced autoimmunity and viral persistence in the body are discussed as potential drivers [3]. Interestingly, even patients who suffered from a mild or moderate acute disease can develop long-lasting symptoms [4,5].

It is known that infectious diseases, especially viral diseases, such as Epstein–Barr virus (EBV) [6], severe acute respiratory syndrome (SARS) in 2003 [7], and the West Nile virus [8], can give rise to long-lasting symptoms. Recovery times vary between individuals and diseases. For example, approximately 10% of individuals have persistent fatigue six months after symptom onset of infectious mononucleosis [9], whereas up to 30% of people with West Nile virus infection have postviral fatigue with an average duration of 5 years [8].

Irrespective of the cause, fatigue is an important factor for quality of life and patients with diagnosed chronic fatigue syndrome showed remarkably lower scores in physical and mental dimensions of HRQoL [10].

Recently, our research group showed that physical- and mental-health-related quality of life (HRQoL) is substantially impaired in patients suffering from post-COVID-19 syndrome after a mild or moderate disease compared with the pre-pandemic general Swiss population [11]. A literature screening review found that at a follow-up at 12 weeks, the median estimate of non-hospitalized patients with ongoing symptoms is approximately 12% (7.5–41%) [12]. The disabilities due to symptoms might come with great economical loss considering the vast amount of affected people and all the potential excessive work absences due to the illness.

Currently, researchers and clinicians lack knowledge about the course of post-COVID-19 symptoms and treatment options are scarce. Our clinical experience suggests that ongoing symptoms might subside over time. Tran et al. demonstrated that the prevalence of most post-COVID-19 symptoms decreases over time before plateauing 6–8 months after onset [13]. However, the evolution of the impact of post-COVID-19 symptoms on HRQoL after mild or moderate acute disease over time has not been thoroughly investigated. Therefore, we followed up on patients and aimed to characterize changes in HRQoL 6 months after an initial assessment.

2. Materials and Methods

2.1. Study Design and Patient Population

The departments of Pulmonology, Cardiology, Neurology and Internal Medicine at the University Hospital Zurich developed an interdisciplinary outpatient clinic for patients suffering from persistent symptoms after developing COVID-19. Questionnaires regarding HRQoL (St. George's Respiratory Questionnaire (SGRQ), EuroQol 5 Dimension 5 Level (EQ-5D-5L) and Short Form-36 (SF-36)) were distributed to the patients during their visit to the outpatient clinic (baseline). For patients who completed the questionnaires at baseline, the same questionnaires were sent by letter to them after six months for a follow-up assessment. Additionally, patients received a questionnaire regarding COVID-19 vaccination at follow-up.

Inclusion criteria were properly completed questionnaires and patients who suffered from ongoing symptoms after developing confirmed or highly suspected acute mild or moderate COVID-19 without hospitalization. Mild illness was defined as any of the various symptoms of COVID-19 (e.g., fever, cough, sore throat, malaise, headache, muscle pain, nausea, vomiting, diarrhea, and loss of taste and smell) but without shortness of breath, dyspnea or abnormal chest imaging. Moderate illness was defined by clinical or radiological evidence of lower respiratory tract involvement but normal oxygen saturation ($SpO_2 \geq 94\%$) with room air. Exclusion criteria were initial severe acute COVID-19 requiring prolonged hospitalization or intensive care treatment and patients with symptoms that were assigned to another diagnosis (e.g., asthma).

Information about demographics, symptoms during acute infection and post-COVID-19 symptoms were drawn from systematically documented medical reports. Pre-existing asthma; pre-pandemic mental health issues; and cardiovascular, rheumatological and thyroid diseases were assessed as comorbidities.

This study was conducted in accordance with the declaration of Helsinki and all subjects provided written informed consent via general consent. The Ethics Committee of the Canton of Zurich approved the study (BASEC 2021-00280), and the study is registered on www.ClinicalTrials.gov as NCT04793269 (accessed on 2 May 2023).

2.2. Questionnaires

All patients received three different questionnaires regarding HRQoL, as well as one self-constructed questionnaire about the COVID-19 vaccination (see Supplementary Materials).

2.2.1. St. George's Respiratory Questionnaire

The St. George's Respiratory Questionnaire (SGRQ) is a validated quality of life assessment tool used to evaluate the impact of respiratory symptoms on everyday life [14,15]. The symptom frequency and severity of respiratory symptoms are measured, and limitations in activity, as well as the social and emotional impacts, due to the disease are covered. Each item is weighted according to the degree of distress. Scores range from 0 to 100, with higher scores indicating worse quality of life. Missing items were handled according to the SGRQ manual [16]. An improvement of 4 points is accepted as the minimal clinically important difference (MCID) in the literature [17].

2.2.2. EuroQol 5 Dimension 5 Level

The EuroQol 5 Dimension 5 Level (EQ-5D-5L) is widely used as a generic measure of health status [18]. The first part (the descriptive system) comprises five dimensions, namely, mobility, self-care, usual activities, pain/discomfort and anxiety/depression. For every dimension, patients are asked to assign a level of severity, ranging from 1 "no problems" to 5 "extreme problems". Patients' responses are then combined to produce a five-digit number describing the participant's health status. Each health state can potentially be assigned a summary index score based on societal preference weights for the health state. Index scores range from less than 0 (dead) to 1 (full health). Index scores were calculated using Germany-specific value sets as we judged the population of Germany to be comparable to the Swiss German population. In the second part of the questionnaire, the self-rated health of patients was recorded using a visual analog scale (VAS) ranging from 0 (worst health) to 100 (best health). The minimally important difference for the EQ index value ranges between 0.03 and 0.069 points [19,20]. For EQ, VAS scores with a difference of 5.0 are suggested to show MCID in fibrotic interstitial lung disease [21].

2.2.3. Short Form-36

The Short Form Health 36 (SF-36) is a multidimensional instrument for measuring HRQoL [22]. It includes eight health dimensions that evaluate physical problems, role limitations due to physical problems, pain, general health, vitality, social functioning, role limitations due to emotional problems and mental health. The health dimensions consist of the summed scores of the assigned questions. Scores range from 0 (worst possible health) to 100 (best possible health). All health dimensions contribute in different proportions to create two summary score components: the physical component summary (PCS) and the mental component summary (MCS). Out of the health dimension scores, a z-score is determined for each dimension by subtracting the dimension mean of the U.S. population from an individual's dimension score and dividing it by the standard deviation from the U.S. general population [23]. Each of the eight z-scores is multiplied by the corresponding factor scoring coefficient (separately for PCS and MCS) for the dimension [24]. Products of the z-scores are summed together, multiplied by 10, and added to 50 to linearly transform the PCS and MCS to T-score metrics. A value of 50 for the norm-based score represents the mean of the respective reference population and higher values mean better HRQoL. For the PCS and MCS T-scores, a 3-point change is suggested for an MCID [25]. Bjorner et al. recommended an MCID of 5 points for the health dimension vitality [26].

2.2.4. Questionnaire about COVID-19 Vaccination

This self-created questionnaire was used to assess the subjective effect of the vaccination on post-COVID-19 symptoms. Besides questions assessing the type, date and adverse events of the vaccine, patients were asked to rate whether the vaccine led to an improvement or worsening of post-COVID-19 symptoms and whether the change in symptom severity was persistent. Moreover, the overall improvement or worsening of symptoms could be displayed using a visual analog scale from 0 (no improvement) to 10 (best possible improvement/no more symptoms).

2.3. Statistical Analysis

Descriptive statistics of baseline patient characteristics are presented as the mean and standard deviation (SD) or median and 25%/75% quartiles (quartiles) for continuous measurements and as the number and percentage of total for categorical measurements. Changes in HRQoL were compared using a paired t-test and Wilcoxon signed rank test for continuous variables. Multivariable regression analysis was performed to test for possible predictors (i.e., sex and subjective effect of vaccination). Missing data were not replaced. All statistical tests were two-tailed and a p-value of <0.05 was considered statistically significant. Statistical analysis was performed using Stata version 16.1 (StataCorp. 2019, College Station, TX, USA). No a priori sample size calculation was performed due to the exploratory study design.

3. Results

3.1. Study Sample

In this observational follow-up study, 112 patients with post-COVID-19 syndrome completed questionnaires at baseline, of whom 69 also completed follow-up questionnaires (38.4% lost to follow-up) (Figure 1). Patients at follow-up did not differ significantly with regard to physical HRQoL in the SF-36 from patients who were not followed up on (PCS mean (95% CI) difference of 1.2 (−2.8, 5.3) points, $p = 0.551$). However, patients who did not complete the follow-up had significantly lower mental HRQoL in the SF-36 compared with patients who completed the follow-up (MCS mean (95% CI) difference of −4.9 (−9.4, −0.4) points, $p = 0.032$). Subjects were predominantly female (80.0%) with a mean (SD) age of 44 (11.9) years. The median (IQR) score for the body mass index was 24.2 (21.5, 26.7) kg/m^2. The median (IQR) time from symptom onset to completing the follow-up questionnaires was 326 (300, 391) days. Before the pandemic, nine (13.0%) patients suffered from asthma, 7 (10.1%) had mental health issues and 14 (20.3%) had at least one relevant comorbidity. The majority of patients (94.2%) suffered from a mild initial COVID-19. Approximately one-third of the patients stated to work less because of long-lasting COVID-19 symptoms. Further patient characteristics are outlined in Table 1.

Table 1. Patient characteristics.

	$n = 69$
Sex	
Female	55 (80.0)
Male	14 (20.0)
Age, mean (SD)	44.2 (11.9)
BMI kg/m^2, median (IQR)	24.2 (21.5, 26.7)
WHO classification	
Mild	65 (94.2)
Moderate	4 (5.8)
Days from first questionnaire to follow-up questionnaire, median (IQR)	182 (174, 192)
Days from symptom onset to follow-up questionnaire, median (IQR)	326 (300, 391)
Smoking history	
Current	6 (8.7)
Former	18 (26.1)
Never	38 (55.2)
Ethnicity	
Caucasian	58 (84)
Not Caucasian	2 (3)
Missing data	9 (13)

Table 1. Cont.

	n = 69
Marital status	
Living with a partner	38 (55.1)
Living alone	10 (14.5)
Missing data	21 (30.4)
Reduced employment due to post-COVID-19	22 (31.9)
Reduced ≥ 50%	10 (14.5)
Reduced < 50%	12 (17.4)
Comorbidities	
Asthma	9 (13.0)
Prepandemic mental health issues	7 (10.1)
Other relevant comorbidities [a]	14 (20.3)

Values are n (%) unless otherwise stated. [a] Other relevant comorbidities were relevant cardiovascular disorders, rheumatological diseases and diseases of the thyroid.

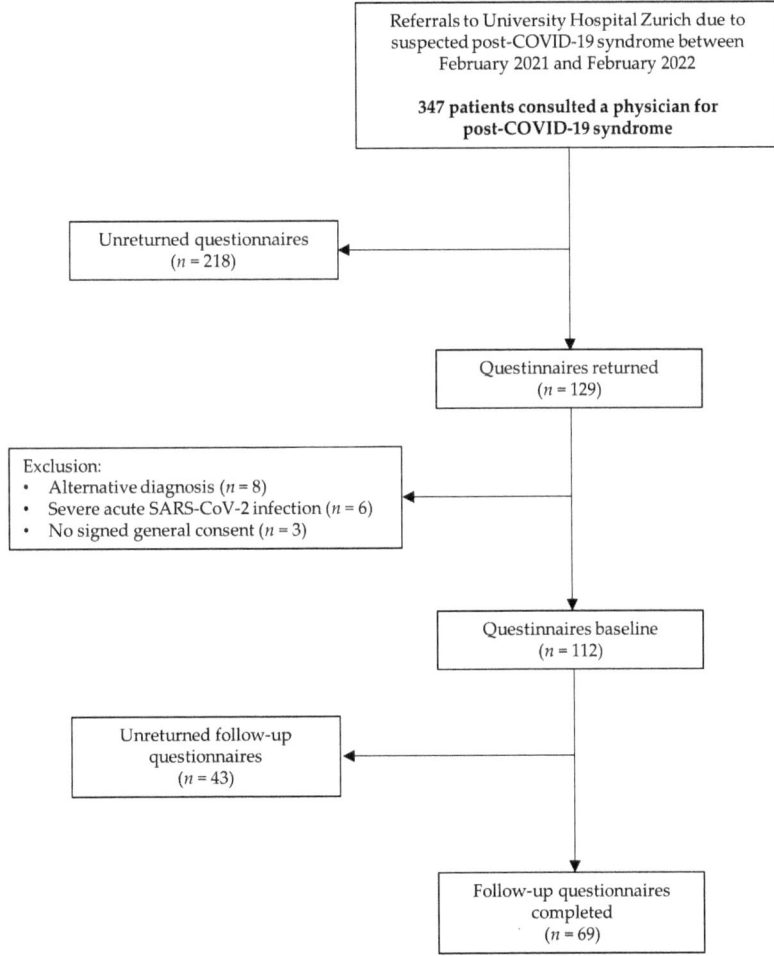

Figure 1. Study flow.

3.2. Symptom Characterization at Baseline

At baseline, patients mostly stated having neurocognitive symptoms, such as fatigue (75.4%) and concentration difficulties (56.5%), as well as cardiorespiratory problems, including dyspnea (59.4%), performance intolerance (55.1%) and thoracic pain (50.7%). See Table S1 (Supplementary Materials) for all symptom frequencies.

3.3. Subjective Effect of Vaccination on Post-COVID-19 Symptoms

A total of 97.1% of patients who completed the follow-up received a COVID-19 vaccine. A median (quartiles) time of 192 (147, 242) days passed from the onset of acute symptoms of COVID-19 to the first shot of the vaccine. About half of the patients received only one vaccine shot. There were 27 patients (40.3%) who had the impression of a persistent improvement of symptoms after a median (quartiles) time of 2 (1, 4) weeks after their vaccination. A persistent worsening of symptoms was stated by 22.4% of patients after a median (quartiles) time of 1 (1, 4) week, and 29.9% of patients neither felt an improvement nor a worsening of symptoms after receiving the vaccine (Table S2, Supplementary Materials).

3.4. SGRQ Questionnaire

Overall, all SGRQ component scores improved significantly after a follow-up of 6 months (Table 2). The largest mean (95% CI) difference of −14.4 (−18.4, −10.3) points was reached in the symptoms score component, whereas the lowest mean (95% CI) difference scores were reached in the impact scores component, with −6.5 (−10.2, −2.7) points. The SGRQ total score component showed a mean (95% CI) difference of −9.4 (−13.3, −5.5) points.

Table 2. SGRQ component scores, EQ-5D-5L index value and EQ-5D-5L VAS scores.

	Baseline, Mean (SD)	Follow-Up, Mean (SD)	Δ *, Mean (95% CI)	p-Value
SGRQ symptom score [a]	40.4 (21.0)	26.0 (21.1)	−14.4 (−18.4, −10.3)	$p < 0.001$
SGRQ activity score [b]	51.3 (25.4)	39.1 (27.6)	−12.2 (−17.4, −7.0)	$p < 0.001$
SGRQ impact score [b]	27.2 (17.7)	20.8 (18.5)	−6.5 (−10.2, −2.7)	$p = 0.001$
SGRQ total score [c]	37.3 (20.2)	27.9 (20.2)	−9.4 (−13.3, −5.5)	$p < 0.001$
EQ index value [d]	0.758 (0.203)	0.818 (0.168)	0.060 (0.019, 0.102)	$p = 0.005$
EQ VAS [e]	59.1 (20.9)	66.0 (20.3)	6.9 (2.7, 11.1)	$p = 0.002$

[a] $n = 69$, [b] $n = 57$, [c] $n = 51$, [d] $n = 66$, [e] $n = 67$. SGRQ: lower scores mean better quality of life. EQ index value and EQ VAS: higher scores mean better quality of life. * Change from baseline.

3.5. EQ-5D-5L

Figure 2 shows the percentage of patients with changes in the dimensions of mobility, self-care, usual activities, pain/discomfort and anxiety/depression. With the exception of the self-care and pain/discomfort dimensions, the majority of patients improved in all EQ-5D-5L health dimensions. At least one in five patients (20%) had an improvement to the level of "no problems" in the dimensions of mobility, usual activities and anxiety/depression. Self-care was the dimension where patients mostly stated having "no problems" at baseline and follow-up. Lower scores at follow-up visits were stated by 15% in the usual activities and anxiety/depression dimensions, 12% in the mobility and pain/discomfort dimensions, and 3% in the self-care dimension. However, there was a significantly greater proportion of patients with improvements compared with worsening in all dimensions, except in the dimension of self-care, where most patients stated having "no problems" at all ($p = 0.003$ for mobility, $p = 0.002$ for usual activities, $p = 0.016$ for pain/discomfort, $p = 0.016$ for anxiety/depression, $p = 0.157$ for self-care). Almost 50% of patients who suffered from pain/discomfort had persistent difficulties in this dimension.

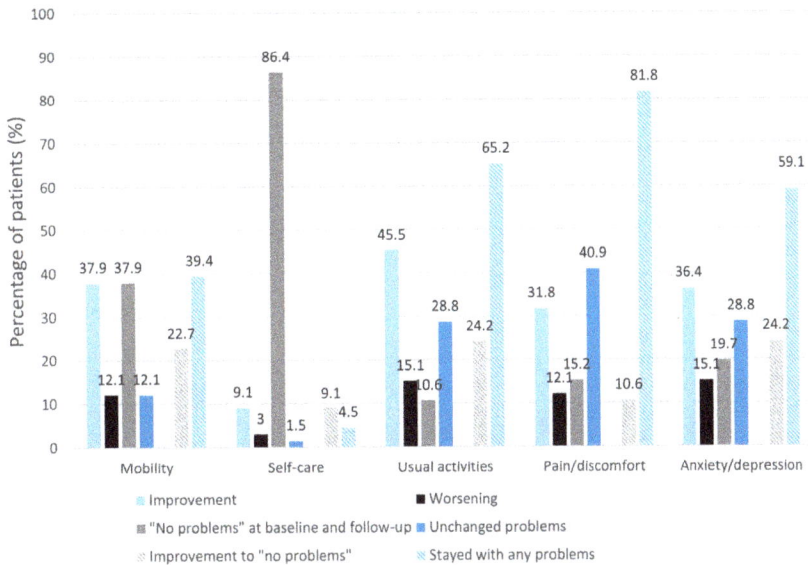

Figure 2. Changes in EQ-5D-5L dimension responses. The figure shows the changes from baseline (improvement/worsening/"no problems" at baseline and follow-up/unchanged problems) in the percentage of patients in the health dimensions of mobility, self-care, usual activities, pain/discomfort and anxiety/depression of the Euroqol-5D-5L questionnaire (EQ-5D-5L). Furthermore, percentages of patients that improved to "no problems" or stayed with any problems are shown. In almost all dimensions (with the exception of self-care), patients stated an improvement. Patients mostly did not report any problems with self-care at baseline, as well as at follow-up.

Dimension scores at baseline and follow-up are displayed in Figure S1 (Supplementary Materials).

Regarding the EQ index value, there was a statistically significant improvement (mean (95% CI) difference of 0.060 (0.019, 0.102), $p = 0.005$) between baseline and follow-up. Furthermore, patients had significantly higher mean (SD) EQ VAS scores at follow-up (59.1 (20.9) vs. 66.0 (20.3), $p = 0.002$) (Table 2).

3.6. SF-36

Mean (SD) scores and mean (95% CI) differences for the eight SF-36 health dimensions and PCS and MCS T-scores are outlined in Table 3. Patients improved significantly in the dimensions of physical functioning, physical role limitations, pain, energy/vitality, emotional role limitations and emotional health at follow-up. The mean (SD) scores of the physical component summary (PCS) score were significantly higher at follow-up (39.2 (10.2) vs. 43.0 (10.9), $p < 0.001$), whereas the mental component summary (MCS) score showed no significant change (41.8 (11.5) vs. 44.1 (11.5), $p = 0.069$). The mean (95% CI) difference scores between follow-up and baseline for the PCS and MCS were 4.9 (2.6, 7.2) and 2.3 (−0.2, 4.8), respectively. No significant difference was found in the dimensions of general health and social functioning between baseline and follow-up. Sex, the subjective effect of the COVID-19 vaccine on post-COVID-19 symptoms, the time from the symptom onset of COVID-19 to the first vaccination and the number of vaccine shots were not independent predictors for the change in the PCS or MCS.

Table 3. SF-36 health domain scores and PCS and MCS T-scores.

	Baseline, Mean (SD)	Follow-Up, Mean (SD)	Δ *, Mean (95% CI)	p-Value
Physical functioning [a]	63.4 (24.6)	75.4 (20.3)	12.1 (7.0, 17.1)	$p < 0.001$
Role limitations (physical) [b]	27.6 (35.7)	48.1 (42.9)	20.5 (10.9, 30.2)	$p < 0.001$
Pain [b]	56.7 (28.9)	67.3 (28.7)	10.7 (4.2, 17.1)	$p = 0.002$
General [c]	54.1 (18.2)	54.7 (19.1)	0.7 (−3.7, 4.9)	$p = 0.795$
Energy/vitality [c]	29.8 (19.4)	40.8 (21.7)	11.0 (6.3, 15.7)	$p < 0.001$
Social functioning [d]	57.9 (28.2)	62.5 (29.7)	4.6 (−2.4, 11.7)	$p = 0.195$
Role limitations (emotional) [b]	57.7 (44.8)	69.2 (41.2)	11.4 (0.98, 21.9)	$p = 0.032$
Emotional health [c]	61.3 (19.1)	66.9 (18.0)	5.6 (1.3, 9.8)	$p = 0.011$
PCS (T-score) [d]	38.2 (10.2)	43.0 (10.9)	4.9 (2.6, 7.2)	$p < 0.001$
MCS (T-score) [d]	41.8 (11.5)	44.1 (11.5)	2.3 (−0.2, 4.8)	$p = 0.069$

[a] $n = 68$, [b] $n = 67$, [c] $n = 66$, [d] $n = 65$. * Change from baseline. SF-36 scores: higher scores mean better quality of life.

4. Discussion

This study investigated the change in health-related quality of life in patients suffering from long-lasting symptoms after mild or moderate acute COVID-19 over time. We found that physical HRQoL, including several aspects of daily living, relevantly improved 6 months from baseline despite treatment options being scarce.

Recently, our research group showed that physical and mental health are substantially impaired in patients referred for a post-COVID-19 consultation compared with the Swiss general population during pre-pandemic times [11]. In particular, the health dimensions "usual activities", "pain" and "anxiety/depression" were affected, whereas "self-care" did not seem to be impaired at all. In patients who were hospitalized due to acute COVID-19, most individuals still reported symptoms 12 months after hospitalization [27]. After an initial mild disease, studies showed persistent symptoms also in this patient group [28,29]. Apart from symptom persistence, little is known about the consequences on HRQoL over time in patients with post-COVID-19 symptoms who suffered an initial mild or moderate COVID-19.

Regarding physical health, patients showed statistically significant and clinically relevant improvements exceeding the recommended 3-point minimal clinically important difference over six months. This was also reflected in the EQ-5D-5L, as one in five patients had improvements to "no problems" in the health dimensions "mobility" and "usual activities", and therefore, this seems to demonstrate potentially higher activity levels in those patients. Our results are contradictory to the findings of Seessle et al. [30], who found decreased physical HRQoL in patients with mild or moderate disease 12 months after the acute disease. This might have been due to the reason that their study cohort consisted of patients, which were considerably older and more patients suffered from an initial moderate disease severity (55.2% vs. 5.8%). Although the pathophysiological mechanisms that might have led to an improvement in symptoms are not available and specific therapies are still missing, physical health relevantly improved over time. It is difficult to say whether time was the key factor for the improvement of physical HRQoL or whether patients learned to cope with their illness, and therefore, did not feel as restricted physically. The considerable proportion of patients (40%) who stated that they had a persistent reduction in symptoms after the COVID-19 vaccine indicated that the severity and/or number of symptoms reduced over time. Complementary to that, Ayoubkhani et al. [31] observed a considerable likelihood of post-COVID-19 symptoms decreasing after COVID-19 vaccination. Further, the SGRQ's symptoms component score, which represents the frequency and severity of respiratory symptoms, showed significantly improved scores. Due to missing evidence-based treatment options, patients try various self-administered or experimental treatment strategies, as well as in- and outpatient rehabilitation programs. Therefore, it is unknown whether and to what extent those therapies or lifestyle changes, such as pacing, also influenced the course of physical HRQoL in a positive way.

No significant improvement was observed in mental health. Mental health might take more time to improve compared with physical health, and thus, the follow-up of 6 months could have been insufficient to detect a significant change. However, as we showed in our previous study [11], mental health was similarly impaired in post-COVID-19 patients and a control group during the first wave of the pandemic compared with the general Swiss population before the pandemic. Subsequently, mental health deterioration might have evolved as a consequence of socio-economical and political changes during the pandemic, and therefore, affect the whole population and not only post-COVID-19 patients. Lastly, it was already reported that physical disabilities might lead to depression [32], and thus, the long period of one year that patients had been suffering from post-COVID-19 symptoms in our cohort might have contributed to persistent mental health issues. Approximately 60% and 45% of patients in the dimensions "pain/discomfort" and "anxiety/depression", respectively, showed a decline or no change, which also might explain the non-significant improvement in mental health.

Future studies are warranted to investigate predictors for improvement or worsening in physical and mental HRQoL so that the course of the disease and its impact on different patient groups can be better understood. In our study cohort, sex, the subjective effect of the SARS-CoV-2-specific vaccination after infection on post-COVID-19 symptoms, the time from symptom onset of COVID-19 disease to the first vaccination, and the amount of vaccine shots were not independent predictors for physical or mental health.

Patients with follow-up showed a higher mental health status at baseline compared with individuals without follow-up. We cannot tell whether these patients did not participate due to remaining impairments or whether other reasons, such as motivational issues, hindered them. However, physical health at baseline was comparable in patients with and without follow-up. Moreover, the response rate to follow-up questionnaires was 61.6%, which can be rated as high enough. There is little literature regarding response rates to follow-up questionnaires, but one randomized trial that compared response rates with and without incentives showed similar results (68.5%) to the group where no incentives were given [33].

This study had some limitations. It is difficult to differentiate what effect can be allocated to time alone and what could be allocated to patients' self-effort or treatment strategies. However, the focus of this study was primarily to assess the change in HRQoL. Additional studies are needed that investigate the course of symptoms over time, as well as treatment strategies on the impact of HRQoL. A previous sample size calculation was not performed due to the exploratory study design, and therefore, the sample size was too small to test for various predictors. However, since the mean PCS was above the MCID and the lower limit was near the MCID, we concluded that our findings have enough power. Further, well-powered studies with bigger sample sizes should be conducted to confirm the findings and to evaluate possible predictors and the influence of different COVID-19 variants on the course of post-COVID-19. Lastly, as this study depicted only a patient collection of the German-speaking part of Switzerland with a generally very stable political situation and labor market, it is difficult to apply our results to other regions of the world.

5. Conclusions

The majority of patients that initially suffered from mild or moderate acute COVID-19 showed significant and clinically relevant improvements in physical-health-related quality of life over 6 months. Future studies are needed to better understand the course of the disease in different patient groups and whether the findings persist over time.

Supplementary Materials: The following supporting information can be downloaded from https://www.mdpi.com/article/10.3390/jcm12124077/s1: Figure S1: EQ-5D-5L dimension responses at baseline and follow-up; Table S1: Prevalence of long COVID symptoms; Table S2: Effect of COVID-19 vaccine on long COVID symptoms.

Author Contributions: Conceptualization, S.M., N.A.S., M.K. and C.F.C.; methodology, S.M., N.A.S., M.K. and C.F.C.; investigation, S.M., N.A.S., D.S., F.V., I.J., M.K. and C.F.C.; writing—original draft preparation, S.M.; writing—review and editing, S.M., N.A.S., D.S., F.V., I.J., M.K. and C.F.C. All authors have read and agreed to the published version of the manuscript.

Funding: This research received no external funding.

Institutional Review Board Statement: This study was conducted in accordance with the Declaration of Helsinki. The Ethics Committee of the Canton of Zurich approved the study (BASEC 2021-00280), and the study is registered on www.ClinicalTrials.gov, NCT04793269 (accessed on 2 May 2023).

Informed Consent Statement: Written informed consent was obtained from all subjects involved in the study.

Data Availability Statement: The data that support the findings of this study are available on request from the corresponding author.

Conflicts of Interest: The authors declare no conflict of interest.

References

1. National Institute for Health and Care Excellence. Clinical Guidelines. In *COVID-19 Rapid Guideline: Managing the Long-Term Effects of COVID-19*; National Institute for Health and Care Excellence (NICE): London, UK, 2020.
2. Aiyegbusi, O.L.; Hughes, S.E.; Turner, G.; Rivera, S.C.; McMullan, C.; Chandan, J.S.; Haroon, S.; Price, G.; Davies, E.H.; Nirantharakumar, K.; et al. Symptoms, complications and management of long COVID: A review. *J. R. Soc. Med.* **2021**, *114*, 428–442. [CrossRef]
3. Mehandru, S.; Merad, M. Pathological sequelae of long-haul COVID. *Nat. Immunol.* **2022**, *23*, 194–202. [CrossRef]
4. Davis, H.E.; Assaf, G.S.; McCorkell, L.; Wei, H.; Low, R.J.; Re'Em, Y.; Redfield, S.; Austin, J.P.; Akrami, A. Characterizing long COVID in an international cohort: 7 months of symptoms and their impact. *Eclinicalmedicine* **2021**, *38*, 101019. [CrossRef]
5. Nasserie, T.; Hittle, M.; Goodman, S.N. Assessment of the Frequency and Variety of Persistent Symptoms among Patients with COVID-19: A Systematic Review. *JAMA Netw. Open* **2021**, *4*, e2111417. [CrossRef]
6. White, P.D.; Thomas, J.M.; Amess, J.; Crawford, D.H.; Grover, S.A.; Kangro, H.O.; Clare, A.W. Incidence, risk and prognosis of acute and chronic fatigue syndromes and psychiatric disorders after glandular fever. *Br. J. Psychiatry* **1998**, *173*, 475–481. [CrossRef] [PubMed]
7. Moldofsky, H.; Patcai, J. Chronic widespread musculoskeletal pain, fatigue, depression and disordered sleep in chronic post-SARS syndrome; A case-controlled study. *BMC Neurol.* **2011**, *11*, 37. [CrossRef] [PubMed]
8. Garcia, M.N.; Hause, A.M.; Walker, C.M.; Orange, J.S.; Hasbun, R.; Murray, K.O. Evaluation of Prolonged Fatigue Post–West Nile Virus Infection and Association of Fatigue with Elevated Antiviral and Proinflammatory Cytokines. *Viral Immunol.* **2014**, *27*, 327–333. [CrossRef] [PubMed]
9. Hickie, I.; Davenport, T.; Wakefield, D.; Vollmer-Conna, U.; Cameron, B.; Vernon, S.D.; Reeves, W.C.; Lloyd, A. Post infective and chronic fatigue syndromes precipitated by viral and non-viral pathogens: Prospective cohort study. *BMJ* **2006**, *333*, 575. [CrossRef]
10. Hardt, J.; Buchwald, D.; Wilks, D.; Sharpe, M.; Nix, W.; Egle, U. Health-related quality of life in patients with chronic fatigue syndrome: An international study. *J. Psychosom. Res.* **2001**, *51*, 431–434. [CrossRef] [PubMed]
11. Malesevic, S.; Sievi, N.A.; Baumgartner, P.; Roser, K.; Sommer, G.; Schmidt, D.; Vallelian, F.; Jelcic, I.; Clarenbach, C.F.; Kohler, M. Impaired health-related quality of life in long-COVID syndrome after mild to moderate COVID-19. *Sci. Rep.* **2023**, *13*, 7717. [CrossRef]
12. Nittas, V.; Puhan, M. Literature screening repport—Update 6. Long COVID: Evolving Definitions, Burden of Disease and Socio-Economic Consequences; Bundesamt für Gesundheit. 2021. Available online: https://www.bag.admin.ch, (accessed on 2 May 2023).
13. Tran, V.-T.; Porcher, R.; Pane, I.; Ravaud, P. Course of post COVID-19 disease symptoms over time in the ComPaRe long COVID prospective e-cohort. *Nat. Commun.* **2022**, *13*, 1812. [CrossRef]
14. Jones, P.W. Quality of life measurement for patients with diseases of the airways. *Thorax* **1991**, *46*, 676–682. [CrossRef]
15. Jones, P.; Quirk, F.; Baveystock, C. The St George's Respiratory Questionnaire. *Respir. Med.* **1991**, *85*, 25–31. [CrossRef]
16. Jones, P.W. St. George's Respiratory Questionnaire Manual. Available online: https://meetinstrumentenzorg.nl/wp-content/uploads/instrumenten/SGRQ-handl-Eng.pdf (accessed on 14 April 2022).
17. Jones, P.W. St. George's Respiratory Questionnaire: MCID. *COPD J. Chronic Obstr. Pulm. Dis.* **2005**, *2*, 75–79. [CrossRef] [PubMed]
18. The EuroQol Group. EuroQol-a new facility for the measurement of health-related quality of life. *Health Policy* **1990**, *16*, 199–208. [CrossRef] [PubMed]
19. McClure, N.S.; Al Sayah, F.; Ohinmaa, A.; Johnson, J.A. Minimally Important Difference of the EQ-5D-5L Index Score in Adults with Type 2 Diabetes. *Value Health* **2018**, *21*, 1090–1097. [CrossRef]

20. McClure, N.S.; Al Sayah, F.; Xie, F.; Luo, N.; Johnson, J.A. Instrument-Defined Estimates of the Minimally Important Difference for EQ-5D-5L Index Scores. *Value Health* **2017**, *20*, 644–650. [CrossRef]
21. Tsai, A.P.Y.; Hur, S.A.; Wong, A.; Safavi, M.; Assayag, D.; Johannson, K.A.; Morisset, J.; Fell, C.; Fisher, J.H.; Manganas, H.; et al. Minimum important difference of the EQ-5D-5L and EQ-VAS in fibrotic interstitial lung disease. *Thorax* **2020**, *76*, 37–43. [CrossRef] [PubMed]
22. Brazier, J.E.; Harper, R.; Jones, N.M.; O'Cathain, A.; Thomas, K.J.; Usherwood, T.; Westlake, L. Validating the SF-36 health survey questionnaire: New outcome measure for primary care. *BMJ* **1992**, *305*, 160–164. [CrossRef]
23. Laucis, N.C.; Hays, R.D.; Bhattacharyya, T. Scoring the SF-36 in Orthopaedics: A Brief Guide. *J. Bone Jt. Surg.* **2015**, *97*, 1628–1634. [CrossRef]
24. Taft, C.; Karlsson, J.; Sullivan, M. Do SF-36 summary component scores accurately summarize subscale scores? *Qual. Life Res.* **2001**, *10*, 395–404. [CrossRef] [PubMed]
25. Frendl, D.; Ware, J.E. Patient-reported Functional Health and Well-Being Outcomes with Drug Therapy: A Systematic Review of Randomized Trials Using the SF-36 Health Survey. *Med. Care* **2014**, *52*, 439–445. [CrossRef]
26. Bjorner, J.B.; Wallenstein, G.V.; Martin, M.C.; Lin, P.; Blaisdell-Gross, B.; Piech, C.T.; Mody, S.H. Interpreting score differences in the SF-36 Vitality scale: Using clinical conditions and functional outcomes to define the minimally important difference. *Curr. Med. Res. Opin.* **2007**, *23*, 731–739. [CrossRef] [PubMed]
27. Comelli, A.; Viero, G.; Bettini, G.; Nobili, A.; Tettamanti, M.; Galbussera, A.A.; Muscatello, A.; Mantero, M.; Canetta, C.; Boneschi, F.M.; et al. Patient-Reported Symptoms and Sequelae 12 Months after COVID-19 in Hospitalized Adults: A Multicenter Long-Term Follow-Up Study. *Front. Med.* **2022**, *9*, 834354. [CrossRef]
28. Peghin, M.; Palese, A.; Venturini, M.; De Martino, M.; Gerussi, V.; Graziano, E.; Bontempo, G.; Marrella, F.; Tommasini, A.; Fabris, M.; et al. Post-COVID-19 symptoms 6 months after acute infection among hospitalized and non-hospitalized patients. *Clin. Microbiol. Infect.* **2021**, *27*, 1507–1513. [CrossRef]
29. Petersen, M.S.; Kristiansen, M.F.; Hanusson, K.D.; Danielsen, M.E.; Steig, B.; Gaini, S.; Strøm, M.; Weihe, P. Long COVID in the Faroe Islands: A Longitudinal Study Among Nonhospitalized Patients. *Clin. Infect. Dis.* **2020**, *73*, e4058–e4063. [CrossRef]
30. Seeßle, J.; Waterboer, T.; Hippchen, T.; Simon, J.; Kirchner, M.; Lim, A.; Müller, B.; Merle, U. Persistent Symptoms in Adult Patients 1 Year After Coronavirus Disease 2019 (COVID-19): A Prospective Cohort Study. *Clin. Infect. Dis.* **2022**, *74*, 1191–1198. [CrossRef]
31. Ayoubkhani, D.; Bermingham, C.; Pouwels, K.B.; Glickman, M.; Nafilyan, V.; Zaccardi, F.; Khunti, K.; Alwan, N.A.; Walker, A.S. Trajectory of long covid symptoms after covid-19 vaccination: Community based cohort study. *BMJ* **2022**, *377*, e069676. [CrossRef] [PubMed]
32. Turner, R.J.; Beiser, M.M. Major Depression and Depressive Symptomatology among the Physically Disabled. Assessing the role of chronic stress. *J. Nerv. Ment. Dis.* **1990**, *178*, 343–350. [CrossRef]
33. Morgan, A.J.; Rapee, R.M.; Bayer, J.K. Increasing response rates to follow-up questionnaires in health intervention research: Randomized controlled trial of a gift card prize incentive. *Clin. Trials* **2017**, *14*, 381–386. [CrossRef]

Disclaimer/Publisher's Note: The statements, opinions and data contained in all publications are solely those of the individual author(s) and contributor(s) and not of MDPI and/or the editor(s). MDPI and/or the editor(s) disclaim responsibility for any injury to people or property resulting from any ideas, methods, instructions or products referred to in the content.

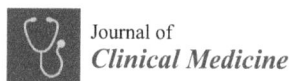

Article

Influence of Clinical and Sociodemographic Variables on Health-Related Quality of Life in the Adult Population with Long COVID

Mª Pilar Rodríguez-Pérez [1], Patricia Sánchez-Herrera-Baeza [1,*], Pilar Rodríguez-Ledo [2], Elisabet Huertas-Hoyas [1], Gemma Fernández-Gómez [1], Rebeca Montes-Montes [1] and Marta Pérez-de-Heredia-Torres [1]

[1] Group in Evaluation and Assessment of Capacity, Functionality and Disability of Universidad Rey Juan Carlos (TO+IDI), Department of Physical Therapy, Occupational Therapy, Physical Medicine and Rehabilitation, Research, Universidad Rey Juan Carlos, 28922 Alcorcón, Spain; pilar.rodriguez@urjc.es (M.P.R.-P.); elisabet.huertas@urjc.es (E.H.-H.); gemma.fernandez@urjc.es (G.F.-G.); rebeca.montes@urjc.es (R.M.-M.); marta.perezdeheredia@urjc.es (M.P.-d.-H.-T.)

[2] COVID Persistent Working Group of the Sociedad Española de Medicos de Familia (SEMG), Department of General Medicine, Lugo, a Mariña and Monforte de Lemos Health Area, 27002 Lugo, Spain; prodriguezl@semg.es

* Correspondence: patricia.sanchezherrera@urjc.es; Tel.: +34-914-888-676

Abstract: Worldwide, about 10 percent of patients affected by long COVID require appropriate follow-up and intervention. The main objective of this study was to analyze the long-term impact of mild long COVID in the adult population, and to determine the effect of clinical and sociodemographic variables on health-related quality of life in those affected. Methods: A cross-sectional descriptive study of a sample of Spanish adult patients with persistent COVID-19 symptoms at least three months after diagnosis. Data collection took place between April and July 2021. The health-related quality of life of the sample was low, with worse results in the physical component summary (PCS) 24.66 (SD = 4.45) compared to the mental component summary (MCS) 45.95 (SD = 8.65). The multi-regression analysis showed significant differences by sex in the dimensions of physical functioning ($p = 0.040$); bodily pain ($p = 0.036$); and health transition ($p = 0.018$). Additionally, a longer time since infection had a significant effect on physical functioning ($p = 0.039$); general health ($p = 0.037$); vitality ($p = 0.034$); and general health transition ($p = 0.002$). The effect of occupational imbalance was significant for all dimensions. Conclusions: people with long COVID have a reduced quality of life. Sex, time since infection, and occupational imbalance are predictors of a worse quality of life.

Keywords: long COVID; quality of life; persistent symptoms; long haulers

Citation: Rodríguez-Pérez, M.P.; Sánchez-Herrera-Baeza, P.; Rodríguez-Ledo, P.; Huertas-Hoyas, E.; Fernández-Gómez, G.; Montes-Montes, R.; Pérez-de-Heredia-Torres, M. Influence of Clinical and Sociodemographic Variables on Health-Related Quality of Life in the Adult Population with Long COVID. *J. Clin. Med.* **2023**, *12*, 4222. https://doi.org/10.3390/jcm12134222

Academic Editor: Mark Van Den Boogaard

Received: 30 May 2023
Revised: 14 June 2023
Accepted: 20 June 2023
Published: 22 June 2023

Copyright: © 2023 by the authors. Licensee MDPI, Basel, Switzerland. This article is an open access article distributed under the terms and conditions of the Creative Commons Attribution (CC BY) license (https:// creativecommons.org/licenses/by/ 4.0/).

1. Introduction

Severe acute respiratory syndrome coronavirus 2 (SARS-CoV-2) is the causative agent that results in acute COVID-19 infection. Research has shown that mild COVID-19 disease is present in up to 80% of cases [1,2]. In addition, long-term complications can occur after the acute phase of COVID-19 disease following recovery from the acute effects of the infection [3]. Some people continue to experience symptoms beyond the initial acute phase of the disease with long term effects from their infection, known as long COVID [2,4]. Thus, Greenhalgh et al. 2020 [5] defined long COVID as the persistence of symptoms beyond 12 weeks of symptom onset. Between 11% and 24% of patients with COVID-19 may experience long-term symptoms even three months after the onset of COVID-19 disease. The hypothesized etiopathogenesis of COVID-19 is that it may be driven by long-term tissue damage or pathological inflammation (due to viral persistence, immune dysregulation, and autoimmunity) [6]. There is scarce evidence for patients who suffered a mild COVID-19 infection and were treated in an outpatient setting. This is potentially contradictory as, according to the available data, most cases of individuals with acute COVID-19 experience a mild disease [7], and therefore, further studies in this population are required. The predominant profile of individuals with long COVID, is that of a woman with a mean age of 43 years and no previous major health problems [8]. Conversely, people with long COVID who were hospitalized in the acute phase of COVID-19 had a higher prevalence of comorbidity and previous pathologies [9]. The impact of the persistence of symptoms beyond the clinical outcome means that the individual's physical, mental, social, and emotional functioning is affected [10], which has a major health and economic impact [11]. Previous research on persistent COVID has focused on characterizing persistent symptoms and the pathophysiology of the disease as well as the need for further research because of the great impact on quality of life [4] and occupational performance [9,12], months after the diagnosis. Thus, it is important to analyze performance limitations, together with the degree of occupational balance, i.e., the ability for a person to distribute their activities, together with time-management and decision-making, as this is fundamental for the individual's autonomy [13]. Occupational balance can be defined as "The individual's subjective experience of having "the right mix" of occupations in his or her occupational pattern. This definition can be used from various perspectives: occupational areas, occupations with different characteristics, and time use" [14]. It has been previously shown that occupational imbalance directly causes high levels of stress and impacts the individual's health, however a balanced participation contributes to the maintenance of people's health and well-being [15].

Due to the novelty of the disease, there is a lack of evidence regarding the evolution of those affected [16]. Thus, previous studies have monitored the number of symptoms [17], the lower health status of those with long COVID compared to that of the control population [18], and the risk factors for long COVID-19, such as being a female, vaccination status, and age [9]. However, the effect of long COVID on quality of life has not yet been sufficiently analyzed; therefore, it is necessary to research the limitations encountered in order to design an appropriate intervention and rehabilitation program to improve both quality of life and autonomy [13].

This study sought to identify the impact of long COVID on health-related quality of life to determine the effect of clinical and sociodemographic variables, and to explore the relationship with the participants' occupational balance by performing a secondary analysis based on the previously published cross-sectional descriptive design by Rodriguez-Perez et al. [19].

2. Materials and Methods

2.1. Design

A descriptive cross-sectional study was conducted on a sample of Spanish adult patients presenting with persistent COVID-19 symptoms for three months or longer. The guidelines of the Strengthening the Reporting of Observational Studies in Epidemiology (STROBE) checklist were followed [20]. This study was approved by the Ethics Committee of University Rey Juan Carlos (170120210212) and is framed within the Spanish Research Network on Persistent COVID (REiCOP). Data collection, processing and transfer were completed in accordance with the provisions of the Declaration of Helsinki [21], and current Spanish regulations on personal data protection. Furthermore, prior to participation, each participant signed an informed consent form.

2.2. Sample

Data collection took place between April to July 2021. The survey method was adopted and applied through videoconference with participants. The sample criteria were determined in consensus with the Spanish Society of General and Family Physicians (SEMG), based on previous international studies [22]. The sample was selected using simple random sampling with all voluntary participants who met the criteria using the 2022 Quick-Calcs GraphPad software system (GraphPad Software, LLC, San Diego, CA, USA). The inclusion criteria consisted of people between 30 and 50 years of age, diagnosed with acute-phase

COVID-19 disease via Polymerase Chain Reaction (PCR) and/or positive serology; who did not require hospitalization in the acute phase of illness; with persistent COVID-19 symptomatology determined by medical diagnosis and not attributed to another cause; for three months or longer; adequate ability to communicate for the purpose of collecting clinical data; and no previous pathologies; additionally, due to the health regulations in place at the time, the participants were non-vaccinated. The exclusion criteria consisted of receiving rehabilitation treatment for COVID-19 at the time of the assessment, not having the necessary technology to conduct the interview, and failure to accept and sign the informed consent form.

2.3. Procedure

Before conducting the study, the researchers established agreements with the Spanish Society of General and Family Physicians (SEMG), the Persistent COVID Association in Spain (ACPE) and representatives of the collective "Long COVID Autonomous Communities Together Spain (ACTS)". Thereafter, Long COVID ACTS conveyed the study information to the regional collectives of each community, who, in turn, disseminated the information to each of the affected patients who voluntarily showed their interest in participating in the study. The form gathered contact and sociodemographic data, COVID-19 diagnostic test data, time of evolution since diagnosis, symptomatology, employment status, and acceptance of the study. Once the participant had completed the form and accepted the informed consent, the investigator conducted a videoconference call. During the interview, both the Occupational Balance Questionnaire and SF-36 health questionnaire were administered. These scales were administered considering the participant's situation at the time, and the same questions were also administered referring to their situation prior to the disease. Subsequently, the data were stored in a digital notebook that was solely available to the principal investigator. The study protocol is published elsewhere in detail [19] (Figure 1).

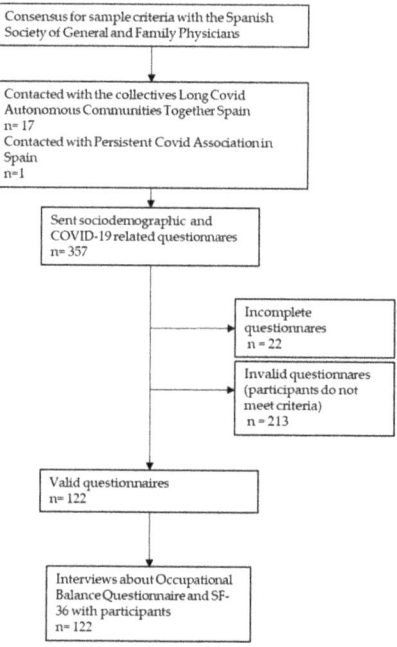

Figure 1. Data collection.

2.4. Measures

The Occupational Balance Questionnaire (OBQ) [23] measures occupational balance in relation to a person's current situation and daily life. Thus, it assesses the ability to manage the amount and variability of tasks within an occupation while preserving personal preferences, as well as the ability to maintain a strong sense of self-identity through participation in meaningful occupations based on personal values. The OBQ particularly focuses a person's satisfaction with the range and variability of occupations and provides a global picture of one's own occupational balance [24]. It consists of 13 items that are scored using an ordinal response scale from 0 to 5 points according to the degree of agreement. The final score ranges from 0 to 65, where a higher score indicates a better occupational balance. A notable advantage of this questionnaire is that it does not focus on a single classification of activities, rather it presents different statements in a global way with several alternatives in reference to a wide range of activities that the individual may have. The main objective is to explore the balance between different types of occupations, the significance of the occupations for the person, the use of time, and how the patient feels about these occupations. Thus, a wide variety of occupations are represented, including physical, social, intellectual, leisure, and other activities [23]. This tool has demonstrated adequate psychometric properties, making it a reliable instrument for measuring occupational balance. Moreover, a Spanish version has been adapted and validated [24].

The impact on health-related quality of life (HRQoL) was measured using the 36-item Short-Form Health Survey (SF-36) [25]. The SF-36 was developed to measure relevant generic health concepts. It is a 36-item scale, measuring the following domains: physical functioning, physical role limitations, bodily pain, general health perceptions, social functioning, emotional role limitations, mental health, and the transformation in health status compared to the previous state. The raw scores are translated into transformed scores and each dimension is given a percentage from 0 to 100, the higher the percentage, the better the health status. The aggregation of the eight subdomain scores enables the calculation of two summary scores: the physical summary component (PCS) scores and the mental summary component (MCS) The PCS is calculated by positively weighting the four subscales in the physical domain (physical functioning, role physical, bodily pain and general health) and the remaining psychological domain subscales negatively [26]. In contrast, the MCS is calculated by positively weighting the four mental domain subscales (mental health, vitality, social functioning and role emotional), and negatively weighting the four physical domain subscales. Previous studies published to date have shown that scores above or below 50 indicate better or worse health status, respectively, than the mean of the reference population [27]. This questionnaire is psychometrically sound and has been validated and adapted to the Spanish population [28]. The SF-36 is designed to be self-administered. Recent studies have used this questionnaire with population affected by the COVID-19 pandemic [29].

2.5. Data Analysis

Concerning qualitative variables, the number of cases present in each category and the corresponding percentages were calculated. In addition, in terms of quantitative variables, the mean and standard deviation were calculated with transformed scores subscales. To calculate PCS and MSC values, scores for each of the eight domains were extracted and standardized using a z-score transformation. They were then multiplied by 10 and added to 50 to generate normalized scores for each domain and aggregated using factor score coefficients and creating normalized scores for each component summary [30]. Correlations between variables were studied using Pearson's correlation coefficient with the raw scores. To determine the possible effect of demographic, clinical and scale variables, multivariable linear regression models were performed for the dimensions scores. The statistical analysis was performed with SPSS 27.0 for Windows (Copyright© 2013 IBM SPSS Corp., Armonk, NY, USA). Statistical significance was set at $p < 0.05$.

3. Results

The final study sample consisted of 122 patients from 35 Spanish territories, presenting with persistent multiple and multisystemic symptomatology. As shown in Table 1, up to 77.9% ($n = 95$) were women and 22.1% ($n = 27$) were men, aged between 30 and 50 years with a mean age of 43.5 years (SD = 5.8). Regarding the time since infection, the mean time was 10.88 months (min.–max.: 4–16, SD = 3.33).

Table 1. Descriptive sociodemographic and clinical variables.

Sociodemographic Variables	n
Sex (n (%))	
Women	95 (77.9)
Men	27 (22.1)
Age (range)	30–50
Age (mean (SD))	43.5 (5.8)
Time since infection (min.–max. months (SD))	4–16 (3.33)

SD: standard deviation.

Table 2 shows the means and standard deviations of the scores for the SF-36 subscales. The health-related quality of life of the sample was low, with worse results in the physical component summary (pcs; 24.66 [sd = 4.45]): physical functioning 27.50 (sd = 20.40); role of physical limitations 5.12 (sd = 16.99); general health 29.51 (sd = 16.23); bodily pain 36.52 (sd = 22.04) than in the mental component summary (mcs; 45.95 [sd = 8.65]): vitality 22.25 (sd = 20.71); mental health 59.30 (sd = 14.94); social functioning 39.45 (sd = 17.53); and role of emotional limitations 62.81 (sd = 46.98). The health transition subscale scored an average of 7.17 (sd = 11.35).

Table 2. Descriptive statistics for the scores on the SF-36 subscales.

	Mean (SD)
Physical Functioning (PF)	27.50 (20.40)
Role of Physical Limitations (RP)	5.12 (16.99)
General Health (GH)	29.51 (16.23)
Bodily Pain (BP)	36.52 (22.04)
Physical Component Summary (Pcs)	24.66 (4.45)
Vitality (V)	22.25 (20.71)
Mental Health (Mh)	59.30 (14.94)
Social Functioning (SF)	39.45 (17.53)
Role of Emotional Limitations (RE)	62.81 (46.98)
Mental Component Summary (MCS)	45.95 (8.65)
Health Transition	7.17 (11.35)

Notes. SD: standard deviation.

Table 3 shows the means (standard deviations) and correlations between the scales (raw scores). Occupational balance measured using the OBQ correlated positively and significantly with all dimensions of the SF36, except with physical role limitations.

Table 3. Means, standard deviations and correlations between scales (raw scores).

		1	2	3	4	5	6	7	8	9	10
1.	Occupational Balance Questionnnaire (OBQ)	1									
2.	Physical Functioning	0.61 *	1								
3.	Role of Physical Limitations	−0.10	0.07	1							

Table 3. Cont.

		1	2	3	4	5	6	7	8	9	10
4.	Role of Emotional Limitations	0.29 *	0.35 *	0.19	1						
5.	Vitality	0.42 *	0.60 *	0.14	0.06	1					
6.	Mental Health	0.28 *	0.39 *	−0.15	0.64 *	−0.05	1				
7.	Social functioning	0.39 *	0.50 *	0.03	0.38 *	0.19 *	0.47 *	1			
8.	Bodily Pain	0.27 *	0.42 *	0.03	0.40 *	0.18 *	0.32 *	0.46 *	1		
9.	General Health	0.53 *	0.58 *	−0.08	0.24 *	0.44 *	0.34 *	0.47 *	0.43 *	1	
10.	Health Transition	0.49 *	0.46 *	0.13	0.27 *	0.38 *	0.12	0.54 *	0.33 *	0.40 *	1

Notes: * $p < 0.05$.

To determine the possible effect of demographic and clinical variables and the OBQ scale on the dimensions of the SF36 scale, multivariable linear regression models were calculated, considering physical functioning, role physical, general health and bodily pain as the dependent variables (Table 4). Regarding physical functioning, the variables with a significant effect were sex ($p = 0.040$), time of evolution ($p = 0.039$), and occupational balance ($p < 0.001$). The results revealed that for general health, time since infection ($p = 0.037$), and occupational balance ($p < 0.001$) were significant. For bodily pain, sex ($p = 0.036$) and OBQ ($p = 0.003$) were significant. None of the independent factors contributed to the role of physical health.

Table 4. Effect of demographic, clinical variables and OBQ on the dimensions related to physical aspects of the SF-36 scale.

		Physical Functioning			Role of Physical Health			General Health			Bodily Pain		
		B (SE)	t	p-Value	B (SE)	t	p-Value	B (SE)	t	p-Value	B (SE)	t	p-Value
Sex (Female vs. Male)		−1.03 (0.44)	−2.08	0.040	−0.07 (0.15)	0.45	0.656	0.44 (0.63)	0.69	0.492	−0.87 (0.41)	−2.12	0.036
Age		−0.01 (0.05)	−0.19	0.851	−0.01 (0.01)	0.65	0.518	0.02 (0.05)	0.52	0.601	0.00 (0.04)	−0.03	0.978
Time since infection		0.05 (0.02)	2.09	0.039	−0.02 (0.02)	1.06	0.291	0.04 (0.02)	2.11	0.037	−0.06 (0.06)	−1.05	0.296
OBQ		0.22 (0.03)	8.08	<0.001	−0.01 (0.01)	1.20	0.231	0.16 (0.02)	6.69	<0.001	0.05 (0.02)	3.00	0.003
	R^2 (%)	36.5			−0.8			26			7.2		
	Model	$F(4; 117) = 18.39$; $p < 0.001$			$F(4; 117) = 0.76$; $p = 0.551$			$F(4; 117) = 11.60$; $p < 0.001$			$F(4; 117) = 3.36$; $p = 0.012$		

B: unstandardized coefficient. SE: standard error.

Regarding the dimensions related to mental health (Table 5), the results showed that time since infection had a statistically significant effect ($p = 0.034$). Additionally, for the four dimensions, the variable with a statistically significant effect was occupational balance, where a lower score was related to greater limitations for the following dimensions: vitality ($p < 0.001$) role of emotional limitations ($p = 0.001$), mental health ($p = 0.005$) and social functioning ($p < 0.001$).

Table 5. Effect of demographic and clinical variables and the OBQ on dimensions related to mental health, according to the SF-36 scale.

	Vitality			Role of Emotional Limitations			Mental Health			Social Functioning		
	B (SE)	t	p-Value	B (SE)	t	p-Value	B (SE)	t	p-Value	B (SE)	t	p-Value
Sex (Female vs. Male)	−1.02 (0.86)	−1.18	0.239	−0.08 (0.31)	−0.27	0.789	0.42 (0.81)	0.52	0.604	−0.23 (0.29)	−0.79	0.432
Age	−0.03 (0.06)	−0.51	0.611	0.02 (0.02)	0.91	0.365	−0.06 (0.06)	−0.98	0.33	0.03 (0.02)	1.38	0.169
Time since infection	−0.03 (0.01)	−2.14	0.034	0.02 (0.04)	0.50	0.616	0.16 (0.10)	1.56	0.121	−0.02 (0.04)	−0.60	0.552
OBQ	0.15 (0.03)	4.75	<0.001	0.04 (0.01)	3.39	0.001	0.09 (0.03)	2.89	0.005	0.05 (0.01)	4.81	<0.001
R^2 (%)	16			8.4			9.2			14.11		
Model	$F_{(4; 117)} = 6.78; p < 0.001$			$F_{(4; 116)} = 3.07; p = 0.019$			$F_{(4; 117)} = 3.35; p = 0.012$			$F_{(4; 117)} = 5.98; p < 0.001$		

B: unstandardized coefficient. SE: standard error.

In the dimension related to health transition (Table 6), the variables with a significant effect were sex ($p = 0.018$), time since infection ($p = 0.002$) and occupational balance ($p < 0.001$).

Table 6. Effect of demographic and clinical variables and OBQ on the health transition of the SF-36 scale.

	Health Transition		
	B (SE)	t	p-Value
Sex (Female vs. Male)	−5.17 (2.16)	−2.40	0.018
Age	0.20 (0.16)	1.26	0.211
Time since infection	−0.86 (0.27)	−3.13	0.002
OBQ	0.52 (0.08)	6.56	<0.001
R^2 (%)	29.5		
Model	$F_{(4; 117)} = 13.66; p < 0.001$		

B: unstandardized coefficient. SE: standard error.

4. Discussion

This study shows the impact of mild persistent COVID on HRQoL. Our findings reveal low HRQOL scores compared to normative data of people in the same age range and similar characteristics [31]. The available evidence regarding the HRQoL of people with Long COVID remains scarce; however, affected individuals continue to present a wide range of symptoms [32], hampering the return to their previous normal life. In line with our results, Garrigues et al. [33] found an impact on quality of life in dimensions measured by the EQ-5D among previously hospitalized patients with persistent symptoms. Similarly, Arnold et al. [29] also administered the SF-36 to hospitalized patients with COVID-19 and showed a decline in HRQoL in all domains compared to age-matched population norms. Similar previous studies [32] have based their analyses on patients with acute COVID-19. However, to date, we have not found any studies focusing on individuals with persistent COVID who presented with mild SARS-CoV-2 infection.

The regression model showed that sex had a significant effect on the domains of physical functioning, bodily pain, and health transitions. Therefore, women had worse scores on the HRQOL compared to men. These scores may be in line with previous studies [34] where men obtained better scores on the HRQOL compared to women. However, these studies were only focused on hospitalized patients. Time since infection was another significant variable for vitality, and general health. Thus, a longer time of disease evolution was significantly correlated with lower HRQOL scores, and worse self-perceived general health. To the best of our knowledge, there is no data on the evolution of HRQOL in people with long-term persistent COVID. Thus, more recent studies have focused on accounting for long-term symptoms [4] and improvement of symptoms [6], and less on analyzing the impact on HRQoL. A recent systematic review [35] concluded that previously hospitalized patients with persistent symptoms beyond 12 weeks still experienced a decline in HRQoL. Meys et al. [36] used the EQ-5D tool to determine HRQoL in non-hospitalized patients with long COVID, and obtained similar conclusions; however, they only analyzed the sample three months after diagnosis. Our study had a longer follow up, with a mean time of evolution of ten months, which may shed light on some hypotheses regarding long-term improvement in this population.

Regarding occupational balance, measured with the OBQ, this was significant for all HRQoL dimensions. Thus, those affected by long COVID showed a decline and imbalance in their occupations, which had a direct impact on their HRQoL. The relationship between occupational balance and health has been analyzed in studies with different populations and has been shown to be associated with quality of life [37]. In line with our results, recent studies have explored the relationship between occupational balance and HRQoL in the context of the pandemic situation due to COVID-19 [11]. Authors such as Messeguer de Pedro et al. [38] found low levels of occupational balance associated with a significant reduction in self-perceived health. However, we are not aware of research that has analyzed this relationship with patients with long COVID-19, even though it may be essential to train people to improve their abilities related to balancing occupational performance in order to produce a positive impact on their health and wellbeing [39]. Although we lack available evidence on the design of rehabilitation programs in this population, authors such as Belhan et al. [40] or Ganesan et al. [41] performed this intervention approach in their rehabilitation program and found improvements in HRQOL in individuals affected by the COVID-19 pandemic.

Practical Implications and Future Lines of Investigation

Our data may be of interest for the design of appropriate and individualized intervention programs for patients with mild long COVID. In the assessment of patients with persistent COVID it is very important to consider aspects such as occupational balance, and it is necessary to design programs aimed at improving occupational balance and autonomy, which will consequently improve the quality of life of those affected.

In the future, longitudinal studies should be conducted to provide data on long-term evolution and follow-up considering other variables such as the long-term effects of vaccines in patients with long COVID who suffered a mild infection during the acute phase of illness.

5. Strengths and Limitations

This study aimed to fill the gap in research regarding occupational balance and its relationship with long COVID and sociodemographic variables. The reported results provide new evidence on occupational balance, a rarely studied variable in this context, and its relationship with quality of life and sociodemographic variables. This relationship has practical implications, the practitioners that attend people diagnosed with long COVID must include occupational interventions aimed to reversing the occupational imbalance, and future research should assess the effects of occupational interventions on quality of life and occupational balance.

The main strength of this research was the participant profile: people who were not vaccinated and did not require hospitalization. In the current literature, different variables related to long-term COVID have been studied in hospitalized patients who have received vaccination; however, few studies have addressed this health condition in people who have not required hospitalization or been vaccinated. In addition, the sample has been collected from different regions of Spain, and therefore, the data is more representative of the national territory. Although, the sample size was estimated to provide reliable data, the results from this study should be further confirmed in future studies with a larger sample size.

This study has several limitations which warrant consideration. Firstly, the sample size and cross-sectional design may limit the generalizability of results. Secondly, the interviews reported information from patients at two different points in time and should therefore be considered with caution to avoid possible measurement or recall bias. In spite of this, the guidelines for this type of observational study [20] were considered to minimize bias as much as possible and the interviews were scheduled soon after their previous situation. In addition, this was a commonly used methodology during pandemic periods [42,43] and at the time of the evaluation movement restrictions were still in place at a national level. Nonetheless, despite these limitations, the present study has enabled us to perform an analysis of HRQOL, as well as to make the first description of the impact of sociodemographic variables, age, sex, time of evolution, and occupational balance in patients with long COVID.

6. Conclusions

The results of this study indicate that people with long COVID present a low HRQOL and occupational imbalance. Furthermore, we have found that female sex, a longer time since infection, and occupational imbalance are influential variables related to a worse HRQOL.

Author Contributions: Conceptualization, M.P.R.-P., M.P.-d.-H.-T. and P.S.-H.-B.; methodology, M.P.R.-P. and P.S.-H.-B.; software, R.M.-M.; validation, E.H.-H., G.F.-G. and P.R.-L.; formal analysis, M.P.R.-P. and M.P.-d.-H.-T.; investigation, G.F.-G.; resources, P.R.-L.; data curation, R.M.-M.; writing—original draft preparation, M.P.R.-P., M.P.-d.-H.-T. and P.S.-H.-B.; writing—review and editing, P.R.-L.; visualization, G.F.-G.; supervision, E.H.-H.; project administration, E.H.-H. All authors have read and agreed to the published version of the manuscript.

Funding: This research received no external funding.

Institutional Review Board Statement: The study was conducted in accordance with the Declaration of Helsinki and approved by the Ethics Committee University Rey Juan Carlos (Code: 170120210212) for studies involving humans.

Informed Consent Statement: Informed consent was obtained from all subjects involved in the study.

Data Availability Statement: All data are available upon request from the corresponding author.

Acknowledgments: We would like to thank the long COVID and SEMG groups, as well as all the people affected, whose participation, help and collaboration was invaluable for this study.

Conflicts of Interest: The authors declare no conflict of interest.

References

1. Mehandru, S.; Merad, M. Pathological sequelae of long-haul COVID. *Nat. Immunol.* **2022**, *23*, 194–202. [CrossRef] [PubMed]
2. Mahase, E. COVID-19: What Do We Know about "Long COVID"? *BMJ* **2020**, *370*, m2815. [CrossRef] [PubMed]
3. Cirulli, E.T.; Barrett, K.M.S.; Riffle, S.; Bolze, A.; Neveux, I.; Dabe, S.; Grzymski, J.J.; Lu, J.T.; Washington, N.L. Long-Term COVID-19 Symptoms in a Large Unselected Population. *medRxiv* **2020**. [CrossRef]
4. Sadat Larijani, M.; Ashrafian, F.; Bagheri Amiri, F.; Banifazl, M.; Bavand, A.; Karami, A.; Asgari Shokooh, F.; Ramezani, A. Characterization of long COVID-19 manifestations and its associated factors: A prospective cohort study from Iran. *Microb. Pathog.* **2022**, *169*, 105618. [CrossRef] [PubMed]
5. Greenhalgh, T.; Knight, M.; A'Court, C.; Buxton, M.; Husain, L. Management of Post-Acute COVID-19 in Primary Care. *BMJ* **2020**, *370*, m3026. [CrossRef] [PubMed]
6. Yong, S.J. Long COVID or Post-COVID-19 Syndrome: Putative Pathophysiology, Risk Factors, and Treatments. *Infect. Dis.* **2021**, *53*, 737–754. [CrossRef] [PubMed]
7. Guan, W.; Ni, Z.; Hu, Y.; Liang, W.; Ou, C.; He, J.; Liu, L.; Shan, H.; Lei, C.; Hui, D.S.C.; et al. Clinical Characteristics of Coronavirus Disease 2019 in China. *N. Engl. J. Med.* **2020**, *382*, 1708–1720. [CrossRef]
8. Moldofsky, H.; Patcai, J. Chronic Widespread Musculoskeletal Pain, Fatigue, Depression and Disordered Sleep in Chronic Post-SARS Syndrome; a Case-Controlled Study. *BMC Neurol.* **2011**, *11*, 37. [CrossRef]
9. Notarte, K.I.; de Oliveira, M.H.S.; Peligro, P.J.; Velasco, J.V.; Macaranas, I.; Ver, A.T.; Pangilinan, F.C.; Pastrana, A.; Goldrich, N.; Kavteladze, D.; et al. Age, Sex and Previous Comorbidities as Risk Factors Not Associated with SARS-CoV-2 Infection for Long COVID-19: A Systematic Review and Meta-Analysis. *J. Clin. Med.* **2022**, *11*, 7314. [CrossRef]

10. Guo, L.; Lin, J.; Ying, W.; Zheng, C.; Tao, L.; Ying, B.; Cheng, B.; Jin, S.; Hu, B. Correlation Study of Short-Term Mental Health in Patients Discharged After Coronavirus Disease 2019 (COVID-19) Infection without Comorbidities: A Prospective Study. *Neuropsychiatr. Dis. Treat.* **2020**, *16*, 2661–2667. [CrossRef] [PubMed]
11. Klok, F.A.; Boon, G.J.A.M.; Barco, S.; Endres, M.; Geelhoed, J.J.M.; Knauss, S.; Rezek, S.A.; Spruit, M.A.; Vehreschild, J.; Siegerink, B. The Post-COVID-19 Functional Status Scale: A Tool to Measure Functional Status over Time after COVID-19. *Eur. Respir. J.* **2020**, *56*, 2001494. [CrossRef]
12. Carfì, A.; Bernabei, R.; Landi, F. Persistent Symptoms in Patients After Acute COVID-19. *JAMA* **2020**, *324*, 603. [CrossRef] [PubMed]
13. Neufeld, K.J.; Leoutsakos, J.-M.S.; Yan, H.; Lin, S.; Zabinski, J.S.; Dinglas, V.D.; Hosey, M.M.; Parker, A.M.; Hopkins, R.O.; Needham, D.M. Fatigue Symptoms During the First Year Following ARDS. *Chest* **2020**, *158*, 999–1007. [CrossRef] [PubMed]
14. Wagman, P.; Håkansson, C. Introducing the Occupational Balance Questionnaire (OBQ). *Scand. J. Occup. Ther.* **2014**, *21*, 227–231. [CrossRef]
15. Backman, C.L. Occupational Balance: Exploring the Relationships among Daily Occupations and Their Influence on Well-Being. *Can. J. Occup. Ther.* **2004**, *71*, 202–209. [CrossRef]
16. Jandhyala, R. Design, Validation and Implementation of the Post-Acute (Long) COVID-19 Quality of Life (PAC-19QoL) Instrument. *Health Qual. Life Outcomes* **2021**, *19*, 229. [CrossRef] [PubMed]
17. Fernández-de-las-Peñas, C.; Notarte, K.I.; Peligro, P.J.; Velasco, J.V.; Ocampo, M.J.; Henry, B.M.; Arendt-Nielsen, L.; Torres-Macho, J.; Plaza-Manzano, G. Long-COVID Symptoms in Individuals Infected with Different SARS-CoV-2 Variants of Concern: A Systematic Review of the Literature. *Viruses* **2022**, *14*, 2629. [CrossRef] [PubMed]
18. Huang, L.; Yao, Q.; Gu, X.; Wang, Q.; Ren, L.; Wang, Y.; Hu, P.; Guo, L.; Liu, M.; Xu, J.; et al. 1-Year Outcomes in Hospital Survivors with COVID-19: A Longitudinal Cohort Study. *Lancet* **2021**, *398*, 747–758. [CrossRef]
19. Rodríguez-Pérez, M.P.; Sánchez-Herrera-Baeza, P.; Rodríguez-Ledo, P.; Serrada-Tejeda, S.; García-Bravo, C.; Pérez-de-Heredia-Torres, M. Headaches and Dizziness as Disabling, Persistent Symptoms in Patients with Long COVID—A National Multicentre Study. *J. Clin. Med.* **2022**, *11*, 5904. [CrossRef]
20. von Elm, E.; Altman, D.G.; Egger, M.; Pocock, S.J.; Gøtzsche, P.C.; Vandenbroucke, J.P. The Strengthening the Reporting of Observational Studies in Epidemiology (STROBE) Statement: Guidelines for Reporting Observational Studies. *Int. J. Surg.* **2014**, *12*, 1495–1499. [CrossRef]
21. World Medical Association Declaration of Helsinki. *JAMA* **2013**, *310*, 2191. [CrossRef] [PubMed]
22. Graham, E.L.; Clark, J.R.; Orban, Z.S.; Lim, P.H.; Szymanski, A.L.; Taylor, C.; DiBiase, R.M.; Jia, D.T.; Balabanov, R.; Ho, S.U.; et al. Persistent Neurologic Symptoms and Cognitive Dysfunction in Non-hospitalized COVID-19 "Long Haulers". *Ann. Clin. Transl. Neurol.* **2021**, *8*, 1073–1085. [CrossRef] [PubMed]
23. Håkansson, C.; Wagman, P.; Hagell, P. Construct Validity of a Revised Version of the Occupational Balance Questionnaire. *Scand. J. Occup. Ther.* **2020**, *27*, 441–449. [CrossRef]
24. Peral-Gómez, P.; López-Roig, S.; Pastor-Mira, M.Á.; Abad-Navarro, E.; Valera-Gran, D.; Håkansson, C.; Wagman, P. Cultural Adaptation and Psychometric Properties of the Spanish Version of the Occupational Balance Questionnaire: An Instrument for Occupation-Based Research. *Int. J. Environ. Res. Public Health* **2021**, *18*, 7506. [CrossRef]
25. Brazier, J.E.; Harper, R.; Jones, N.M.; O'Cathain, A.; Thomas, K.J.; Usherwood, T.; Westlake, L. Validating the SF-36 Health Survey Questionnaire: New Outcome Measure for Primary Care. *BMJ* **1992**, *305*, 160–164. [CrossRef] [PubMed]
26. Mishra, G.D.; Hockey, R.; Dobson, A.J. A comparison of SF-36 summary measures of physical and mental health for women across the life course. *Qual. Life Res.* **2014**, *23*, 1515–1521. [CrossRef]
27. Ware, J.E., Jr.; Kosinski, M.; Keller, S.D. *SF-36 Physical and Mental Health Summary Scales: A Manual for Users of Version 1*, 2nd ed.; Quality Metric Incorporated: Lincoln, RI, USA, 2005.
28. Alonso, J.; Prieto, L.; Antó, J.M. Adaptación Versión Española de SF-36v2TM Health Survey©. *Med. Clin.* **1995**, *104*, 771–776.
29. Arnold, D.T.; Hamilton, F.W.; Milne, A.; Morley, A.J.; Viner, J.; Attwood, M.; Noel, A.; Gunning, S.; Hatrick, J.; Hamilton, S.; et al. Patient Outcomes after Hospitalisation with COVID-19 and Implications for Follow-up: Results from a Prospective UK Cohort. *Thorax* **2021**, *76*, 399–401. [CrossRef]
30. Taft, C.; Karlsson, J.; Sullivan, M. Do SF-36 summary component scores accurately summarize subscale scores? *Qual. Life Res.* **2001**, *10*, 395–404. [CrossRef]
31. Mills, S.D.; Fox, R.S.; Bohan, S.; Roesch, S.C.; Sadler, G.R.; Malcarne, V.L. Psychosocial and Neighborhood Correlates of Health-Related Quality of Life: A Multi-Level Study among Hispanic Adults. *Cult. Divers. Ethn. Minor Psychol.* **2020**, *26*, 1–10. [CrossRef]
32. Fernández-de-las-Peñas, C.; Palacios-Ceña, D.; Gómez-Mayordomo, V.; Florencio, L.L.; Cuadrado, M.L.; Plaza-Manzano, G.; Navarro-Santana, M. Prevalence of post-COVID-19 symptoms in hospitalized and non-hospitalized COVID-19 survivors: A systematic review and meta-analysis. *Eur. J. Intern. Med.* **2021**, *92*, 55–70. [CrossRef] [PubMed]
33. Garrigues, E.; Janvier, P.; Kherabi, Y.; le Bot, A.; Hamon, A.; Gouze, H.; Doucet, L.; Berkani, S.; Oliosi, E.; Mallart, E.; et al. Post-Discharge Persistent Symptoms and Health-Related Quality of Life after Hospitalization for COVID-19. *J. Infect.* **2020**, *81*, e4–e6. [CrossRef] [PubMed]
34. Chen, K.-Y.; Li, T.; Gong, F.-H.; Zhang, J.-S.; Li, X.-K. Predictors of Health-Related Quality of Life and Influencing Factors for COVID-19 Patients, a Follow-Up at One Month. *Front. Psychiatry* **2020**, *11*, 668. [CrossRef] [PubMed]

35. Poudel, A.N.; Zhu, S.; Cooper, N.; Roderick, P.; Alwan, N.; Tarrant, C.; Ziauddeen, N.; Yao, G.L. Impact of COVID-19 on Health-Related Quality of Life of Patients: A Structured Review. *PLoS ONE* **2021**, *16*, e0259164. [CrossRef] [PubMed]
36. Meys, R.; Delbressine, J.M.; Goërtz, Y.M.J.; Vaes, A.W.; Machado, F.V.C.; van Herck, M.; Burtin, C.; Posthuma, R.; Spaetgens, B.; Franssen, F.M.E.; et al. Generic and Respiratory-Specific Quality of Life in Non-Hospitalized Patients with COVID-19. *J. Clin. Med.* **2020**, *9*, 3993. [CrossRef]
37. Håkansson, C.; Lissner, L.; Björkelund, C.; Sonn, U. Engagement in Patterns of Daily Occupations and Perceived Health among Women of Working Age. *Scand. J. Occup. Ther.* **2009**, *16*, 110–117. [CrossRef]
38. Meseguer de Pedro, M.; Fernández-Valera, M.M.; García-Izquierdo, M.; Soler Sánchez, M.I. Burnout, Psychological Capital and Health during COVID-19 Social Isolation: A Longitudinal Analysis. *Int. J. Environ. Res. Public Health* **2021**, *18*, 1064. [CrossRef]
39. Park, S.; Lee, H.J.; Jeon, B.-J.; Yoo, E.-Y.; Kim, J.-B.; Park, J.-H. Effects of Occupational Balance on Subjective Health, Quality of Life, and Health-Related Variables in Community-Dwelling Older Adults: A Structural Equation Modeling Approach. *PLoS ONE* **2021**, *16*, e0246887. [CrossRef] [PubMed]
40. Belhan Çelik, S.; Özkan, E.; Bumin, G. Effects of Occupational Therapy via Telerehabilitation on Occupational Balance, Well-Being, Intrinsic Motivation and Quality of Life in Syrian Refugee Children in COVID-19 Lockdown: A Randomized Controlled Trial. *Children* **2022**, *9*, 485. [CrossRef] [PubMed]
41. Ganesan, B.; Fong, K.N.K.; Meena, S.K.; Prasad, P.; Tong, R.K.Y. Impact of COVID-19 Pandemic Lockdown on Occupational Therapy Practice and Use of Telerehabilitation—A Cross Sectional Study. *Eur. Rev. Med. Pharmacol.* **2021**, *25*, 3614–3622.
42. Fridman, A.; Gershon, R.; Gneezy, A. COVID-19 and Vaccine Hesitancy: A Longitudinal Study. *PLoS ONE* **2021**, *16*, e0250123. [CrossRef] [PubMed]
43. Hay, J.W.; Gong, C.L.; Jiao, X.; Zawadzki, N.K.; Zawadzki, R.S.; Pickard, A.S.; Xie, F.; Crawford, S.A.; Gu, N.Y. A US Population Health Survey on the Impact of COVID-19 Using the EQ-5D-5L. *J. Gen. Intern. Med.* **2021**, *36*, 1292–1301. [CrossRef] [PubMed]

Disclaimer/Publisher's Note: The statements, opinions and data contained in all publications are solely those of the individual author(s) and contributor(s) and not of MDPI and/or the editor(s). MDPI and/or the editor(s) disclaim responsibility for any injury to people or property resulting from any ideas, methods, instructions or products referred to in the content.

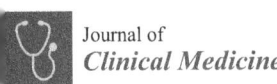

Article

Immediate and Long-Term Effects of Hyperbaric Oxygenation in Patients with Long COVID-19 Syndrome Using SF-36 Survey and VAS Score: A Clinical Pilot Study

Joerg Lindenmann [1,*], Christian Porubsky [1], Lucija Okresa [1], Huberta Klemen [1], Iurii Mykoliuk [1], Andrej Roj [1], Amir Koutp [1], Eveline Kink [2], Florian Iberer [2], Gabor Kovacs [3,4], Robert Krause [5], Josef Smolle [6] and Freyja Maria Smolle-Juettner [1]

1. Division of Thoracic Surgery and Hyperbaric Surgery, Department of Surgery, Medical University of Graz, 8036 Graz, Austria
2. Department of Internal and Respiratory Medicine, Hospital Graz II, Academic Teaching Hospital of the Medical University of Graz, 8036 Graz, Austria
3. Ludwig Boltzmann Institute for Lung Vascular Research, Medical University of Graz, 8036 Graz, Austria
4. Division of Pulmonology, Department of Internal Medicine, Medical University of Graz, 8036 Graz, Austria
5. Division of Infectious Diseases, Department of Internal Medicine, Medical University of Graz, 8036 Graz, Austria
6. Institute of Medical Informatics, Statistics and Documentation, Medical University of Graz, 8036 Graz, Austria
* Correspondence: jo.lindenmann@medunigraz.at; Tel.: +43-316-385-13302; Fax: +43-316-385-14679

Abstract: (1) Background: Long COVID syndrome (LCS) is a heterogeneous long-standing condition following COVID-19 infection. Treatment options are limited to symptomatic measures, and no specific medication has been established. Hyperbaric oxygenation (HBO) has been found to have a positive impact on the treatment of COVID-19 infection. This study evaluates both the feasibility and outcome of supportive HBO in patients with LCS. (2) Methods: Within 17 months, 70 patients with proven LCS were prospectively included. Each patient underwent a cycle of 10 subsequent HBO treatment sessions administered for 75 min at 2.2 atmospheres. Evaluation of the patients was performed before the first and after the last HBO session and 3 months afterwards. Statistical evaluation was based on an intention-to-treat analysis using Fisher's exact test and Student's t-test for paired samples. (3) Results: In total, 59 patients (33 females, 26 males; mean age: 43.9 years; range: 23–74 years; median: 45.0) were evaluable. After HBO, a statistically significant improvement of physical functioning ($p < 0.001$), physical role ($p = 0.01$), energy ($p < 0.001$), emotional well-being ($p < 0.001$), social functioning ($p < 0.001$), pain ($p = 0.01$) and reduced limitation of activities ($p < 0.001$) was confirmed. (4) Conclusions: Physical functioning and both the physical and emotional role improved significantly and sustainably, suggesting HBO as a promising supportive therapeutic tool for the treatment of LCS.

Keywords: long COVID; hyperbaric oxygenation; long-term effect; improvement; physical function; pain; fatigue; energy; general perception of health

1. Introduction

1.1. Background

Long COVID syndrome (LCS), also called post-COVID-19 syndrome or long-haul coronavirus disease 2019 (COVID-19) [1], is a heterogenous condition affecting patients following COVID-19 infections.

Though a variety of defining criteria have been proposed, the most common description is symptoms extending for more than 12 weeks beyond the initial COVID-19 infection [1]. Among individuals with LCS 3 months after symptomatic severe acute respiratory syndrome coronavirus type 2 (SARS-CoV-2) infection, an estimated 15.1% continued to experience symptoms at 12 months [2].

LCS evolves either directly from the initial COVID-19 infection or develops after a symptom-free interval and affects patients regardless of the severity of the COVID-19 disease. Though LCS is predominantly found in younger, female individuals, it relates to all age groups and both sexes. The array of symptoms varies individually and derives from three LCS symptom clusters: (a) persistent fatigue, mood swings, body pain; (b) cognitive impairment; and (c) ongoing respiratory problems [2]. The dimension of the problem is considerable. Wulf-Hanson et al. reviewed reports of 1.2 million formerly symptomatic COVID-19 patients. They estimated that at least 6.2% of them experienced at least one out of the three LCS symptom clusters [2].

Physical symptoms relating to the cardiorespiratory system are common and, in many cases, they persist despite normal objective parameters [2]. In addition, mental disorders, headaches, smell and taste dysfunction, hair loss, insomnia, rhinorrhea and gastrointestinal issues are frequently experienced in LCS. In some cases, the condition is highly debilitating, resulting in an inability to return to work or even perform household chores [3], not only because of the physical symptoms but also due to the psychic impact of LCS [4].

Treatment options are currently limited to symptomatic measures including physical rehabilitation, and support by mental and social services alongside monitoring of symptoms. Since there is insufficient understanding of the mechanisms underlying LCS, no specific medication has been established yet [3,5].

Hyperbaric oxygenation (HBO) denotes the inhalation of 100% oxygen at pressures exceeding one atmosphere absolute, thus enhancing the amount of oxygen dissolved in the body tissues. During HBO, the arterial oxygen (O_2) tension typically exceeds 100 mmHg.

Depending on the pressure applied, arterial O_2 tension reaches 1300 to 2000 mmHg, equaling 200–400 mmHg in tissues. Even though many of the beneficial effects of HBO can be explained by the improvement of tissue oxygenation, it is now understood that the combined action of hyperoxia and hyperbaric pressure triggers both oxygen- and pressure-sensitive genes, resulting in inducing regenerative processes. These include stem cell proliferation and mobilization, enhancement of anti-apoptotic and anti-inflammatory factors, and downregulation of inflammatory cascades [6].

For acute COVID-19 infection, there are anecdotal reports about compassionate use [7,8] and first prospective studies [9,10] of HBO, showing accelerated improvement of hypoxemia but no effect on mortality. Based on an unadjusted meta-analysis of data from 36 cases, Jansen et al. concluded that HBO might add therapeutic benefits in treating COVID-19 induced hypoxia as an adjunct to standard care [11].

The short existence of COVID-19 and of LCS notwithstanding, there are already a few reports about the successful application of HBO to post-COVID-19 syndrome. Bhaiat et al. published a case of successful HBO treatment of LCS in a former athlete who dramatically improved cognition deficits and cardiopulmonary function as documented by elaborate pre- and post-treatment workup, including spiro-ergometry and functional magnetic resonance imaging (MRI) [12].

The six LCS patients treated by Zant et al. suffered predominantly from muscle pain, joint pain, and dyspnea. Five out of six experienced improvements to pre-infection levels whilst the remaining patient reported significant relief [13].

Robbins et al. treated 10 consecutive patients in 10 sessions of HBO at 2.4 atmospheres over 12 days, focusing on fatigue and cognitive impairments. HBO yielded a statistically significant improvement of fatigue, global cognition, executive function, attention, information processing and verbal function [14].

Turova et al. performed a prospective, observational trial on HBO as an adjunctive measure in 45 patients participating in an outpatient rehabilitation program for LCS. They found the use of HBO beneficial in terms of improvement of functional and laboratory parameters [15].

Recently, in a large, prospectively randomized study, Zilberman et al. described the improvement of neuropsychological and neurocognitive symptoms in LCS [16] and the same group analyzed the neuro-structural background of the HBO action on LCS [17].

Based on the encouraging results mentioned above, we initiated an opportunistic and exploratory study on HBO in LCS focusing on both feasibility and outcome according to self-reporting by patients with symptoms from all three LCS clusters.

1.2. Hypothesis and Objectives

The overall hypothesis to be evaluated is that HBO is a safe and feasible treatment to alleviate symptoms associated with LCS.

The primary objective is to evaluate if HBO improves physical functioning, physical role, energy, emotional role, emotional well-being, social functioning, pain, general perception of health and limitation of activities.

The secondary objective is to evaluate if HBO has a beneficial impact on blood pressure, heart rate and peripheral oxygen saturation.

2. Materials and Methods

2.1. Study Design

This clinical, prospective, observational single-center pilot study was approved by the Local Institutional Review Board of the Medical University of Graz (No. 33-308 ex 20/21). Written informed consent was obtained from each patient before participation in the study. The study was conducted in accordance with the Declaration of Helsinki and according to good clinical practice.

2.2. Patient Characteristics

Seventy patients aged between 18 and 90 years with proven LCS were enrolled in the study between April 2021 and August 2022. All of them had had COVID-19 infection proven by a polymerase chain reaction (PCR)-test and an at least 3 months' history of a minimum of two typical symptoms such as fatigue, dyspnea, dizziness, muscle weakness, insomnia, joint pain, myalgia or headache.

Patients with active malignancy, chest pathology incompatible with pressure changes such as pulmonary emphysema or moderate to severe asthma and pathological findings on electrocardiogram (ECG), spirometry, ear, or sinus pathology incompatible with pressure changes, pregnant or breast-feeding patients and those who had been administered HBO due to other reasons were excluded from the study. Patients unable to give informed consent and those with an active phase of COVID-19 infection were not included in the present study.

2.3. HBO Treatment

HBO treatment was carried out on an outpatient basis in a large walk-in, drive-in hyperbaric chamber. Each patient underwent a cycle of 10 subsequent HBO treatment sessions. HBO sessions were carried five times a week with a weekend break (two series of five compressions were performed). Each session lasted 75 min for a scheduled total time of 12 h and 30 min per patient. HBO was administered at a pressure of 2.2 atmospheres using medical oxygen. During compression the patients breathed 100% oxygen.

2.4. Patient Evaluation

Patient evaluation was carried out at three defined time points: immediately before HBO, immediately after the 10th HBO session and after 3 months.

These three evaluations were conducted in the same structured manner during the forenoon and consisted of the collection of both the patient's circulation parameters and the data from self-reporting questionnaires about their health-related quality of life (HRQoL).

Among the patient´s circulation parameters, measurement of the blood pressure and the heart rate using a standardized electronic blood pressure meter was carried out. Measurement of the peripheral oxygen saturation was performed using a standardized pulse oximeter finger device.

With regard to their quality of life, the patients were asked to fill in the Short-Form-36 questionnaire (SF-36) and the visual analog scale (VAS).

The SF-36 survey is a widely used standardized questionnaire consisting of 36 self-reported items that are grouped into 8 dimensions [18]. These eight dimensions (physical functioning; physical role; energy; emotional role; emotional well-being; social functioning; pain; general perception of health) were used as main outcome measures in our exploratory analysis. In addition, the SF-36 questionnaire comprises a list of 38 everyday activities, where patients have to judge whether they were limited in performing these activities. The question proposed for the visual analogue scale was "How would you rank your present health and fitness by using this scale?", where the scale extended across a distance of 100 mm. The mark set by the patient was measured with a ruler and recorded as mm from 0, where 0 indicated the worst case and 100 the best case [19–21].

The VAS has been widely used in medical research for several decades, especially for the measurement of pain. This numeric score describes the patients' general perception of the severity of the disease on a 10-piece scale, with 10 indicating the highest severity [22].

2.5. Statistical Analysis

Descriptive statistics included mean, standard deviation, range and absolute and relative frequency where appropriate. For statistical analysis of pre- and post-treatment values, we used Student's *t*-test for paired samples and—when there was no normal distribution—the Wilcoxon matched pairs signed rank test. Testing for normality was performed using the Shapiro–Wilk test. Since it is an exploratory study, we did not apply any correction for multiple comparisons. As far as multiple independent variables were concerned, however, we applied a multivariable statistical test. The evaluation was based on an intention-to-treat analysis.

Regarding power analysis using G*Power [23], a sample size of 45 cases is large enough to detect an effect size of 0.5 between pre- and post-treatment values with alpha = 0.05 and power (1-beta) = 0.95.

In addition, we used stepwise multivariable regression analysis. As independent parameters, we included age, sex, respiratory support during the acute COVID-19 episode, comorbidity of any type, diabetes, hypertension, body mass index and time between onset of the acute disease and the implementation of HBO therapy. We tested the relationship of these independent variables for each of the dependent variables. These were systolic and diastolic blood pressure, heart rate, O2 saturation, the eight dimensions of the SF-36 questionnaire, limitations in 38 different activities, and the results of the visual analogue scale. For each dependent variable, the difference between the values after HBO and the values before HBO were used. A negative difference indicates improvement, and a positive difference indicates worsening of the particular parameter. $p < 0.05$ was considered to indicate statistical significance.

3. Results

3.1. Study Population

After the dropout of 11 patients (9 due to non-compliance, 1 because of barotrauma to the middle ear and 1 because of an anxiety attack during treatment) 59 patients (33 females, 26 males; mean age: 43.9 years; range: 23–74 years; median: 45.0) were evaluable for the study and had the planned number of HBO sessions. Thirty-seven patients wished to continue the HBO treatment beyond the 10th session due to subjective improvement of symptoms. They had a varying number of further HBO sessions and were excluded from the statistical evaluation beyond this time point. Out of the 22 remaining patients, 18 entered the final evaluation at 3 months, whilst 4 declined to show up for the investigation (Figure 1).

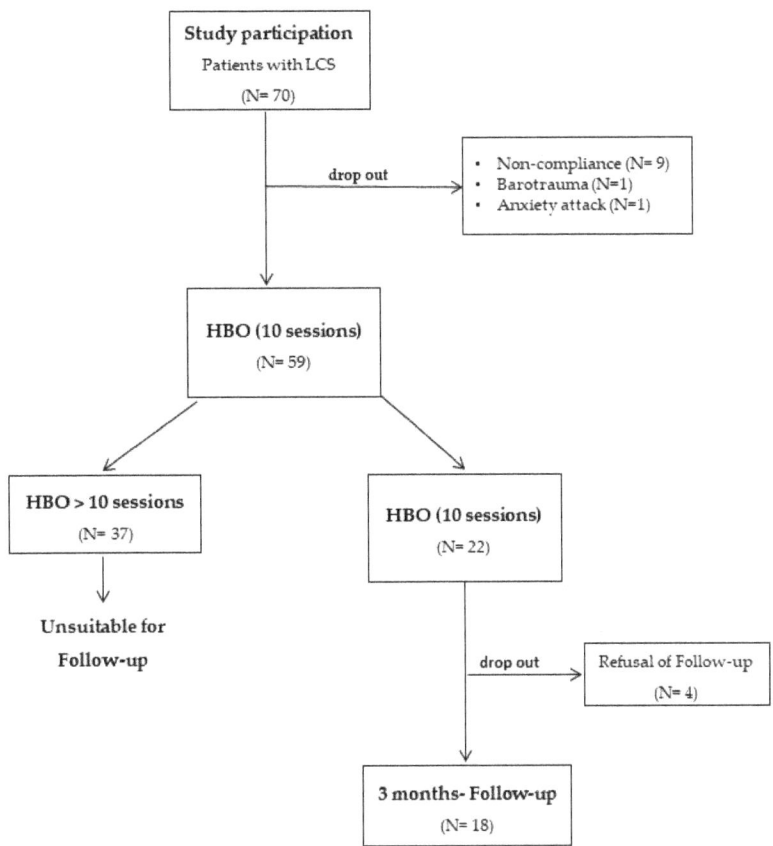

Figure 1. Study flow chart. Abbreviations: LCS: long COVID syndrome; HBO: hyperbaric oxygenation.

3.2. Severity of COVID-19 Infection

Fifty-three patients had had mild COVID-19 symptoms treated at home, and two had been hospitalized for medication and oxygen administration via a facemask. Four patients had required intensive care unit (ICU) treatment with intubation in one and tracheotomy in three of them. In stepwise multivariable regression analysis, the severity of the initial COVID-19 infection, as indicated by the requirement of oxygen or respiratory support measures, showed a more pronounced reduction of systolic blood pressure (t = −2.17, $p = 0.03$) and of pain (t = −2.76, $p = 0.01$) during the course of HBO therapy. The degree of improvement of all other parameters was not affected by the severity of the acute COVID-19 disease. The time between onset of acute COVID-19 and implementation of HBO therapy did not influence the degree of improvement of any of the outcome parameters.

3.3. Biometrical Data and Co-Morbidity

Mean body mass index (BMI) at the time of admission to the study was 25.3 (range: 18.6–38.2). Forty-one patients (69.4%) had some type of comorbidity with hypercholesterinemia (N = 21; 35.5%), found most frequently followed by hypertension (N = 20; 33.9%), obesity (N = 14; 23.7%) diabetes (N = 3; 5.0%) or coronary heart disease (N = 2; 3.3%). Twenty-five patients (42.3%) had further relevant preexisting disease such as allergic asthma, depression, disorders of the thyroid, or migraines. Neither age, sex nor co-morbidities had any statistically significant influence on the effect of HBO treatment measured by the outcome parameters. Only a high BMI slightly reduced the HBO treatment effect on the number of impaired activities (t = 2.04, $p = 0.05$). The two subgroups (those treated on schedule and those who continued HBO beyond 10 sessions) did not show any statistically significant differences concerning sex, age, biometrical data and co-morbidity.

3.4. Collective of Patients Finishing HBO Treatment (10 Sessions) without Follow-Up

Among these 59 patients, a slight, but statistically not significant decrease of the mean blood pressure was observed, whereas the mean heart rate decreased significantly ($p = 0.03$). Mean peripheral oxygen saturation remained nearly unchanged.

Physical functioning improved significantly ($p < 0.001$) after treatment and so did the physical role ($p = 0.01$). The same was true for social functioning, which improved significantly ($p < 0.001$). The limitation of activities according to SF-36 also decreased significantly after treatment ($p < 0.001$). Patients felt significant improvement also for energy ($p < 0.001$), emotional well-being ($p < 0.001$) and pain ($p = 0.01$). Improvement that failed to reach statistical level of significance was found for emotional role ($p = 0.26$) and general perception of health ($p = 0.07$).

The mean pre-therapeutic VAS score describing the patients' general perception of the severity of their actual disease was $5.85 +/- 2.01$ on a 10-piece scale, with 10 indicating the highest severity. After HBO, the score decreased significantly to $3.79 +/- 2.11$ ($p < 0.001$).

The details are given in Table 1.

Table 1. Circulation parameters, peripheral oxygen saturation and data from self-assessment; pairwise comparison of pre- and post-treatment data. Total collective that finished 10 HBO treatment sessions.

	Pre-HBO (N = 59)	Post-HBO (N = 59)	p Compared with Pre
Mean systolic blood pressure (mm Hg)	131.9 +/− 20.0	130.6 +/− 15.8	0.46
Mean diastolic blood pressure (mm Hg)	81.3 +/− 12.1	79.3 +/− 10.2	0.09
Mean heart rate (bpm)	80.3 +/− 12.9	76.8 +/− 11.4	**0.03**
Peripheral oxygen saturation (%)	96.0 +/− 1.5	96.2 +/− 1.5	0.35
Physical functioning	43.9 +/− 24.6	52.4 +/− 24.6	**<0.001**
Physical role	10 +/− 27.4	16.8 +/− 30.4	**0.01 (0.02)**
Energy	22.3 +/− 20.2	30.4 +/− 20.4	**<0.001 (<0.001)**
Emotional role	45.0 +/− 48.1	51.2 +/− 46.5	0.26
Emotional well-being	54.0 +/− 18.5	64.0 +/− 18	**<0.001**
Social functioning	32.6 +/− 26.6	43.7 +/− 25.9	**<0.001**
Pain	42.7 +/− 25.0	50.1 +/− 22.1	**0.01**
General perception of health	39.5 +/− 16.8	42.9 +/− 16.3	0.07
Limitation of activities	12.8 +/− 5.5	9.4 +/− 7.9	**<0.001**
VAS score	5.85 +/− 2.01	3.79 +/− 2.11	**<0.001**

t-test for paired samples; p values in parenthesis were calculated using the Wilcoxon matched pairs signed rank test. Abbreviations: HBO: hyperbaric oxygenation; mmHg: millimeters of mercury; bpm: beats per minute; %: percent; VAS: visual analog scale.

3.5. Collective of Patients Finishing HBO Treatment (10 Sessions) without Follow-Up

Among these 22 patients, the circulation parameters changed but without reaching statistical significance. The mean systolic blood pressure slightly decreased, whereas the mean diastolic blood pressure nearly remained unchanged. Mean heart rate and mean peripheral oxygen saturation slightly decreased.

Physical functioning ($p < 0.001$), energy ($p = 0.02$), social functioning ($p = 0.02$) and limitation of activities ($p < 0.001$) improved significantly after 10 sessions. All other parameters ascertained by the SF-36 survey also showed an improvement after HBO treatment but without statistical significance.

The mean VAS score reported pre-treatment decreased significantly from 5.5 to 3.3 ($p < 0.001$).

The details are presented in Table 2.

Table 2. Circulation parameters, peripheral oxygen saturation and data from self-assessment; pairwise comparison of pre-treatment data, post-treatment data after 10 HBO sessions and data after 3 months.

	Pre-HBO (N = 22)	Post-HBO (N = 22)	p Compared with Pre	Pre-HBO (N = 18)	After 3 Months (N = 18)	p Compared with Pre
Mean systolic blood pressure (mm Hg)	135.3 +/− 23.8	131.5 +/− 15.6	0.25	141.4 +/− 24.1	131.3 +/− 11.8	0.06
Mean diastolic blood pressure (mm Hg)	82.8 +/− 10.9	82.5 +/− 10.3	0.79	86.1 +/− 10.9	81.4 +/− 8.9	0.09
Mean heart rate (bpm)	82.2 +/− 12.7	80.7 +/− 12.4	0.47	81.9 +/− 13.0	80.1 +/− 10.4	0.45
Peripheral oxygen saturation (%)	96.0 +/− 1.4	95.7 +/− 1.5	0.38	96.1 +/− 1.7	96.7 +/− 1.7	0.41
Physical functioning	46.8 +/− 25.6	57.3 +/− 26.4	**<0.001**	44.1 +/− 26.7	58.3 +/− 24.7	**<0.001**
Physical role	14.4 +/− 32.6	21.0 +/− 35.6	0.14 (0.25)	16.1 +/− 34.7	30.9 +/− 41.9	0.07 (0.13)
Energy	26.8 +/− 25.1	36.5 +/− 20.9	**0.02 (0.01)**	30.8 +/− 26.0	38.0 +/− 25.9	0.15 (0.13)
Emotional role	41.6 +/− 48.2	50 +/− 48.9	0.06	42.6 +/− 49.6	50.0 +/− 46.1	0.16
Emotional well-being	54.1 +/− 22.4	61.4 +/− 21.1	0.07	58.3 +/− 46.7	64.4 +/− 24.5	0.09
Social functioning	38.1 +/− 31.2	48.1 +/− 29.3	**0.02**	39.6 +/− 32.7	60.4 +/− 32.4	**<0.001**
Pain	49.3 +/− 28.1	53.5 +/− 24.0	0.42	52.9 +/− 28.2	58.2 +/− 30.2	0.17
General perception of health	38.3 +/− 20.7	42.7 +/− 20.3	0.17	43.2 +/− 19.6	46.2 +/− 23.9	0.49
Limitation of activities	13.0 +/− 6.9	9.2 +/− 5.7	**<0.001**	12.2 +/− 7.1	9.2 +/− 6.8	**0.02**
VAS score	5.5 +/− 2.3	3.3 +/− 2.4	**<0.001**	5.2 +/− 2.3	2.6 +/− 1.9	**<0.001**

t-test for paired values; p-values in parenthesis were calculated using the Wilcoxon matched pairs signed rank test. Abbreviations: HBO: hyperbaric oxygenation; mmHg: millimeters of mercury; bpm: beats per minute; %: percent; VAS: visual analog scale.

3.6. Collective of Patients Finishing HBO Treatment (10 Sessions) with Follow-Up

Among these 18 patients, mean systolic blood pressure, mean diastolic blood pressure and mean heart rate continued to decrease after 3 months compared to pre-HBO values. The mean peripheral oxygen saturation slightly increased, but none of these changes showed statistical significance at long-term follow-up.

Among the ascertained SF-36 parameters, physical functioning ($p = 0.05$), social functioning ($p < 0.001$) and limitation of activities ($p = 0.02$) improved even after 3 months as compared to their pre-HBO values, reaching statistical significance. The other SF-36-related parameters also showed an improvement after HBO treatment but without statistical significance.

Regarding the mean VAS, the change from the pre-treatment 5.2 to 2.6 post-treatment was still significant even after 3 months ($p < 0.001$).

The details are given in Table 2.

3.7. Collective of Patients Exceeding 10 HBO Sessions without Follow-Up

Among these 37 patients, the pre-treatment mean systolic blood pressure was slightly elevated and the mean diastolic pressure decreased slightly, but both without statistical significance. The mean heart rate decreased significantly ($p = 0.04$), whereas mean peripheral oxygen saturation remained nearly unchanged within the normal range.

Physical functioning improved significantly after 10 HBO sessions ($p < 0.001$). Physical role improved significantly ($p = 0.05$). The same was true for energy ($p < 0.001$), emotional well-being ($p < 0.001$), social functioning ($p < 0.001$) and limitation of activities ($p < 0.001$). All further SF-36 parameters also improved, yet without reaching statistical significance.

The mean VAS score improved statistically significantly from 6.06 +/− 1.84 to 4.08 +/− 1.9 ($p < 0.001$).

The details are given in Table 3.

Table 3. Circulation parameters, peripheral oxygen saturation and data from self-assessment; pair-wise comparison of pre- and post-treatment data. Collective non-eligible for 3-months evaluation due to continuation of HBO beyond 10 treatment sessions.

	Pre-HBO (N = 37)	Post-HBO (N = 37)	p Compared with Pre
Mean systolic blood pressure (mm Hg)	129.9 +/− 17.3	130.1 +/− 16.1	0.94
Mean diastolic blood pressure (mm Hg)	80.4 +/− 12.8	77.4 +/− 9.8	0.08
Mean heart rate (bpm)	79.2 +/− 13.1	74.4 +/− 10.2	**0.04**
Peripheral oxygen saturation (%)	96.1 +/− 1.5	96.6 +/− 1.5	0.09
Physical functioning	42.2 +/− 24.2	49.5 +/− 23.3	**<0.001**
Physical role	7.6 +/− 24.5	14.6 +/− 27.6	**0.05** (0.05)
Energy	19.8 +/− 16.8	27.1 +/− 19.7	**<0.001** (<0.001)
Emotional role	47.0 +/− 48.6	51.9 +/− 45.8	0.56
Emotional well-being	54.0 +/− 16.3	65.6 +/− 15.9	**<0.001**
Social functioning	29.4 +/− 23.4	41.2 +/− 23.7	**<0.001**
Pain	38.9 +/− 22.6	48.2 +/− 21.1	**<0.001**
General perception of health	40.1 +/− 14.7	43 +/− 14.1	0.22
Limitation of activities	12.6 +/− 4.6	9.6 +/− 5.7	**<0.001**
VAS score	6.06 +/− 1.84	4.08 +/− 1.9	**<0.001**

t-test for paired values; *p*-values in parenthesis were calculated using the Wilcoxon matched pairs signed rank test. Abbreviations: HBO: hyperbaric oxygenation; mmHg: millimeters of mercury; bpm: beats per minute; %: percent; VAS: visual analog scale.

3.8. Side Effects

Three patients experienced problems in pressurization of the middle ear, which were overcome by decongestant nose drops in one case and insertion of a vent tube in the eardrum in the second case. The third patient declined eardrum venting and had to discontinue the treatment. Another patient experienced an anxiety attack during treatment, which also led to discontinuation. There were neither acute nor prolonged side effects of HBO.

4. Discussion

This clinical prospective, observational pilot study demonstrates that HBO may provide a safe and feasible therapeutic tool for mitigation of LCS-related symptoms in both the short-term and long-term follow-up. After 10 HBO treatment sessions, a statistically significant improvement in 80% of the ascertained items of the SF-36 survey together with a significant decrement of the VAS were obtained immediately. Even after 3 months, the statistically significant improvement in physical and social functioning and the reduction of limitations persisted. The subjective perception of the severity of disease mirrored by the VAS also remained significantly decreased.

HBO has been applied for decades for various indications requiring tissue repair in the broadest sense. They cover a wide range of acute and chronic diseases from ischemia-reperfusion injury to impaired wound healing, radiation-induced tissue damage and central nervous injury [24]. Since the turn of the millennium, the underlying mechanisms have gradually been elucidated. HBO affects various molecular pathways including transcription, vascular signaling and the response to oxidative stress. In addition, structural cellular components involved in angiogenesis, epithelization or collagen formation, cell-to-cell contacts, adhesion and transmigration are modified. The regulatory effects of HBO on apoptosis, autophagy, and cell death are further assets in regenerative processes. Additionally, HBO is a potent regulatory effector of inflammatory mechanisms [6].

There are numerous hypotheses about the causes of LCS. Although some findings indicate that LCS may result from prolonged organ damage mainly due to hypoxemia and coagulation disorders during the acute infection, specific processes following initial COVID-19 could trigger immune dysregulation, autoimmunity phenomena and endothelial dysfunction [5]. It is also plausible that neuronal damage, inflammation, or disturbance of transcription processes caused by occult viral persistence may play a role in this multisystem disease.

With regard to the neurophysiological characteristics of LCS, sub-optimal executive function associated with increased fatigue related to significantly reduced intracortical neurotransmission was confirmed [25]. These finding were corroborated by Ortelli and colleagues. They showed that patients with fatigue and cognitive disorders after COVID-19 infection presented altered excitability and neurotransmission with deficits in executive functions and attention [26]. Significant cerebral hypoperfusion affecting the frontal, parietal and temporal cortex leading to cognitive complaints could be detected as another causative in LCS [27]. These findings correlate with proven intracerebral hypometabolism verified by Positron emission tomography (PET). The affected cerebral regions ranged from the olfactory gyrus and connected (para-)limbic regions to the cerebellum and the brain steam and resulted in significantly increased functional complaints and clinical symptoms, i.e., hyposmia/anosmia, cognitive impairment, pain and insomnia [28].

In this context, HBO was shown to increase brain perfusion in the insula, hippocampus, putamen, and prefrontal and cingulate cortex. A further feature of HBO is its potential for stem-cell mobilization, neuro-regeneration and induction of neuroplasticity, which may mitigate neurological symptoms in LCS [16]. Based on these mechanisms, HBO can improve physical, neurocognitive and psychiatric symptoms related to LCS [29]. We could confirm these findings in the present study. After 10 HBO treatment sessions, we found immediate significant improvement of physical functioning, physical role, energy, emotional well-being, social functioning, and pain as well as significantly reduced limitation of activities as reported according to the SF-36 questionnaire. The subjective perception of the severity of disease mirrored by the VAS improved significantly, as displayed in Table 1.

Though patients with LCS may display objective pathological findings [29–31], many cases with pronounced symptoms show normal function tests, laboratory parameters and imaging. Authors have therefore suggested including LCS in the "unexplained post-infection syndromes" [32]. Accordingly, none of our patients had abnormal circulation parameters. Blood pressure, heart rate and peripheral oxygen saturation were within normal range, as displayed in Tables 1–3.

In consideration of this astonishing discrepancy between proven organ damage and inconspicuous function tests, the effectiveness of treatment in LCS is difficult to assess. Many patients are unable to describe their symptoms distinctly, though they do perceive them as severely debilitating. Fatigue is a common finding and so are memory issues, brain fog, attention disorder and sleep disturbance. Secondary anxiety and even psychiatric manifestations such as depression [33] contribute to subjective aggravation of symptoms. Because of the inherent vagueness of symptom descriptions by the patients, we solely relied on the self-reporting SF-36 survey [18–21] and on the 10-piece VAS [22] for evaluation of treatment effects. In this context, the methodology of the current study is in accordance with other authors who also used the SF-36 survey [16] and other standardized self-reporting questionnaires to assess the patient´s quality of life [13,14,17,21,29,33].

Of note, pain in LCS is refractory to most analgetic treatments [34] and to some degree resembles fibromyalgia, a central sensitization syndrome. The positive impact of HBO on pain, as shown in our study, resembles the effect of HBO on fibromyalgia as demonstrated by various authors [35,36]. As in our investigation, Zant et al. [13] and Zilberman et al. [16] reported significant pain relief in LCS. We could corroborate this findings in the current study. After HBO, a significant relief of pain according to the SF-36 survey and a significant decrease of the VAS could be confirmed, as shown in Tables 1–3. Due to these HBO-induced analgetic effects, 37/59 patients (63%) insisted on continuing the HBO treatment exceeding the scheduled 10 sessions, leaving only 18 patients evaluable for long-term assessment after 3 months, as shown in Figure 1.

To preclude differences in treatment response between the group that continued HBO and the one that adhered to the scheduled 10 sessions, we evaluated not only the total collective but also both groups separately. After 10 HBO treatments, the 37 patients who insisted on continuing HBO showed a statistically significant response for heart rate, and otherwise the same significant responses for SF-36 parameters and VAS as the total collective. By contrast, at the same time point, the 18 patients who finished HBO according to schedule displayed no statistically significant effect on heart rate, physical role, emotional well-being and pain, whereas the other positive effects of HBO as found in the total collective were present. Thus, the group that continued HBO had improvement in nine categories, whereas the "on-schedule" patients improved in only five categories.

The subjective impression of pronounced improvement that triggered the wish for continuation of treatment in the former group is confirmed by these data. Since there were no differences in the baseline criteria such as age, sex, biometrical data, severity of COVID-19 infection, or duration of symptoms, it is unclear why this group had a better response after 10 sessions.

In addition to the proven short-term effects induced by HBO in the present study, we were able to demonstrate the following long-term effects. In the subgroup of on-schedule patients we could show that the effect of HBO remained stable within 3 months following treatment. The statistically significant improvement in physical and social functioning and the reduction of limitations persisted. The subjective perception of the severity of disease mirrored by the VAS also remained significantly decreased. This proven long-term effect of HBO represents one strength of the current study in comparison to recent literature without evaluation of long-term data [14,16].

However, the second strength of the present study is the number of patients undergoing HBO treatment (N = 59). To the best of our knowledge, our study is the second-largest reported up to this time. In this context, Zilberman and colleagues investigated a larger collective consisting of 73 patients [16].

Despite applying only 10 HBO treatment sessions, our results resemble those of the prospectively randomized, sham control, double-blind study by Zilberman et al., who administered 40 HBO sessions per patient [16]. This enormous series of HBO sessions is the largest number documented in recent literature. Based on the assumption that an increasing number of HBO sessions could have a beneficial impact on the mitigation of LCS-related symptoms, the subgroup of 37 patients from the present study might confirm this suspicion. Feeling subjective improvement of their well-being during HBO, they insisted on continuing HBO treatment exceeding 10 sessions. However, according to our findings in comparison to matchable literature [14,16], we share the opinion that the optimal number of HBO sessions for maximal therapeutic effect has yet not be determined. However, Zilberman and co-workers were able to demonstrate significant improvement in global cognitive function, attention, executive function, the energy domain, sleep, psychiatric symptoms and pain. These findings are favorably in line with the results of the present study, which show a statistical significant improvement of clinical symptoms of the physical, the neurocognitive and the psychiatric areas, as documented in Tables 1–3. In contrast to our current study, the clinical features were mirrored by improvement in brain MRI perfusion and functional magnetic resonance changes in the respective areas. These findings suggest a change of the functional connectivity and organization of neural pathways by induction of neuroplasticity following HBO treatment [16,17].

Recently, the same group investigated the effect of HBO on left ventricular function in patients with LCS in a prospective, randomized study. Despite normal ejection fraction, almost half of the collective of 60 patients had reduced global longitudinal strain (GLS) at baseline. Following HBO, GLS increased significantly as a sign that HBO promotes myocardial recovery. This could at least in part explain the positive effect of HBO on physical function and energy [37], as we could confirm in the findings of the current study with significant improvements of both physical function and energy, as displayed in Tables 1–3.

However, our study has two limitations that have to be addressed: The most prominent feature was the prospective, observational study design without a control group. Due to technical issues (because of the lack of a gas blender), it is not possible to deliver hyperbaric sham treatment in our hyperbaric chamber. This is why we had to conduct the current study without a control group. Another shortcoming was the fact that about two thirds of the patients had wanted to continue HBO treatment beyond the planned 10 sessions after they had noticed a subjective improvement of their well-being during HBO. For this reason they were unfortunately unsuitable for the scheduled 3 months' evaluation. In consequence, the latter is based on only 18 cases, as displayed in Figure 1.

5. Conclusions

In conclusion, though the pathogenesis of LCS is still unclear, and hence the specific mechanisms of HBO must remain speculative, HBO may provide a safe and feasible therapeutic tool for mitigation of LCS-related symptoms. Regarding the findings of the present clinical pilot study, we are able to conclude that after administration of HBO, physical functioning and both the physical and emotional role improved significantly and sustainably even during long-term follow-up. However, there is a strong need for further, prospectively randomized studies focusing on dose-finding, duration of HBO, elucidation of mechanisms and duration of the treatment effects.

Author Contributions: Conceptualization, J.L. and F.M.S.-J.; formal analysis, J.S. and F.M.S.-J.; statistical analysis, J.S.; patient acquisition, F.I., E.K. and R.K.; investigation, C.P., L.O., H.K., I.M., A.R., A.K., G.K. and R.K.; data curation, writing—original draft preparation, J.L. and F.M.S.-J.; writing—review and editing, J.L., C.P., L.O., H.K., I.M., A.R., A.K., E.K., F.I., G.K., R.K., J.S. and F.M.S.-J.; final approval, J.L., C.P., L.O., H.K., I.M., A.R., A.K., E.K., F.I., G.K., R.K., J.S. and F.M.S.-J.; supervision, J.L. and F.M.S.-J.; project administration, J.L., F.M.S.-J., F.I. and E.K. All authors have read and agreed to the published version of the manuscript.

Funding: This research received no external funding.

Institutional Review Board Statement: The study was conducted in accordance with the Declaration of Helsinki, and approved by the local Ethics Committee of the Medical University of Graz, Austria (33–308 ex 20/21).

Informed Consent Statement: Informed consent was obtained from all subjects involved in the study.

Data Availability Statement: The data presented in this study are available upon request from the corresponding author.

Conflicts of Interest: The authors declare no conflict of interest.

References

1. Yong, S.J. Long COVID or post-COVID-19 syndrome: Putative pathophysiology, risk factors, and treatments. *Infect. Dis.* **2021**, *53*, 737–754. [CrossRef] [PubMed]

2. Wulf Hanson, S.; Abbafati, C.; Aerts, J.G.; Al-Aly, Z.; Ashbaugh, C.; Ballouz, T.; Blyuss, O.; Bobkova, P.; Bonsel, G.; Borzakova, S.; et al. Estimated Global Proportions of Individuals with Persistent Fatigue, Cognitive, and Respiratory Symptom Clusters Following Symptomatic COVID-19 in 2020 and 2021. *JAMA* **2022**, *328*, 1604–1615. [PubMed]
3. Aiyegbusi, O.L.; Hughes, S.E.; Turner, G.; Rivera, S.C.; McMullan, C.; Chandan, J.S.; Haroon, S.; Price, G.; Davies, E.H.; Nirantharakumar, K.; et al. Symptoms, complications and management of long COVID: A review. *J. R. Soc. Med.* **2021**, *114*, 428–442. [CrossRef] [PubMed]
4. Joli, J.; Buck, P.; Zipfel, S.; Stengel, A. Post-COVID-19 fatigue: A systematic review. *Front. Psychiatry* **2022**, *13*, 947973. [CrossRef]
5. Castanares-Zapatero, D.; Chalon, P.; Kohn, L.; Dauvrin, M.; Detollenaere, J.; Maertens de Noordhout, C.; Primus-de Jong, C.; Cleemput, I.; Van den Heede, K. Pathophysiology and mechanism of long COVID: A comprehensive review. *Ann. Med.* **2022**, *54*, 1473–1487. [CrossRef]
6. Lindenmann, J.; Smolle, C.; Kamolz, L.P.; Smolle-Juettner, F.M.; Graier, W.F. Survey of Molecular Mechanisms of Hyperbaric Oxygen in Tissue Repair. *Int. J. Mol. Sci.* **2021**, *22*, 11754. [CrossRef]
7. Guo, D.; Pan, S.; Wang, M.; Guo, Y. Hyperbaric oxygen therapy may be effective to improve hypoxemia in patients with severe COVID-2019 pneumonia: Two case reports. *Undersea Hyperb. Med.* **2020**, *47*, 181–187. [CrossRef]
8. Thibodeaux, K.; Speyrer, M.; Raza, A.; Yaakov, R.; Serena, T.E. Hyperbaric oxygen therapy in preventing mechanical ventilation in COVID-19 patients: A retrospective case series. *J. Wound Care* **2020**, *29*, S4–S8. [CrossRef]
9. Cannellotto, M.; Duarte, M.; Keller, G.; Larrea, R.; Cunto, E.; Chediack, V.; Mansur, M.; Brito, D.M.; García, E.; Di Salvo, H.E.; et al. Hyperbaric oxygen as an adjuvant treatment for patients with COVID-19 severe hypoxaemia: A randomised controlled trial. *Emerg. Med. J.* **2022**, *39*, 88–93. [CrossRef]
10. Gorenstein, S.A.; Castellano, M.L.; Slone, E.S.; Gillette, B.; Liu, H.; Alsamarraie, C.; Jacobson, A.M.; Wall, S.P.; Adhikari, S.; Swartz, J.L.; et al. Hyperbaric oxygen therapy for COVID-19 patients with respiratory distress: Treated cases versus propensity-matched controls. *Undersea Hyperb. Med.* **2020**, *47*, 405–413. [CrossRef]
11. Jansen, D.; Dickstein, D.R.; Erazo, K.; Stacom, E.; Lee, D.C.; Wainwright, S.K. Hyperbaric oxygen for COVID-19 patients with severe hypoxia prior to vaccine availability. *Undersea Hyperb. Med.* **2022**, *49*, 295–305. [CrossRef] [PubMed]
12. Bhaiyat, A.M.; Sasson, E.; Wang, Z.; Khairy, S.; Ginzarly, M.; Qureshi, U.; Fikree, M.; Efrati, S. Hyperbaric oxygen treatment for long coronavirus disease-19: A case report. *J. Med. Case Rep.* **2022**, *16*, 80. [CrossRef] [PubMed]
13. Zant, A.E.; Figueroa, X.A.; Paulson, C.P.; Wright, J.K. Hyperbaric oxygen therapy to treat lingering COVID-19 symptoms. *Undersea Hyperb. Med.* **2022**, *49*, 333–339. [CrossRef] [PubMed]
14. Robbins, T.; Gonevski, M.; Clark, C.; Baitule, S.; Sharma, K.; Magar, A.; Patel, K.; Sankar, S.; Kyrou, I.; Ali, A.; et al. Hyperbaric oxygen therapy for the treatment of long COVID: Early evaluation of a highly promising intervention. *Clin. Med.* **2021**, *21*, e629–e632. [CrossRef]
15. Turova, E.A.; Shchikota, A.M.; Pogonchenkova, I.V.; Golovach, A.V.; Tagirova, D.I.; Gusakova, E.V. Hyperbaric oxygenation in outpatient rehabilitation of COVID-19 convalescents. *Vopr. Kurortol. Fizioter. Lech. Fiz. Kult.* **2021**, *98*, 16–21. [CrossRef]
16. Zilberman-Itskovich, S.; Catalogna, M.; Sasson, E.; Elman-Shina, K.; Hadanny, A.; Lang, E.; Finci, S.; Polak, N.; Fishlev, G.; Korin, C.; et al. Hyperbaric oxygen therapy improves neurocognitive functions and symptoms of post-COVID condition: Randomized controlled trial. *Sci. Rep.* **2022**, *12*, 11252. [CrossRef]
17. Catalogna, M.; Sasson, E.; Hadanny, A.; Parag, Y.; Zilberman-Itskovich, S.; Efrati, S. Effects of hyperbaric oxygen therapy on functional and structural connectivity in post-COVID-19 condition patients: A randomized, sham-controlled trial. *Neuroimage Clin.* **2022**, *36*, 103218. [CrossRef]
18. Hussain, R.; Wark, S.; Dillon, G.; Ryan, P. Self-reported physical and mental health of Australian carers: A cross-sectional study. *BMJ Open* **2016**, *6*, e011417. [CrossRef]
19. Ware, J.E., Jr.; Sherbourne, C.D. The MOS 36-item short-form health survey (SF-36): I. Conceptual framework and item selection. *Med. Care* **1992**, *30*, 473–483. [CrossRef]
20. Lins, L.; Carvalho, F.M. SF-36 total score as a single measure of health-related quality of life: Scoping review. *SAGE Open Med.* **2016**, *4*, 2050312116671725. [CrossRef]
21. Poudel, A.N.; Zhu, S.; Cooper, N.; Roderick, P.; Alwan, N.; Tarrant, C.; Ziauddeen, N.; Yao, G.L. Impact of Covid-19 on health-related quality of life of patients: A structured review. *PLoS ONE* **2021**, *16*, e0259164. [CrossRef]
22. Weigl, K.; Forstner, T. Design of Paper-Based Visual Analogue Scale Items. *Educ. Psychol. Meas.* **2021**, *81*, 595–611. [CrossRef]
23. Faul, F.; Erdfelder, E.; Buchner, A.; Lang, A.G. Statistical power analyses using G* Power 3.1: Tests for correlation and regression analyses. *Behav. Res. Methods* **2009**, *41*, 1149–1160. [CrossRef]
24. Mathieu, D.; Marroni, A.; Kot, J. Tenth European Consensus Conference on Hyperbaric Medicine: Recommendations for accepted and non-accepted clinical indications and practic of hyperbaric oxygten treatment. *Diving Hyperb. Med.* **2017**, *47*, 24–32. [CrossRef] [PubMed]
25. Manganotti, P.; Michelutti, M.; Furlanis, G.; Deodato, M.; Buoite Stella, A. Deficient GABABergic and glutamatergic excitability in the motor cortex of patients with long-COVID and cognitive impairment. *Clin. Neurophysiol.* **2023**, *151*, 83–91. [CrossRef] [PubMed]
26. Ortelli, P.; Ferrazzoli, D.; Sebastianelli, L.; Maestri, R.; Dezi, S.; Spampinato, D.; Saltuari, L.; Alibardi, A.; Engl, M.; Kofler, M.; et al. Altered motor cortex physiology and dysexecutive syndrome in patients with fatigue and cognitive difficulties after mild COVID-19. *Eur. J. Neurol.* **2022**, *29*, 1652–1662. [CrossRef] [PubMed]

27. Ajčević, M.; Iscra, K.; Furlanis, G.; Michelutti, M.; Miladinović, A.; Buoite Stella, A.; Ukmar, M.; Cova, M.A.; Accardo, A.; Manganotti, P. Cerebral hypoperfusion in post-COVID-19 cognitively impaired subjects revealed by arterial spin labeling MRI. *Sci. Rep.* **2023**, *13*, 5808. [CrossRef]
28. Guedj, E.; Campion, J.Y.; Dudouet, P.; Kaphan, E.; Bregeon, F.; Tissot-Dupont, H.; Guis, S.; Barthelemy, F.; Habert, P.; Ceccaldi, M.; et al. ^{18}F-FDG brain PET hypometabolism in patients with long COVID. *Eur. J. Nucl. Med. Mol. Imaging* **2021**, *48*, 2823–2833. [CrossRef]
29. Rosenberg, K. Hyperbaric Oxygen Improves Neurocognitive Function and Symptoms of Post-COVID Condition. *Am. J. Nurs.* **2022**, *122*, 61–62. [CrossRef]
30. Nopp, S.; Moik, F.; Klok, F.A.; Gattinger, D.; Petrovic, M.; Vonbank, K.; Koczulla, A.R.; Ay, C.; Zwick, R.H. Outpatient Pulmonary Rehabilitation in Patients with Long COVID Improves Exercise Capacity, Functional Status, Dyspnea, Fatigue, and Quality of Life. *Respiration* **2022**, *101*, 593–601. [CrossRef]
31. Raman, B.; Bluemke, D.A.; Lüscher, T.F.; Neubauer, S. Long COVID: Post-acute sequelae of COVID-19 with a cardiovascular focus. *Eur. Heart J.* **2022**, *43*, 1157–1172. [CrossRef] [PubMed]
32. Choutka, J.; Jansari, V.; Hornig, M.; Iwasaki, A. Unexplained post-acute infection syndromes. *Nat. Med.* **2022**, *28*, 911–923. [CrossRef] [PubMed]
33. Premraj, L.; Kannapadi, N.V.; Briggs, J.; Seal, S.M.; Battaglini, D.; Fanning, J.; Suen, J.; Robba, C.; Fraser, J.; Cho, S.M. Mid and long-term neurological and neuropsychiatric manifestations of post-COVID-19 syndrome: A meta-analysis. *J. Neurol. Sci.* **2022**, *434*, 120162. [CrossRef]
34. Shanthanna, H.; Nelson, A.M.; Kissoon, N.; Narouze, S. The COVID-19 pandemic and its consequences for chronic pain: A narrative review. *Anaesthesia* **2022**, *77*, 1039–1050. [CrossRef] [PubMed]
35. Hadanny, A.; Bechor, Y.; Catalogna, M.; Daphna-Tekoah, S.; Sigal, T.; Cohenpour, M.; Lev-Wiesel, R.; Efrati, S. Hyperbaric Oxygen Therapy Can Induce Neuroplasticity and Significant Clinical Improvement in Patients Suffering from Fibromyalgia with a History of Childhood Sexual Abuse-Randomized Controlled Trial. *Front. Psychol.* **2018**, *9*, 2495. [CrossRef]
36. Curtis, K.; Katz, J.; Djaiani, C.; O'Leary, G.; Uehling, J.; Carroll, J.; Santa Mina, D.; Clarke, H.; Gofeld, M.; Katznelson, R. Evaluation of a Hyperbaric Oxygen Therapy Intervention in Individuals with Fibromyalgia. *Pain. Med.* **2021**, *22*, 1324–1332. [CrossRef]
37. Leitman, M.; Fuchs, S.; Tyomkin, V.; Hadanny, A.; Zilberman-Itskovich, S.; Efrati, S. The effect of hyperbaric oxygen therapy on myocardial function in post-COVID-19 syndrome patients: A randomized controlled trial. *Sci. Rep.* **2023**, *13*, 9473. [CrossRef]

Disclaimer/Publisher's Note: The statements, opinions and data contained in all publications are solely those of the individual author(s) and contributor(s) and not of MDPI and/or the editor(s). MDPI and/or the editor(s) disclaim responsibility for any injury to people or property resulting from any ideas, methods, instructions or products referred to in the content.

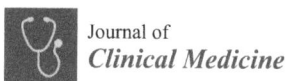

Article

Pulmonary Evaluation in Children with Post-COVID-19 Condition Respiratory Symptoms: A Prospective Cohort Study

Einat Shmueli [1,2,*], Ophir Bar-On [1], Ben Amir [2], Meir Mei-Zahav [1,2], Patrick Stafler [1,2], Hagit Levine [1,2], Guy Steuer [1], Benjamin Rothschild [1], Lior Tsviban [1], Nofar Amitai [1,2], Miri Dotan [1,2], Gabriel Chodick [2], Dario Prais [1,2,†] and Liat Ashkenazi-Hoffnung [2,3,†]

[1] Pulmonology Institute, Schneider Children's Medical Center of Israel, 14 Kaplan Street, Petach Tikva 49202, Israel; ophirbo@clalit.org.il (O.B.-O.); meir_zahav@clalit.org.il (M.M.-Z.); patrickst@clalit.org.il (P.S.); hagitlevine@clalit.org.il (H.L.); guysh2@clalit.org.il (G.S.); binyaminro@clalit.org.il (B.R.); liorts@clalit.org.il (L.T.); nofaram2@clalit.org.il (N.A.); mirido@clalit.org.il (M.D.); prais@tauex.tau.ac.il (D.P.)

[2] Faculty of Medicine, Tel Aviv University, Tel Aviv 69978, Israel; benami@clalit.org.il (B.A.); hodik_g@mac.com (G.C.); liat.ashkenazi@clalit.org.il (L.A.-H.)

[3] Department of Day Hospitalization, Schneider Children's Medical Center of Israel, Petach Tikva 49202, Israel

* Correspondence: einatsh3@clalit.org.il; Tel.: +972-3-9253654; Fax: +972-3-9253308

† These authors contributed equally to this work.

Abstract: Background: Studies on post-COVID-19 condition (PCC) in adults have shown deterioration in pulmonary function tests (PFTs), mainly a diffusion limitation. Among the pediatric population, data are scarce. **Aim:** To characterize PFTs in children with PCC, including changes over time. **Methods:** A prospective longitudinal study of children with defined PCC and respiratory complaints who were referred to a designated multidisciplinary clinic from 11/2020 to 12/2022. **Results:** Altogether, 184 children with a mean age of 12.4 years (SD 4.06) were included. A mild obstructive pattern was demonstrated in 19/170 (11%) at presentation, as indicated by spirometry and/or positive exercise challenge test and/or reversibility post bronchodilators, only three had a previous diagnosis of asthma. Lung volumes and diffusion were normal in all but one patient (1/134, 0.7%). Exhaled nitric oxide levels were elevated in 32/144 (22%). A total of 33 children who had repeated PFTs had normal or near-normal PFTs on follow-up testing, including seven (21.2%) who had mild obstructive PFTs at presentation. Multivariate analysis identified older age [OR 1.36 (95% CI:1.07–1.75)], specific imaging findings (prominent bronchovascular markings (OR 43.28 (95% CI: 4.50–416.49)), and hyperinflation (OR 28.42, 95% CI: 2.18–370.84)] as significant predictors of an obstructive pattern on PFTs. **Conclusions:** In children with PCC and respiratory symptoms, the most common impairment was a mild obstructive pattern; most were without a history of asthma. Improvement was witnessed in long-term follow-up. In contrast to the adult population, no diffusion limitation was found. Empirical periodic inhaler therapy may be considered in children with factors associated with PFT abnormalities.

Keywords: post-COVID-19 condition; long COVID; pulmonary function tests; lung clearance index; SARS-CoV-2

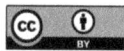

1. Introduction

Since coronavirus disease 2019 (COVID-19) has emerged, many studies have reported long-lasting symptoms after recovery, commonly known as 'Long COVID' or 'post COVID-19 condition') PCC(, the latter being the preferred terminology by the World Health Organization (WHO) [1]. The definition of PCC in children includes a history of confirmed SARS-CoV-2 infection, with at least one persisting physical symptom for a minimum duration of 12 weeks after initial testing that cannot be explained by an alternative diagnosis. The symptoms have an impact on everyday functioning, may continue or develop after

COVID infection, and may fluctuate or relapse over time [2]. These symptoms include dyspnea, chronic cough, and chest tightness, as well as cognitive dysfunction and extreme fatigue [3,4].

Studies monitoring post-COVID pulmonary function tests (PFTs) in adults have shown altered respiratory function, with abnormal diffusion capacity being the most prevalent finding, appearing in 40% to more than 50% of patients in most studies [5–7]. These studies found restrictive patterns to be much less common and only a small minority of patients demonstrated an obstructive pattern [6].

It is well known that acute COVID-19 infection in children is less severe than in adult patients [8–10], with cough as a dominant feature of acute illness [11], but little is known about the prevalence and severity of pediatric PCC [12–14].

To date, only a few studies monitoring PFTs in children with PCC and respiratory symptoms have been published [12–15]. These studies included mostly children with asymptomatic mild acute COVID-19 infection, with a follow-up of up to 8 months post infection, and showed mixed results, ranging from no abnormalities to an obstructive pattern seen in a large proportion of patients. In a systemic review and meta-analysis by Martino et al. the [16] authors have found that children can develop persistent respiratory symptoms after SARS-CoV-2 infection; however, the methodological variabilities of the analyzed studies did not allow them to provide firm conclusions about the rate, type and best diagnostics for children with persistent respiratory symptoms. Furthermore, long-term follow-up data on children are scarce and guidelines regarding the management of these cases are lacking.

In November 2020, a designated multidisciplinary clinic was implanted at our tertiary pediatric center for children with complaints associated with PCC symptoms [17].

In the current study we followed children presenting to this designated clinic with respiratory complaints after recovery from microbiologically confirmed COVID-19 who prospectively performed PFTs. The aims of our study were to evaluate whether PFT abnormalities are present in pediatric PCC, as seen in the adult population, and to characterize those abnormalities. In addition, the study aimed to evaluate longitudinal changes in PFTs over time in this population. Characterization of the respiratory abnormalities in these children may elucidate the underlying pathophysiology and potentially provide a basis for treatment for this chronic condition.

2. Methods

2.1. Study Design and Population

This prospective cohort study included children referred to a designated multidisciplinary clinic for PCC at Schneider Children's Medical Center of Israel (SCMCI), a tertiary pediatric center, between November 2020 and December 2022. Inclusion criteria included the following: (a) children ≤18 years of age AND (b) SARS-CoV-2 infection microbiologically confirmed by PCR during acute infection or by subsequent serology AND (c) symptoms suggestive of PCC >12 weeks from acute illness that cannot be explained by an alternative diagnosis AND (d) respiratory complaints (exercise intolerance, dyspnea, cough, etc.) [2].

All referred patients underwent an evaluation including baseline chest X-ray and a structured interview which included demographic data, medical history, and acute COVID-19 infection symptoms, as well as assessment of PCC symptoms and their impact on daily activities. The presence of atopy was determined by anamnesis as well as review of electronic medical records and included personal or familial history of atopic manifestations (dermatitis, asthma, or allergic rhinitis). Past respiratory comorbidities were evaluated based on self-report and medical records.

The subset of children with cardio-respiratory complaints (e.g., dyspnea, cough, chest tightness, and exercise intolerance) underwent additional investigation, including electrocardiography (ECG) echocardiography, and comprehensive PFTs according to age, which included baseline spirometry, exercise challenge test (ECT), bronchodilator response, lung plethysmography, diffusion capacity, fractional exhaled nitric oxide (FeNO), and multiple breath washout (MBW). In cases of severe continuous complaints and based on clinical judgment, a cardiopulmonary exercise test (CPET) was performed. Following this investigation, children with abnormal PFTs were assessed by a pediatric pulmonologist; if indicated, specific treatment was prescribed and further investigation, including repeated PFTs and methacholine challenge testing (MCT), was performed when clinically appropriate (Figure 1).

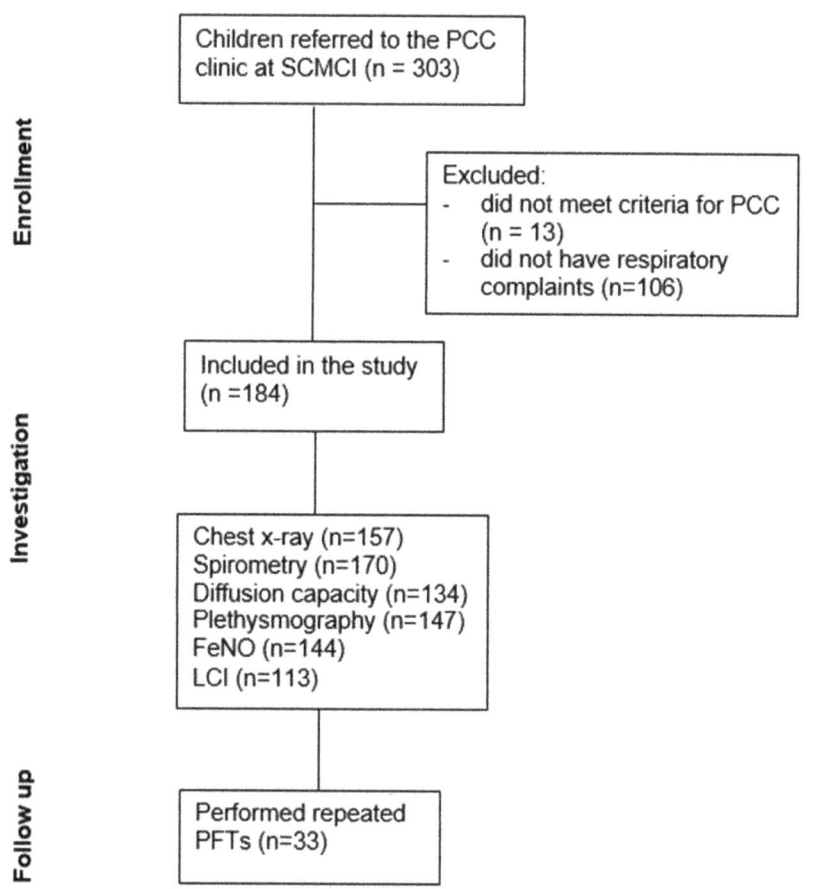

Figure 1. Consort flow diagram of the study.

2.2. Microbiology

A positive SARS-CoV-2 PCR test was defined according to the Israeli Ministry of Health guidelines [18]. Testing methods included the Real-Time Fluorescent PCR kit (BGI) and the SARS-CoV-2 PCR kit (Seegene, Seoul, Republic of Korea). Anti-spike receptor-binding domain IgG antibodies were measured using an in-house enzyme-linked immunosorbent assay (The Central Virology Laboratory of the Ministry of Health at Sheba Medical Center, Tel Hashomer, Israel) until mid-March 2021 and the SARS-CoV-2 IgG II Quant assay (Abbott) thereafter.

2.3. Pulmonary Function Testing

PFTs were measured in the lung function laboratory of the SCMCI's pulmonary institute.

2.3.1. Spirometry and Exercise Challenge

Spirometry was obtained using Smart PFT UI (Medical Equipment Europe GmbH, Hammelburg, Germany) according to the American Thoracic Society (ATS)/European Respiratory Society (ERS) consensus guidelines [19].

ECT was performed while running on a treadmill for 6 min, with speed and slope adjusted to achieve a target heart rate of $(220 - age) \times 0.8$ for a minimum of 4 min, according to ATS/ERS guidelines [20,21]. Heart rate and oxygen saturation were monitored continuously during running. Post-exercise spirometry was performed at 1, 3, 5, 10, 15, and 20 min after ceasing exercise. Any fall in FEV_1 of 10% or greater from baseline FEV_1 was considered as positive [20]. A bronchodilator (4 puffs of salbutamol metered-dose inhaler 100 mcg) was administered when the ECT was positive or when FEV_1 was <95% predicted. Reversibility was defined by a rise of 10% or greater in FEV_1 [21].

2.3.2. Plethysmography and Diffusion Capacity

Plethysmography and diffusion capacity for carbon monoxide were obtained using Smart PFT body box (Medical Equipment Europe GmbH, Hammelburg, Germany) according to the ATS/ERS guidelines [22]. Carbon monoxide diffusion was corrected for alveolar volume and hemoglobin level, indicated as KCO. Spirometry and lung volumes were expressed as percent of predicted normal values with the use of the equations of Polgar and Varuni [23]. KCO percent predicted was calculated as described by Weng and Levinson [24].

2.3.3. Exhaled Nitric Oxide Levels (FeNo)

FeNo was measured using a chemiluminescence analyzer (CLD 77 AM; EcoMedics AG, Duernten, Switzerland) according to ATS/ERS recommendations [25]. Normal values were considered ≤20 parts per billion (ppb) for single-breath or ≤8 ppb for multiple-breath test.

2.3.4. Lung Clearance Index (LCI)

MBW, expressed as the Lung Clearance Index (LCI), was performed with an ultrasonic flow meter (Spiroson 1; EcoMedics AG, Switzerland) according to ATS/ERS consensus statement [26]. Normal values were considered < 7.91 [27].

2.3.5. Methacholine Testing

MCT was obtained using Smart PFT UI (Medical Equipment Europe GmbH, Germany) using a triple-dose accelerated protocol of fresh methacholine solutions in normal saline solution [28]. A positive methacholine test was defined as provocative concentration causing 20% decline in FEV_1 (PC20) of <4 mg/mL [21]. A bronchodilator (4 puffs of salbutamol metered-dose inhaler 100 mcg) was administered when the methacholine challenge test was positive or when FEV_1 at the end of the test was <80% predicted.

2.4. Statistical Methods

Descriptive statistics were used to define the demographic and clinical characteristics of the cohort. Multivariate logistic regression was used to assess the association between clinical patient characteristics (pre-defined independent variables selected on the basis of clinical evaluation) and an obstructive pattern on pulmonary function testing (dependent variable). The Wald test was used for CI calculation. A probability value of ≤0.05 was considered significant. Results are presented based on the full data set. Interactions were systematically searched for. Data were analysed using IBM SPSS Statistics for Windows, version 27.0 (IBM Corp. Released 2020 and R Core Team, 2016, Armonk, NY, USA).

3. Results

3.1. Patient Characteristics

Altogether 303 Children were assessed for PCC at our multidisciplinary clinic between November 2020 and December 2022. Of those, 184 reported respiratory symptoms at enrolment and thus were included in this study.

3.1.1. Demographic and Clinical Parameters

The mean age of the participants was 12.6 years (SD 4.06, range 2–18 years), with 33/184 children (17.9%) under 10 years old; of those, 111 (60.3%) were female and mean BMI% was 60.8% (SD 31.7%). Most children had no underlying diseases (137, 74.5%). Previous asthma diagnosis was reported in 11 (5.4%) and depression/anxiety disorders in eight (4.3%). In total, 17 (9.2%) were diagnosed with attention deficit disorder (ADHD), and 24 (13%) were competitive athletes. Most participants had mild or asymptomatic acute SARS-CoV-2 infection (170, 92.4%), with only five children (2.7%) hospitalized due to O_2 saturation <94%, with disease defined as "severe" by the National Institutes of Health (NIH) [29] (Table 1).

Table 1. Demographic and clinical characteristics of 184 children with post-COVID-19 condition and respiratory symptoms.

Age, mean ± SD, years	12.64 ± 4.06
Female, n (%)	111 (60.3%)
BMI%, mean ± SD	60.8% ± 31.7%
Underlying disease, n (%) *	45 (24.5%)
Asthma	11 (5.4%)
Depression/anxiety	8 (4.3%)
Gastrointestinal disease	5 (2.7%)
Rheumatologic disease	4 (2.2%)
Immunodeficiency **	4 (2.2%)
Neurological impairment ***	4 (2.2%)
Nephrological disease	3 (1.6%)
Other ****	9 (4.9%)
Prematurity (<37 weeks)	4 (2.2%)
Atopic background by history, n (%)	
Personal	50 (27.2%)
Familial	32 (17.4%)
Attention deficit disorder (ADHD), n (%)	17 (9.2%)
Competitive athletes, n (%)	24 (13%)
Severity of acute COVID-19 illness according to NIH *****, n (%)	
Asymptomatic	9 (4.9%)
Mild	161 (87.5%)
Moderate	9 (4.9%)
Severe	5 (2.7%)

* Including 3 children with two underlying diseases. ** Neurological impairment, including developmental delay and epilepsy. *** Immunodeficiency, including congenital immunodeficiency, solid organ transplantation, and hematopoietic stem cell transplantation. **** Other, including migraine/headache, kidney disease, and hematologic disease. ***** National Institutes of Health (NIH) [29].

3.1.2. Post-COVID Respiratory Symptoms and Consequences

Evaluation was done at a mean time of 25.1 weeks (IQR 13.7–34.9) after acute COVID infection. The most common respiratory symptom was dyspnea (136, 73.9%), followed by chest pain (89, 48.4%), and cough (19, 10.3%). In all, 104 (56.5%) reported mild functional impairment, with moderate and severe impairment in 74 (40.2%) and six (3.3%), respectively. Activities of daily living were significantly affected in 116 (63%) and 142 (77.2%) reported impaired physical activity (Table 2).

Table 2. Chronic respiratory symptoms in 184 children with post-COVID-19 condition.

Respiratory Complaint, n (%)	
Dyspnea	136 (73.9%)
Chest pain	89 (48.4%)
Cough	19 (10.3%)
Functional status, n (%)	
Mild	104 (56.5%)
Moderate	74 (40.2%)
Severe	6 (3.3%)
Influence ADL *, n (%)	116 (63%)
Physical activity effected, n (%)	142 (77.2%)

* ADL = Activities of Daily Living.

3.2. Cardio-Pulmonary Evaluation

- Among patients who performed PFTs, 170/184 (92%) performed spirometry, with a mean FEV_1 of 92.6% (SD 10.6%, Table 3); 19/170 (11%) patients had FEV_1 < 80%, of which FEV_1/FVC was <80% in three of them, one with a rheumatologic disease and two previously healthy, and one with a personal history of atopy; the latter two also had a positive ECT and all had significant reversibility post bronchodilators.
- ECT was performed by 133 children (Table 3), of whom four had a positive test; all four had complete post bronchodilator reversibility, three were previously healthy, and one had a background gastrointestinal disease; none had a history of asthma, but three had personal atopy. Eleven other children had negative ECT but a rise of $\geq 10\%$ in FEV_1 post bronchodilators; one had asthma and six of the remaining 10 had either a personal or familial history of asthma. All the participants who performed ECT maintained normal O_2 saturations during the test.
- Following baseline spirometry with FEV_1 < 90% or FEV_1/FVC < 90%, 11 children were evaluated for bronchodilator responsiveness, of whom three showed FEV_1 improvement of $\geq 10\%$. All three had no previous history of asthma or atopy.
- Overall, 19/175 (11%) children had an obstructive pattern, as indicated by FEV_1/FVC <80%, and/or positive ECT, and/or post bronchodilator reversibility—of whom only one had a previous asthma diagnosis.
- Altogether, 144 children underwent FeNO testing (Table 3), of whom 32 (22%) had elevated values, and 4/34 had a previous diagnosis of asthma as well as personal atopy. Another four children with elevated FeNO levels also demonstrated an obstructive pattern on spirometry: two with FEV1/FVC < 80% and two more with positive ECT. All four had personal atopy, and 14 others had either a personal or family history of atopy.
- In all of the 147 children who performed plethysmography lung volume testing, TLC was normal ($\geq 80\%$ predicted, Table 3); RV/TLC > 150% was found in 27 (18%), of whom one had a history of asthma.
- In all, 111 children performed MBW test, with a mean LCI of 7.48 (SD 0.9, Table 3); 27/111 (24.3%) had a value of >7.9, of whom two had known asthma, seven more

had personal atopy and three had familial atopy; none had a history of prematurity and baseline spirometry was normal in all but one, who also had a significant post bronchodilator reversibility.
- Of the 134 children who performed a lung diffusion test (Table 3) KCO was >75% predicted in all but one patient with a rare genetic syndrome, post kidney transplantation, without a previous known lung disease.
- Overall, abnormal PFTs—including an obstructive pattern, elevated FeNO, air trapping, elevated LCI, or diffusion limitation—were documented in 85 children (46.2%); of those, 20/85 had at least two abnormal tests, and 17/20 demonstrated an obstructive pattern.

Table 3. Pulmonary function tests in 184 children with post-COVID-19 condition and respiratory complaints.

Test	n	Result, Mean (SD)
FEV_1% predicted	170	92.6% (10.6)
FVC% predicted	170	95.9% (11.4)
FEV_1/FVC%	170	90.38% (6.9)
FEV_1% post exercise	133	91.7% (10.6)
FEV_1% post BD *	96	93.9 (9.5)
FeNO		
SBT **, ppb (normal < 8 ppb)	128	15.1 (14.6)
MBT **, ppb (normal < 20 ppb)	16	13.5 (8.4)
TLC% predicted	147	105.2 (12.9)
RV/TLC%	146	118.5 (32.7)
KCO% predicted	134	104.3 (14.2)
LCI	113	7.48 (0.9)
MCT ** (n = 7)		
Positive/borderline	3	
Negative	4	

Either post ECT or post spirometry alone. * BD = Bronchodilator. ** SBT = Single Breath Test, MBT = Multiple Breath Test, MCT = Methacholine Challenge Test, CXR = Chest X-ray.

- As part of their assessment, chest X-ray was performed on 157/184, of whom results were normal in 122 (78%), while 13 (8%) exhibited peribronchial cuffing, seven (4%) prominent bronchovascular markings, and 10 had other abnormalities, as detailed in Table 4.

Table 4. Chest X-ray results in 157 children with post-COVID-19 condition and respiratory complaints.

Result	n (%)
Normal	122 (77.7%)
Peribronchial cuffing	13 (8.3%)
Prominent bronchovascular markings	7 (4.5%)
Residual pulmonary infiltrate	6 (3.8%)
Hyperinflation	2 (1.3%)
Enlarged cardiac silhouette	1 (0.6%)
Minimal effusion unilateral	1 (0.6%)

- ECG testing was done in 167 children; nine (5.4%) had abnormal results that were previously identified and were not COVID-related.
- Echocardiography was performed in 145 children, showing mild abnormalities in six (4.1%), all detected previous to SARS-CoV-2 infection.
- CPET testing was performed in six children due to continuous severe complaints of exercise intolerance at a median time of 38.8 weeks after acute COVID infection (range 32.8–115.8 weeks); five were previously healthy individuals and one had known asthma. In all cases, CPET demonstrated normal cardio-respiratory function.

3.2.1. Pulmonary Evaluation in Children with Moderate to Severe Acute COVID-19

- Among the 9 children with moderate acute COVID-19 infection according to the NIH criteria [29], one demonstrated an obstructive pattern on PFTs without a previous asthma diagnosis; three had elevated FeNO values, of whom two had either a personal or a familial history of atopy; two had elevated LCI values, one with known asthma.
- Among the 5 children with severe acute COVID-19 infection, none had abnormal spirometry, two had elevated FeNO values, of whom one had a personal history of atopy, and two had elevated LCI values. One child, post kidney transplantation, had diffusion limitation.

3.2.2. Pulmonary Evaluation in Children Previously Vaccinated against SARS-CoV-2

Overall, three children (1.6%) in our cohort were previously vaccinated against COVID-19. All had normal spirometry upon evaluation, one had mildly elevated FeNO and one had an elevated LCI.

3.2.3. Multivariate Logistic Regression Analysis for Factors Associated with an Obstructive Pattern on Pulmonary Function Testing

Upon evaluation of predicting factors for an obstructive pattern, defined as $FEV_1/FVC < 80\%$ and/or positive ECT and/or reversibility post bronchodilators, the following were found to have a significant predictive value: older age (OR 1.36 (95% CI:1.07–1.75)), CXR findings of prominent bronchovascular markings (OR 43.28 (95% CI: 4.50–416.49) and hyperinflation (OR 28.42, 95% CI: 2.18–370.84), as detailed in Table 5.

Table 5. Multivariate analysis of predicting factors for obstructive pattern on pulmonary function testing.

	OR	95%CI	p-Value
Age	1.36	1.07–1.75	0.014
Chest pain	2.97	0.88–10.08	0.080
CXR			
Prominent bronchovascular markings	43.28	4.50–416.49	0.001
Hyperinflation	28.42	2.18–370.84	0.011
Peribronchial cuffing	4.06	0.84–19.77	0.082

Multivariate logistic regression was used to assess the association between clinical patient characteristics and an obstructive pattern on pulmonary function testing. Results are presented based on the full data set. There are missing data for 7 patients. Interactions were systematically searched for.

3.3. Interventions and Drug Therapy

In all, 17 children with an obstructive pattern on PFTs were evaluated by a pediatric pulmonologist and 16 of them received a trial of inhaler therapy with a combination of inhaled corticosteroid (ICS) and long-acting beta agonists (LABA).

3.4. Pulmonary Long-Term Follow-Up

A total of 33 children performed repeated PFTs at least 30 days after the first test, due to previous abnormal PFTs and/or continuous respiratory complaints. The second evaluation was done at a mean time of 13.6 weeks (IQR 6.3–21.7 weeks) after the first evaluation. At baseline evaluation 7/33 (21.2%) had abnormal PFTs, demonstrating a mild obstructive pattern. Seventeen of the 33 (51.5%) were followed in the pulmonary institute, of which 16 received inhaler therapy as previously detailed. Upon follow-up, all 33 children had normal or near-normal PFTs on repeated testing. Four of them underwent CPET with normal results. All 33 had reported clinical improvement in their respiratory symptoms upon follow-up.

4. Discussion

This prospective cohort study of children with PCC respiratory symptoms provides comprehensive data on their PFTs and the change over time. Respiratory function abnormalities were seen in 85 (46.2%) of the participants, of whom 17 (20%) had reversible obstructive pattern—most of them without known asthma. Repeated PFTs 1–6 months later have demonstrated normalization of PFTs in all children re-tested after presenting with an obstructive pattern, most of them (16/17) treated with inhaled corticosteroids. Furthermore, unlike adults with PCC [5–7], diffusion capacity and exercise O_2 saturation remained within normal limits in our study population.

Previous reports on PCC in the pediatric population [9,10,15] suggest a different pathogenesis than in adult PCC: while in adults, pulmonary interstitial or vascular changes are the cause of diffusion limitation [5], it seems that in children the disease does not cause these changes. One possible mechanism of respiratory PCC in children, which may explain the majority of symptomatic children with normal PFTs, is autonomic dysfunction—as suggested by Morrow et al. [30]. This mechanism is also supported by the study by Knoke et al. [14] in which the PFTs of children with PCC and respiratory complaints, including MBW, body plethysmography, and diffusion capacity testing, were all within normal limits.

Another mechanism, which may explain the reversible obstructive pattern seen in some children in our cohort as well as in the studies by Leftin Dobkin et al. [13] and by Palacios et al. [12], might be post-inflammatory changes causing airway hyper-responsiveness. Post-viral wheezing is a known phenomenon after RSV and Rhinovirus infection in early childhood [31] and similar mechanisms might also explain airway hyper-responsiveness in our study and support the notion of inhaled beta-agonists and corticosteroids as possible treatment for PCC respiratory symptoms. A meta-analysis by Tau et al. has demonstrated a large proportion of co-infection with *influenza* virus among children with COVID-19 compared to adults [32]; this fact might also contribute to the high prevalence of the presumed post-inflammatory reaction causing airway hyper-responsiveness.

As opposed to the studies by Leftin Dobkin et al. [13] and Palacios et al. [12], which reported high rates of children with asthma diagnosis suffering from PCC respiratory symptoms, only 2.5% of the children in our cohort had a previous diagnosis of asthma. These results are in keeping with some reports on PCC in adults, which found a low asthma rate in their cohorts [33], but there are also reports suggesting a higher incidence of PCC among asthmatics [34]. One theory is that enhanced Th-2 immune responsiveness, while having a protective effect against acute-COVID, increases the risk of PCC [35]. This theory might be supported by the fact that 45% of our cohort had a history of personal or familial atopy and also by the high FeNO values seen in 22% of the children performing the test, most, but not all, with an atopic background (22/32, 69%).

A high proportion of competitive athletes was found in our study, in keeping with the study by Palacios et al. [12]. This may be explained by the fact that physical activity is a known trigger of bronchial hyperreactivity, and while most children kept a sedentary lifestyle during the COVID-19 outbreak, competitive athletes were still engaged in physical activity during the quarantines or early after social distancing provisions were withdrawn [36].

Repeated PFTs in children with continuous respiratory complaints and normal baseline PFTs did not change in the follow-up test. Furthermore, in all children who presented with reversible obstructive pattern at first visit, repeated PFTs had demonstrated normalization, including negative MCT. Palacios et al. also reported clinical improvement as well as improvement in spirometry and 6 min walk test in their patients at follow-up, although to a smaller degree [12]; other observational studies also showed clinical improvement over time [37].

As older age and specific abnormalities on chest X-ray were significant predictors of obstructive PFTs in our cohort, it might be beneficial to perform PFTs, mainly ECT, in this subset of patients, as well as to consider inhaler therapy for these children.

Treatment options for children with PCC remain extremely limited. In the current cohort, 16/17 children with obstructive pattern on PFTs received inhaler therapy with ICS-LABA; all improved over time. Clinical improvement was also noted in the 17 children who did not receive inhaler therapy. Although treatment was not specifically addressed in the present study, it may be suggested that bronchodilators or inhaled corticosteroids can be a transitory treatment option for the period of severe respiratory symptoms.

The main limitation of our study is the lack of prior PFTs in study participants, so some may have had undiagnosed asthma prior to COVID-19; however, these children had no respiratory symptoms prior to COVID (13% were participating in competitive sports) and also, in those with repeated testing, improvement in their PFTs was apparent with time. Another limitation is that follow-up testing was only available for some of the cohort; nevertheless, in the majority PFTs improved, supporting the notion of a temporary phenomenon.

In conclusion, PCC respiratory symptoms were associated with mild abnormal findings in almost half of the children tested; of them, 20% had an obstructive pattern that resolved with time. Therefore, bronchodilators or inhaled corticosteroids can be considered as a transitory treatment option for the period of severe respiratory symptoms. Unlike adults, PFTs did not show diffusion limitation. Future studies should focus on the effectiveness of various treatments for this population.

Author Contributions: Conceptualization, E.S., D.P. and L.A.-H.; investigation, E.S., O.B.-O., M.M.-Z., P.S., H.L., G.S., B.R., L.T., N.A. and M.D.; data curation, E.S. and B.A.; formal analysis, G.C.; writing—original draft preparation, E.S., D.P. and L.A.-H.; writing—review and editing, E.S., D.P. and L.A.-H. All authors have read and agreed to the published version of the manuscript.

Funding: This research received no external funding.

Institutional Review Board Statement: The study was approved by the institutional ethics research board (RMC 20-0085).

Informed Consent Statement: Informed consent was obtained from all subjects involved in the study.

Data Availability Statement: The data presented in this study are available on request from the corresponding author. The data are not publicly available due to privacy restrictions.

Conflicts of Interest: The authors declare no conflict of interest.

References

1. Crook, H.; Raza, S.; Nowell, J.; Young, M.; Edison, P. Long COVID—Mechanisms, Risk Factors, and Management. *BMJ* **2021**, *374*, n1648. [CrossRef]
2. Stephenson, T.; Allin, B.; Nugawela, M.D.; Rojas, N.; Dalrymple, E.; Pereira, S.P.; Soni, M.; Knight, M.; Cheung, E.Y.; Heyman, I.; et al. Long COVID (post-COVID-19 condition) in children: A modified Delphi process. *Arch. Dis. Child.* **2022**, *107*, 674–680. [CrossRef] [PubMed]
3. *COVID-19 Rapid Guideline: Managing the Long-Term Effects of COVID-19*; National Institute for Health and Care Excellence (NICE): London, UK, 2020.
4. Shachar-Lavie, I.; Shorer, M.; Segal, H.; Fennig, S.; Ashkenazi-Hoffnung, L. Mental health among children with long COVID during the COVID-19 pandemic. *Eur. J. Pediatr.* **2023**, *182*, 1793–1801. [CrossRef] [PubMed]
5. Qin, W.; Chen, S.; Zhang, Y.; Dong, F.; Zhang, Z.; Hu, B.; Zhu, Z.; Li, F.; Wang, X.; Wang, Y.; et al. Diffusion Capacity Abnormalities for Carbon Monoxide in Patients with COVID-19 At Three-Month Follow-up. *Eur. Respir. J.* **2021**, *58*, 2003677. [CrossRef]

6. Torres-Castro, R.; Vasconcello-Castillo, L.; Alsina-Restoy, X.; Solis-Navarro, L.; Burgos, F.; Puppo, H.; Vilaró, J. Respiratory function in patients post-infection by COVID-19: A systematic review and meta-analysis. *Pulmonology* **2020**, *27*, 328–337. [CrossRef] [PubMed]
7. Lee, J.H.; Yim, J.-J.; Park, J. Pulmonary function and chest computed tomography abnormalities 6–12 months after recovery from COVID-19: A systematic review and meta-analysis. *Respir. Res.* **2022**, *23*, 233. [CrossRef] [PubMed]
8. Martins, M.M.; Prata-Barbosa, A.; da Cunha, A.J.L.A. Update on SARS-CoV-2 infection in children. *Paediatr. Int. Child Health* **2021**, *41*, 56–64. [CrossRef]
9. Berg, S.K.; Palm, P.; Nygaard, U.; Bundgaard, H.; Petersen, M.N.S.; Rosenkilde, S.; Thorsted, A.B.; Ersbøll, A.K.; Thygesen, L.C.; Nielsen, S.D.; et al. Long COVID symptoms in SARS-CoV-2-positive children aged 0–14 years and matched controls in Denmark (LongCOVIDKidsDK): A national, cross-sectional study. *Lancet Child Adolesc. Health* **2022**, *6*, 614–623. [CrossRef]
10. Borch, L.; Holm, M.; Knudsen, M.; Ellermann-Eriksen, S.; Hagstroem, S. Long COVID symptoms and duration in SARS-CoV-2 positive children—A nationwide cohort study. *Eur. J. Pediatr.* **2022**, *181*, 1597–1607. [CrossRef]
11. Cui, X.; Zhao, Z.; Zhang, T.; Guo, W.; Guo, W.; Zheng, J.; Zhang, J.; Dong, C.; Na, R.; Zheng, L.; et al. A systematic review and meta-analysis of children with coronavirus disease 2019 (COVID-19). *J. Med. Virol.* **2020**, *93*, 1057–1069. [CrossRef]
12. Palacios, S.; Krivchenia, K.; Eisner, M.; Young, B.; Ramilo, O.; Mejias, A.; Lee, S.; Kopp, B.T. Long-term pulmonary sequelae in adolescents post-SARS-CoV-2 infection. *Pediatr. Pulmonol.* **2022**, *57*, 2455–2463. [CrossRef]
13. Dobkin, S.C.L.; Collaco, J.M.; McGrath-Morrow, S.A. Protracted respiratory findings in children post-SARS-CoV-2 infection. *Pediatr. Pulmonol.* **2021**, *56*, 3682–3687. [CrossRef]
14. Knoke, L.; Schlegtendal, A.; Maier, C.; Eitner, L.; Lücke, T.; Brinkmann, F. Pulmonary Function and Long-Term Respiratory Symptoms in Children and Adolescents After COVID-19. *Front. Pediatr.* **2022**, *10*, 851008. [CrossRef] [PubMed]
15. Doležalová, K.; Tuková, J.; Pohunek, P. The respiratory consequences of COVID-19 lasted for a median of 4 months in a cohort of children aged 2–18 years of age. *Acta Paediatr.* **2022**, *111*, 1201–1206. [CrossRef] [PubMed]
16. Martino, L.; Morello, R.; De Rose, C.; Buonsenso, D. Persistent respiratory symptoms associated with post-covid condition (Long covid) in children: A systematic review and analysis of current gaps and future perspectives. *Expert Rev. Respir. Med.* **2023**. [CrossRef] [PubMed]
17. Ashkenazi-Hoffnung, L.; Shmueli, E.; Ehrlich, S.; Ziv, A.; Bar-On, O.; Birk, E.; Lowenthal, A.; Prais, D. Long COVID in Children. *Pediatr. Infect. Dis. J.* **2021**, *40*, e509–e511. [CrossRef]
18. Testing—Corona Traffic Light Model (Ramzor) Website. Available online: https://corona.health.gov.il/en/testing-lobby/ (accessed on 1 December 2022).
19. Graham, B.L.; Steenbruggen, I.; Miller, M.R.; Barjaktarevic, I.Z.; Cooper, B.G.; Hall, G.L.; Hallstrand, T.S.; Kaminsky, D.A.; McCarthy, K.; McCormack, M.C.; et al. Standardization of Spirometry 2019 Update. An Official American Thoracic Society and European Respiratory Society Technical Statement. *Am. J. Respir. Crit. Care Med.* **2019**, *200*, e70–e88. [CrossRef]
20. American Thoracic Society Guidelines for Methacholine and Exercise Challenge. Available online: www.atsjournals.org (accessed on 4 August 2023).
21. Coates, A.L.; Wanger, J.; Cockcroft, D.W.; Culver, B.H.; Carlsen, K.-H.; Diamant, Z.; Gauvreau, G.; Hall, G.L.; Hallstrand, T.S.; Horvath, I.; et al. ERS technical standard on bronchial challenge testing: General considerations and performance of methacholine challenge tests. *Eur. Respir. J.* **2017**, *49*, 1601526. [CrossRef]
22. Wanger, J.; Clausen, J.L.; Coates, A.; Pedersen, O.F.; Brusasco, V.; Burgos, F.; Casaburi, R.; Crapo, R.; Enright, P.; van der Grinten, C.P.M.; et al. Standardisation of the measurement of lung volumes. *Eur. Respir. J.* **2005**, *26*, 511–522. [CrossRef]
23. Polgar, G.; Varuni, P. *Pulmonary Function Testing in Children: Techniques and Standards*; Saunders Limited: Collingwood, ON, Canada, 1971.
24. Weng, T.R.; Levison, H. Standards of pulmonary function in children. *Am. Rev. Respir. Dis.* **1969**, *99*, 879–894.
25. Dweik, R.A.; Boggs, P.B.; Erzurum, S.C.; Irvin, C.G.; Leigh, M.W.; Lundberg, J.O.; Olin, A.-C.; Plummer, A.L.; Taylor, D.R. American Thoracic Society Committee on Interpretation of Exhaled Nitric Oxide Levels (FENO) for Clinical Applications. An Official ATS Clinical Practice Guideline: Interpretation of Exhaled Nitric Oxide Levels (FeNO) for Clinical Applications. *Am. J. Respir. Crit. Care Med.* **2011**, *184*, 602–615. [CrossRef]
26. Robinson, P.D.; Latzin, P.; Verbanck, S.; Hall, G.L.; Horsley, A.; Gappa, M.; Thamrin, C.; Arets, H.G.; Aurora, P.; Fuchs, S.I.; et al. Consensus statement for inert gas washout measurement using multiple- and single- breath tests. *Eur. Respir. J.* **2013**, *41*, 507–522. [CrossRef] [PubMed]
27. Anagnostopoulou, P.; Latzin, P.; Jensen, R.; Stahl, M.; Harper, A.; Yammine, S.; Usemann, J.; Foong, R.E.; Spycher, B.; Hall, G.L.; et al. Normative data for multiple breath washout outcomes in school-aged Caucasian children. *Eur. Respir. J.* **2019**, *55*, 1901302. [CrossRef] [PubMed]
28. Izbicki, G.; Bar-Yishay, E. Methacholine inhalation challenge: A shorter, cheaper and safe approach. *Eur. Respir. J.* **2001**, *17*, 46–51. [CrossRef] [PubMed]
29. COVID-19 Treatment Guidelines 2. Available online: https://www.covid19treatmentguidelines.nih.gov/ (accessed on 4 August 2023).
30. Morrow, A.K.; Malone, L.A.; Kokorelis, C.; Petracek, L.S.; Eastin, E.F.; Lobner, K.L.; Neuendorff, L.; Rowe, P.C. Long-Term COVID 19 Sequelae in Adolescents: The Overlap with Orthostatic Intolerance and ME/CFS. *Curr. Pediatr. Rep.* **2022**, *10*, 31–44. [CrossRef] [PubMed]

31. Narayanan, D.; Grayson, M.H. Comparing respiratory syncytial virus and rhinovirus in development of post-viral airway disease. *J. Asthma* **2020**, *59*, 434–441. [CrossRef] [PubMed]
32. Dao, T.L.; Hoang, V.T.; Colson, P.; Million, M.; Gautret, P. Co-infection of SARS-CoV-2 and influenza viruses: A systematic review and meta-analysis. *J. Clin. Virol. Plus* **2021**, *1*, 100036. [CrossRef] [PubMed]
33. Palmon, P.A.; Jackson, D.J.; Denlinger, L.C. COVID-19 Infections and Asthma. *J. Allergy Clin. Immunol. Pract.* **2021**, *10*, 658–663. [CrossRef]
34. Cervia, C.; Zurbuchen, Y.; Taeschler, P.; Ballouz, T.; Menges, D.; Hasler, S.; Adamo, S.; Raeber, M.E.; Bächli, E.; Rudiger, A.; et al. Immunoglobulin signature predicts risk of post-acute COVID-19 syndrome. *Nat. Commun.* **2022**, *13*, 1–12. [CrossRef]
35. Warner, J.O.; Warner, J.A.; Munblit, D. Hypotheses to explain the associations between asthma and the consequences of COVID-19 infection. *Clin. Exp. Allergy* **2022**, *52*, 7–9. [CrossRef]
36. Neville, R.D.; Lakes, K.D.; Hopkins, W.G.; Tarantino, G.; Draper, C.E.; Beck, R.; Madigan, S. Global Changes in Child and Adolescent Physical Activity During the COVID-19 Pandemic. *JAMA Pediatr.* **2022**, *176*, 886–894. [CrossRef]
37. Say, D.; Crawford, N.; McNab, S.; Wurzel, D.; Steer, A.; Tosif, S. Post-acute COVID-19 outcomes in children with mild and asymptomatic disease. *Lancet Child Adolesc. Health* **2021**, *5*, e22–e23. [CrossRef] [PubMed]

Disclaimer/Publisher's Note: The statements, opinions and data contained in all publications are solely those of the individual author(s) and contributor(s) and not of MDPI and/or the editor(s). MDPI and/or the editor(s) disclaim responsibility for any injury to people or property resulting from any ideas, methods, instructions or products referred to in the content.

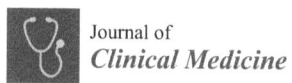

Article

Effects of COVID-19 Lockdown on Heart Failure Patients: A Quasi-Experimental Study

Juan Luis Sánchez-González [1], Luis Almenar-Bonet [2,3,4], Noemí Moreno-Segura [5], Francisco Gurdiel-Álvarez [6], Hady Atef [7], Amalia Sillero-Sillero [8,9,10], Raquel López-Vilella [2], Iván Santolalla-Arnedo [11,*], Raúl Juárez-Vela [11], Clara Isabel Tejada-Garrido [11] and Elena Marques-Sule [12]

1. Department of Nursing and Physiotherapy, University of Salamanca, 37007 Salamanca, Spain; juanluissanchez@usal.es
2. Heart Failure and Transplantation Unit, Department of Cardiology, La Fe University and Polytechnic Hospital, 46026 Valencia, Spain; lualmenar@gmail.com (L.A.-B.); lopez_raqvil@gva.es (R.L.-V.)
3. Centro de Investigación Biomédica en Red de Enfermedades Cardiovasculares (CIBERCV), Instituto de Salud Carlos III, 28933 Madrid, Spain
4. Department of Medicine, Universidad de Valencia, 46010 Valencia, Spain
5. Department of Physiotherapy, Faculty of Physiotherapy, University of Valencia, 46010 Valencia, Spain; noemi.moreno@uv.es
6. Escuela Internacional de Doctorado, Department of Physical Therapy, Occupational Therapy, Reha-Bilitation and Physical Medicine, Universidad Rey Juan Carlos, 28933 Alcorcón, Spain
7. School of Allied Health Professions (SAHP), Keele University, Keele, Staffordshire ST5 5BG, UK; hady612@hotmail.com
8. University School of Nursing and Physiotherapy "Gimbernat", Autonomous University of Barcelona, Avd de la Generalitat, 202-206, Sant Cugat del Vallès, 08174 Barcelona, Spain; amaliasillero@hotmail.com
9. ESIMar (Mar Nursing School), Parc de Salut Mar, Universitat Pompeu Fabra Affiliated, 08018 Barcelona, Spain
10. SDHEd (Social Determinants and Health Education Research Group), IMIM (Hospital del Mar Medical Research Institute), 08003 Barcelona, Spain
11. Nursing Department, Faculty of Health Sciences, Research Group GRUPAC, University of La Rioja, 26004 Logroño, Spain; raul.juarez@unirioja.es (R.J.-V.); clara-isabel.tejada@unirioja.es (C.I.T.-G.)
12. Physiotherapy in Motion, Multispeciality Research Group (PTinMOTION), Department of Physiotherapy, Faculty of Physiotherapy, University of Valencia, 46010 Valencia, Spain
* Correspondence: ivan.santolalla@unirioja.es

Abstract: Introduction: The COVID-19 lockdown has been associated with reduced levels of physical activity, quality of life, and sleep quality, but limited evidence exists for its impact on heart failure patients. This study examined the influence of the COVID-19 lockdown on these aspects in heart failure patients, with specific comparisons by age and sex. Methods: A quasi-experimental cross-sectional study of patients with heart failure was conducted. The assessment involved two time points: during the COVID-19 lockdown (March to June 2020) and post-lockdown (July to October 2020). A total of 107 HF patients participated, with assessments of overall PA (using the International Physical Activity Questionnaire), QoL (employing the Cantril Ladder of Life), and sleep quality (utilizing the Minimal Insomnia Symptom Scale) conducted during and after the COVID-19 lockdown. Results: HF patients reported lower levels of total PA ($p = 0.001$) and walking PA ($p < 0.0001$) during lockdown than after lockdown, whilst no differences were observed in QoL nor sleep quality. In addition, both younger and older patients reported lower walking PA and total PA during lockdown than after lockdown, while older patients reported lower QoL during lockdown than after lockdown. Moreover, both men and women reported lower walking PA and total PA during lockdown than after lockdown, whilst women reported lower QoL. Conclusions: HF patients need improved PA programs during lockdowns, as these programs can elevate PA levels and enhance QoL, especially when faced with the risk of decompensation during health crises.

Keywords: COVID-19; heart failure; physical activity; quality of life; sleep quality

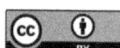

1. Introduction

At the beginning of the pandemic in 2020, many countries opted to contain the spread of COVID-19 by shutting down most significant activities to reduce the pressure on the national health system and avoid increasing deaths [1]. In Spain, the first case of COVID-19 was reported on 1 January 2020, and on 14 March 2020, the government approved a nationwide lockdown. That action prohibited wandering in public spaces except under exceptional circumstances from March to June 2020. These lockdown measures interfered with the general population's daily life and physical and psychological health [2,3], including health professionals and university students [4]. Furthermore, previous studies have demonstrated that this situation has had several consequences on the cardiometabolic system, morbidity, and mortality levels, even in healthy subjects [5]. The situation was even worse with older adults [6] and patients with cardiovascular diseases such as heart failure (HF) [7]. However, Spain was not the only country affected; Asia, Europe, and America were also affected both by the infection itself and by the measures adopted [8,9].

Heart failure HF is a lifelong condition in which the heart cannot pump enough blood to meet the body's needs for blood and oxygen [10]. The same happened to all people during the COVID-19 lockdown, and HF patients had similarly experienced a reduction of physical activity and lockdown-related psychological affection [2,11]. Moreover, this population is more vulnerable to suffering severe COVID-19 and its complications. A recent review by Harrison et al. [12] indicated that cardiovascular disease, specifically HF, is associated with an increased risk of severe COVID-19 and mortality from COVID-19 [12]. This higher proportion of adverse effects could be explained by underlying changes (such as lifestyle), which affect inflammatory pathways and immune and pulmonary functions [12].

The primary variable affected during the pandemic was the physical activity (PA) performed due to the inability to walk regularly outside during the prolonged lockdown [5]. This sedentary behavior can also increase the risk of suffering health problems such as diabetes [13], cancer [14], or osteoporosis [15]. Considering that patients with cardiovascular diseases such as HF have shown lower values of PA than healthy adults [16] may explain why these patients' clinical condition may have been aggravated during the mandatory COVID-19 lockdowns [17,18]. Moreover, in the study performed by Vetrovsky et al. [2], the number of daily steps in 26 patients with HF was analyzed for six weeks, and three of these weeks were during the COVID-19 lockdown period. They found a significant decrease of 1134 daily steps during the lockdown. In parallel, the study of Brasca et al. [19] showed a reduction of 6.5% in PA levels during the COVID-19 lockdown in a cohort of 405 HF patients. Previous studies have demonstrated that the reduction of PA levels tended to be more significant and maintained post-lockdown in those patients who were less physically active before the COVID-19 lockdown and had a more significant NYHA classification [19,20]. The study of Bakel et al. [17] explained that the lack of social contact limited the possibilities of performing PA, whilst younger age was independently associated with a higher sedentary behavior during lockdown.

The consequences of this reduction of the PA levels in HF patients went beyond physical and cardiometabolic sequelae. Previous studies have explained that decreased levels of PA could also affect mental health and quality of life [21–23]. For example, the review of Brooks et al. [3] showed that those who underwent forced lockdown had an increased risk of experiencing some episode of stress, decreasing their emotional quality of life. Sang et al. [22] showed that the COVID-19 lockdown created various psychological impacts, negatively impacting the emotional status due to depression and anxiety. Other studies showed an increased incidence of sleep disturbances in the general population during the first months of the pandemic [16,17]. For example, Voitsidis et al. [24] showed that 37.6% of the Greek general population presented alterations in sleep quality.

Furthermore, the literature has strong evidence that sleep quality disturbance has been associated with an increased risk of cardiovascular events [25]. In addition, people with chronic illnesses such as HF have an increased risk of mood and sleep disturbances that affect their quality of life [26–28]; thus, a more in-depth study of these aspects would be necessary. In consistency with these studies, Quintana et al. [29] evaluated the influence of the COVID-19 lockdown on the quality of life in HF patients. They concluded that during the COVID-19 lockdown, participants showed reduced ability to enjoy daily activities and self-confidence and decreased quality of life.

However, the population with HF is very heterogeneous regarding sociodemographic characteristics. Previous studies on the general population during the COVID-19 lockdown have been performed in this regard. Faulkner et al. [30] assessed physical activity, mental well-being, and quality of life among adults in the United Kingdom, Ireland, New Zealand, and Australia during the COVID-19 lockdown. Their findings revealed that women experienced more favorable physical activity and mental health improvements than men. Additionally, younger participants reported more adverse changes in these aspects than their older counterparts. Beck et al. [31] showed, in a cohort of more than 1000 participants, that approximately 75% of the subjects reporting sleep quality problems were women. Young participants were the ones who presented more sleep issues. Thus, it is evident that the pandemic has affected such outcomes differently depending on age and sex.

Therefore, there is enough evidence to report the changes in PA, quality of life, and sleep quality in the general population during the COVID-19 lockdown. The evidence on HF patients is scarce, and, to the best of our knowledge, no literature makes a differentiation based on sex and age in HF patients in this regard; therefore, this research is novel in this field. The present study explored the PA, quality of life, and sleep quality in HF patients during and after the COVID-19 lockdown and compared the results by sex and age.

The hypotheses of the study are as follows:

H1: *The physical activity in HF patients during the COVID-19 lockdown was lower than after the lockdown.*

H2: *The quality of life in HF patients during the COVID-19 lockdown was lower than after the lockdown.*

H3: *The sleep quality in HF patients during the COVID-19 lockdown was lower than after the lockdown.*

H4: *Physical activity, quality of life, and sleep quality are different when comparing women with HF with men during the COVID-19 lockdown.*

H5: *Physical activity, quality of life, and sleep quality are different when comparing those aged $\geq$ 65 years old with those aged < 65 years old.*

2. Materials and Methods

2.1. Design and Setting

This study employed a cross-sectional, pre-post, quasi-experimental design without a control group. Patient recruitment occurred from March 2020 to October 2020 in Valencia, Spain. Written informed consent was obtained from all participants.

2.2. Sample

This study was completed with a total of 107 participants with HF at different outpatient clinics in Valencia, Spain. Inclusion criteria were as follows: (1) participants above 18 years of age (2) who have a clinical diagnosis of HF and (3) who are cognitively capable of completing the assessments. Participants with cognitive and neuropsychiatric disorders were excluded from this study.

2.3. Procedure

Participants were clinically diagnosed with heart failure (HF) based on electronic medical records. The assessment involved two time points: during the COVID-19 lockdown (March to June 2020) and post-lockdown (July to October 2020), as depicted in Figure 1.

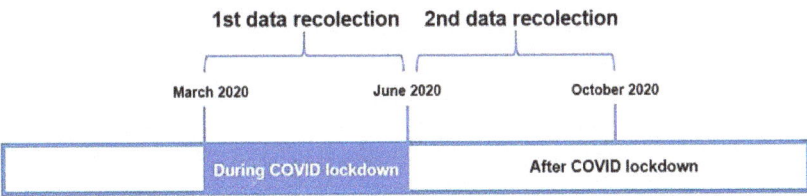

Figure 1. Timeline.

Due to the unique circumstances posed by the COVID-19 pandemic, our data collection strategy was adapted. Despite the initial recruitment being carried out in a face-to-face setting, we opted for telephone interviews to ensure the safety and well-being of our participants. These interviews were conducted by a trained researcher who adhered to a structured and standardized approach.

2.4. Outcomes and Measures

A patient information form was developed to collect data regarding demographic and clinical variables: Our study encompassed a range of sociodemographic and clinical variables, including gender, age, marital status, working status, education, time since diagnosis, weight, height, and body mass index (BMI). Additionally, we assessed the following variables:

(1) Overall physical activity: This was measured with the Spanish version of the International Physical Activity Questionnaire (IPAQ) [32]. The IPAQ contains seven questions to determine the duration and frequency of light activity (<600 metabolic minutes: walking at home and at work or any walking that can be done solely for leisure); moderate activity (between 600 and 3000 MET minutes/week such as cycling, playing tennis, or carrying light loads); and vigorous activity (>3000 MET minutes/week: doing aerobic exercise, digging, or heavy lifting). It also assesses the inactivity of the last week. The total PA score is the sum of vigorous, moderate, and light PA in MET minutes/week [32,33]. The questionnaire presents a total intra-observer reliability of 0.914 and 0.900 in the three dimensions of the questionnaire separately. Moreover, the questionnaire presents an internal consistency of Cronbach's alpha = 0.51 [34].

(2) Quality of life (QoL): QoL was assessed using the Cantril Ladder of Life [35]. This questionnaire has been employed in previous cardiovascular studies and is considered a valid measure of global quality of life [36–38]. It does not cover quality of life as a multidimensional concept, although it is related to aspects of quality of life such as psychosocial adjustment and functional capabilities [39]. Patients were asked about their quality of life on a scale from 0 to 10 (scores of 10 reflected the best quality of life and 0 reflected the worst). The scale shows good convergent validity [40] and presents a total intra-observer reliability of 0.914 [40,41]. This scale was translated to Spanish by a native Spanish speaker and was back-translated by another independent bilingual researcher.

(3) Quality of sleep: Sleep quality was assessed by the Minimal Insomnia Symptom Scale (MISS) [42,43], which consists of three items with five response categories (no, minor, moderate, severe, and very severe problems) that are scored from 0 to 4, respectively. The total score ranged from 0 to 12, with higher scores representing higher sleeping difficulties. The questionnaire asks about difficulties falling asleep, nighttime awakenings, and rest during sleep. The reliability and validity of the MISS have been established among the elderly with a high intraclass correlation coefficient of 0.79 with an internal consistency

of Cronbach's alpha = 0.73 [43]. This questionnaire was translated to Spanish by a native Spanish speaker and was back-translated by another independent bilingual researcher.

Reliability and validity of the questionnaires shows in Table 1.

Table 1. Reliability and validity of the questionnaires.

	Intra-Observer Reliability	Internal Consistency
Physical activity (IPAQ)	0.900–0.914	0.51
Quality of life (Cantril Ladder of Life)	0.914	-
Quality of sleep (MISS)	0.79	0.73

2.5. Data Analysis

Statistical analyses were performed using the statistical package SPSS version 24 (IBM SPSS, Inc., Chicago, IL, USA). Mean, standard deviation, and percentage were used to describe the sample data. Sample size calculation: We determined the required sample size before the study. With an estimated alpha risk of 0.05 and a beta risk of less than 0.2 in a bilateral contrast, we aimed to have sufficient statistical power to detect differences of 15% or more. Based on these criteria and assuming a standard deviation of 60 for the difference between measurements taken before and after the lockdown, we determined that a sample size of 100 subjects was necessary for our analysis. This ensured that the study would have the statistical strength to identify significant changes in the variables of interest. The Kolmogorov–Smirnov test was used to verify the normality of the continuous data. Paired t-tests for the Cantril Ladder of Life, MISS, and IPAQ were employed to compare the differences between COVID-19 lockdown and after-lockdown periods within matched pairs. The effect size was calculated using Cohen's d for the paired t-test. Subgroup analyses were also performed for age (<65 years and ≥65 years) and sex. For the subgroup analysis, paired t-tests were used to compare between time events and Student t-tests were used to compare between groups. Statistical significance was considered when p-values were <0.05.

2.6. Ethical Considerations

Approval was obtained from the Regional Ethics Committee (Approval No. IE1529273). All procedures were conducted strictly within the principles of the Declaration of Helsinki (October 2013, Fortaleza, Brazil). The researchers explained the research aims to all participants. Stringent measures were taken to ensure the privacy and confidentiality of participant data. The anonymity of the participants was guaranteed, and informed consent to participate was obtained prior to data collection. These ethical measures were implemented to safeguard the rights and well-being of the study participants.

3. Results

A total of 107 HF patients were assessed during and after the COVID-19 lockdown. The characteristics of the 107 participants are shown in Table 2.

Regarding PA, HF patients reported significantly lower levels of walking PA during lockdown than after lockdown (r = 0.49, p < 0.001). In addition, significantly lower levels of total PA were also found when comparing during lockdown and after lockdown periods (r = 0.46, p < 0.001). Nevertheless, no differences were found in vigorous PA (p = 0.181) or moderate PA (p = 0.068) levels or in sedentary time (p = 0.872). With regards to quality of life, no differences were found during lockdown compared to after lockdown (p = 0.091). Regarding sleep quality, no differences were found during lockdown compared to after lockdown (difficulties falling asleep, p = 0.897; night awakenings, p = 1.000; not being rested by sleep, p = 0.495) (Table 3).

Table 2. Clinical and demographic characteristics of the participants.

Variables	Total (n = 107)	By Sex Male	By Sex Female	By Age <65	By Age ≥65
Age, (years), mean (SD)	73.18 (12.68)	73.54 (12.91)	72.70 (12.51)	53.48 (8.78) *	77.99 (7.95) *
Sex, n (%)					
Male	61.00 (57.00)	61.00 (100.00)	0.00 (0.00)	12.00 (57.10)	49.00 (57.00)
Female	46.00 (43.00)	0.00 (0.00)	46.00 (100.00)	9.00 (42.90)	37.00 (43.00)
Marital status, n (%)					
Married	90.00 (84.10)	52.00 (85.20)	38.00 (82.60)	70.00 (81.40)	70.00 (81.40)
Single	2.00 (1.90)	2.00 (3.30)	0.00 (0.00)	1.00 (1.20)	1.00 (1.20)
Widowed	15.00 (14.00)	7.00 (11.5)	8.00 (17.40)	15.00 (17.40)	15.00 (17.40)
Working status, n (%)					
Employed	1.00 (10.20)	7.00 (11.40)	4.00 (8.70)	10.00 (47.70)	1.00 (1.20)
Unemployed	4.00 (3.70)	2.00 (3.30)	2.00 (4.30)	4.00 (19.00)	0.00 (0.00)
Housekeeper	14.00 (13.10)	5.00 (8.20)	9.00 (19.60)	0.00 (0.00)	14.00 (16.30)
Retired	78.00 (72.90)	47.00 (77.00)	31.00 (67.40)	7.00 (33.30)	71.00 (82.50)
Education, n (%)					
None	17.00 (15.80)	7.00 (11.40)	10.00 (21.70)	0.00 (0.00)	17.00 (19.80)
Primary education	39.00 (36.40)	24.00 (39.30)	15.00 (32.60)	2.00 (9.50)	37.00 (43.00)
Secondary education	38.00 (35.50)	20.00 (32.80)	13.00 (28.30)	14.00 (66.60)	24.00 (27.90)
University	13.00 (12.10)	8.00 (13.10)	5.00 (10.90)	5.00 (23.80)	8.00 (9.30)
Time since diagnosis, months, mean (SD)	96.54 (134.81)	82.75 (121.87)	114.83 (149.69)	64.38 (76.85)	104.40 (144.76)
LVEF, %, mean (SD)	43.36 (15.44)	40.51 (15.00) *	47.12 (15.38) *	41.74 (13.60)	43.75 (15.91)
NYHA Classification, n (%)					
I	7.00 (6.50)	5.00 (8.20)	2.00 (4.30)	1.00 (4.80)	6.00 (7.00)
II	73.00 (68.2)	43.00 (70.50)	30.00 (65.20)	15.00 (71.40)	58.00 (67.40)
III	22.00 (20.6)	10.00 (16.40)	12.00 (26.10)	5.00 (23.80)	17.00 (19.80)
IV	5.00 (4.70)	3.00 (4.90)	2.00 (4.30)	0.00 (0.00)	5.00 (5.80)
Weight, kilograms, mean (SD)	71.78 (14.11)	75.59 (13.80) *	66.72 (13.02) *	74.38 (14.64)	71.14 (13.99)
BMI, mean (SD)	26.42 (4.73)	26.51 (4.58)	26.30 (4.97)	27.45 (4.42)	26.17 (4.79)

Note: SD = standard deviation; BMI = body mass index; LVEF = left ventricular ejection fraction; NYHA = New York Heart Association. * $p < 0.05$.

Table 3. Results of physical activity, quality of life, and sleep quality during and after the COVID-19 lockdown.

	During Lockdown Mean (SD)	After Lockdown Mean (SD)	T Student p Value
Physical activity (IPAQ)			
Vigorous PA, METS minute/week	0.00 (0.00)	26.92 (206.74)	0.181
Moderate PA, METS minute/week	87.48 (329.90)	129.35 (424.27)	0.068
Walking, METS minute/week	302.61 (371.98)	871.23 (931.94)	<0.001 *
Sedentary time, hours/day	5.88 (5.41)	5.80 (4.66)	0.872
Total score, METS minute/week	386.85 (581.69)	999.16 (10)	<0.001 *
Quality of life (Cantril Ladder of Life)	5.61 (2.32)	5.84 (2.31)	0.091
Quality of sleep (MISS)			
Difficulties falling asleep	1.40 (1.46)	1.41 (1.45)	0.897
Night awakenings	1.51 (1.29)	1.51 (1.33)	1.000
Not being rested by sleep	0.63 (1.04)	0.59 (1.00)	0.495

Note: SD = standard deviation; IPAQ = International Physical Activity Questionnaire; MISS = Minimal Insomnia Symptom Scale; *: $p < 0.05$.

When comparing by age, both those aged <65 years old and those aged ≥65 years old reported significantly lower levels during a lockdown than after lockdown in walking PA (<65 years: r = 0.52, $p = 0.001$; ≥65 years: r = −0.48, $p < 0.001$), as well as in total PA (<65 years: r = 0.52, $p = 0.003$; ≥65 years: r = 0.45, $p < 0.001$), whilst there were no differences in the rest of the IPAQ variables. In addition, when comparing age subgroups (<65 years old vs. ≥65 years) during lockdown, we did not find significant differences in any of the IPAQ variables (vigorous PA ($p = 1.000$), moderate PA ($p = 0.451$), walking PA ($p = 0.256$), sedentary time ($p = 0.264$), total PA ($p = 0.203$)). When comparing the quality of life by age, those aged ≥ 65 years old reported significantly lower quality of life (r = 0.15, $p = 0.039$) during lockdown than after lockdown. When comparing sleep quality by age, we did not find differences between groups or intra-groups (Table 4).

Table 4. Comparison of physical activity, quality of life, and sleep quality during and after the COVID-19 lockdown by age.

	<65 Years Old Mean (SD)			≥65 Years Old Mean (SD)		
	During Lockdown	After Lockdown	p Value	During Lockdown	After Lockdown	p Value
Physical activity (IPAQ)						
Vigorous PA, METS/min/week	0.00 (0.00)	91.43 (418.98)	0.329	0.00 (0.00)	11.16 (103.52)	0.320
Moderate PA, METS/min/week	80.00 (366.61)	80.00 (366.61)	1.000	89.30 (322.62)	141.40 (438.29)	0.068
Walking PA, METS/min/week	196.43 (244.12)	891.79 (899.75)	<0.001 *	328.85 (394.03)	866.15 (944.86)	<0.001 *
Sedentary time	7.10 (5.30)	7.38 (3.58)	0.788	5.58 (5.42)	5.42 (4.83)	0.756
Total score, METS/min/week	276.43 (488.48)	1063.21 (1180.22)	0.003 *	413.81 (601.73)	983.52 (1069.83)	<0.001 *
Quality of life (Cantril Ladder of Life)	6.33 (2.31)	6.24 (1.90)	0.776	5.43 (2.30)	5.74 (2.40)	0.039 *
Sleep quality (MISS)						
Difficulties falling asleep	1.33 (1.53)	1.48 (1.66)	0.526	1.42 (1.45)	1.40 (1.40)	0.748
Night awakenings	1.24 (1.22)	1.38 (1.28)	0.379	1.58 (1.31)	1.55 (1.34)	0.671
Not being rested by sleep	0.43 (0.81)	0.43 (0.81)	1.000	0.67 (1.09)	0.63 (1.04)	0.436

Note: Md = median; IQ range = interquartile range; SD = standard deviation; MISS = Minimal Insomnia Symptom Scale; IPAQ = International Physical Activity Questionnaire; *: $p < 0.05$.

When comparing by sex, both men and women reported significantly lower levels during lockdown than after lockdown in walking PA (men: r = 0.57, $p < 0.001$; women: r = 0.47, $p < 0.001$), as well as in total PA (men: r = 0.54, $p < 0.001$; women: r = 0.07, $p < 0.001$), while there were no differences in the rest of the IPAQ variables. In addition, when comparing by sex during lockdown, we did not find significant differences in vigorous PA ($p = 1.000$), moderate PA ($p = 0.289$), walking PA ($p = 0.069$), sedentary time ($p = 0.071$), or total PA ($p = 0.135$). When comparing the quality of life by sex, women reported a significantly lower quality of life (r = 0.21, $p = 0.046$) during lockdown than after lockdown. When comparing sleep quality by sex, we did not find any difference between women and men (Table 5).

Table 5. Comparison of physical activity, quality of life, and sleep quality during and after the COVID-19 lockdown by sex.

	Men Mean (SD)			Women Mean (SD)		
	During Lockdown	After Lockdown	p Value	During Lockdown	After Lockdown	p Value
Physical activity (IPAQ)						
Vigorous PA, METS/min/week	0.00 (0.00)	47.21 (273.01)	0.182	0.00 (0.00)	0.00 (0.00)	1.000
Moderate PA, METS/min/week	78.69 (324.14)	106.23 (343.70)	0.366	99.13 (340.64)	160 (514.60)	0.084
Walking PA, METS/min/week	347.33 (374.82)	929.14 (880.67)	<0.001 *	242 (393.44)	792.73 (1002.01)	<0.001 *
Sedentary time	6.72 (5.36)	6.57 (4.34)	0.815	4.76 (5.32)	4.78 (4.92)	0.975
Total score, METS/min/week	426.18 (527.38)	1082.58 (1060.86)	<0.001 *	334.70 (649.09)	888.54 (1123.06)	<0.001 *
Quality of life (Cantril Ladder of Life)	5.70 (2.25)	5.87 (2.22)	0.450	5.48 (2.43)	5.80 (2.46)	0.046 *
Sleep quality (MISS)						
Difficulties falling asleep	1.44 (1.50)	1.49 (1.49)	0.643	1.35 (1.41)	1.30 (1.40)	0.642
Night awakenings	1.57 (1.35)	1.56 (1.37)	0.874	1.43 (1.22)	1.46 (1.28)	0.830
Not being rested by sleep	0.61 (1.05)	0.61 (1.05)	0.471	0.59 (0.98)	0.57 (0.94)	0.811

Note: SD = standard deviation; MISS = Minimal Insomnia Symptom Scale; IPAQ = International Physical Activity Questionnaire; *: $p < 0.05$.

4. Discussion

In this study, we investigated the physical activity (PA), quality of life, and sleep quality in heart failure (HF) patients during and after the COVID-19 lockdown, with a focus on differences related to age and sex.

4.1. Physical Activity (PA) during Lockdown

Our study findings reveal that HF patients, both men and women, irrespective of age (above or below 65 years), experienced a decline in their PA levels during the COVID-19 lockdown. However, once the lockdown restrictions were lifted, there was an increase in PA. Notably, participants exhibited higher sedentary behavior during the lockdown, validating our initial hypothesis (H1: The PA in HF patients during the COVID-19 lockdown was lower than after the lockdown). These results are consistent with previous research, such as that of Tison et al. [44], who noted an increase in daily steps post-lockdown, and Van Bakkel et al. [18], who observed progressively increasing sedentary behavior as restrictions eased. Nevertheless, a recent systematic review emphasized a significant decrease in PA levels among patients with cardiovascular diseases, particularly HF patients, during the COVID-19 lockdown [45]. Subgroup analysis indicated that the decrease in PA was consistent across gender and age, leading us to reject hypotheses H4 (differences in PA between women and men with HF during the lockdown) and H5 (differences in PA between those aged $\geq$ 65 and <65 years). Kim et al. [46] found different results in the sex difference in a sample of 229,099 subjects. They observed that men engaged in more moderate-intensity PA than women before and during COVID-19. On the other hand, Punia et al. [47] observed that men showed lower physical activity levels during the pandemic in a sample of 1992 subjects. Therefore, there seems to be too much discrepancy between BP levels between the two genders.

4.2. Quality of Life during Lockdown

Contrary to our expectations (H2), the overall quality of life among HF patients did not exhibit any significant changes during the COVID-19 lockdown in our study. However, variations were observed when examining different age and gender groups, leading us to accept hypotheses H4 (differences in quality of life between women and men with HF during the lockdown) and H5 (differences in quality of life between those aged $\geq$65 and <65 years). Specifically, adults older than 65 and women reported a lower quality of life during the lockdown than those younger than 65 years and men. It is important to note that an HF diagnosis can substantially impact a patient's quality of life [29]. These results differ from a recent epidemiological study [29], which reported that patients with HF had difficulties enjoying daily activities during the COVID-19 lockdown, although no post-lockdown assessments were conducted. As such, it is crucial to emphasize self-care behaviors and provide practical self-care management information to HF patients and their families. To our knowledge, this is the first study that reports the results about the quality of life of HF patients during lockdown, but previous studies were performed on other health problems such as the study of van Erck et al. [48], who found an increase in the quality of life during lockdown in patients awaiting transcatheter aortic valve implantation. In contrast, Banerjee et al. [49] showed that the quality of life of patients with Parkinson's Disease and their caregivers was decreased. This lack of differences could be due to the fact that patients with HF have a chronic clinical condition that limits their quality of life; therefore, the modifications in quality of life due to confinement could be more subtle. Then, future studies that explored the changes in quality of life in diseases that already had a reduced quality of life should be performed in order to understand these results better.

4.3. Sleep Quality during Lockdown

Our study showed no discernible differences in sleep quality between different periods, genders, or age groups. As a result, hypotheses H3 (that sleep quality in HF patients during the COVID-19 lockdown was lower than after lockdown), H4 (that sleep quality differed between women and men with HF during the COVID-19 lockdown), and H5 (that sleep quality varied between those aged ≥ 65 years and <65 years) were not supported. However, various studies have highlighted the severe impact of the COVID-19 pandemic on multiple aspects of human life and its substantial threat to the mental and physical health of the general population [50]. Our results do not align with a study by Okely et al. [51], who investigated changes in sleep quality among elderly individuals during the COVID-19 lockdown. They also explored whether participant characteristics were related to positive or negative changes in sleep quality, ultimately concluding that participants with a history of cardiovascular disease had worse sleep quality during the lockdown. As with the quality of life, to our knowledge, this is the first study that analyzes the quality of sleep of HF patients during lockdown, but studies performed in patients with pulmonary hypertension [52], women with polycystic ovary syndrome [53], and also in the general population [54] showed a reduced quality of sleep during lockdown [52]. A reason for these results could be the fact that the HF patients had a reduced PA in normal conditions; therefore, although a reduction in PA was evidenced in the lockdown period, it could be insufficient to reduce the quality of sleep.

Study limitations: Our study had several limitations to consider. First, the relatively small sample size and the predominance of male participants introduced potential gender bias, limiting the generalizability of findings to a broader heart failure (HF) population. Second, the exclusive focus on HF patients within a single country restricted the generalizability of results across diverse international contexts. Additionally, the reliance on self-reported questionnaires for assessing physical activity (PA) may have introduced recall bias and overestimation. We recognize the need for validity and reliability testing on the questionnaires to enhance the study's robustness. Furthermore, the absence of data quality checks may imply potential data quality issues. It is also worth noting that socioeconomic status and mental health are possible factors that could influence the PA levels in this population, which, in conjunction with the study design, account for a causal inference problem in the results. Nonetheless, future investigations can explore data accuracy, completeness, reliability, relevance, and timeliness.

Strengths: Our study offered a comprehensive assessment of PA, quality of life, and sleep quality changes in HF patients during and after the COVID-19 lockdown, which were areas with limited prior research. Conducting measurements at two time points provided valuable insights into the impact of the pandemic and lockdown measures on these aspects of patients' lives. In summary, despite these limitations, our study contributes significant insights into the experiences of HF patients during and after the COVID-19 lockdown, and future research should aim to address these constraints and further enrich our understanding of this critical issue.

4.4. Implications and Future Lines of Action

Physical activity (PA) constitutes a pivotal intervention in heart failure (HF) management, with research underscoring its significant impact on patient survival rates, including reduced all-cause mortality and HF-related mortality [55,56]. Therefore, addressing the risk of HF decompensation due to physical inactivity remains a paramount concern, necessitating the encouragement of HF patients to uphold substantial PA levels and minimize prolonged sedentary behavior, especially in contexts like the COVID-19 lockdown. This underscores the imperative need for developing home-based PA programs and implementing routine follow-up assessments for HF patients, emphasizing monitoring their PA levels.

Furthermore, preserving the high quality of life and overall health in the HF population is essential for averting decompensation and fostering well-being. To this end, a compelling strategy involves the integration of eHealth initiatives, specializing in medical care and cardiac telerehabilitation, thus offering PA-centric programs and services tailored to HF patients [57–59]. These eHealth initiatives should closely align with the exercise guidelines set forth by the American Heart Association [60] because they emphasize activities like moderate aerobic exercise for a minimum of 150 min per week, bi-weekly muscle strengthening routines, regular stretching, and a medical consultation before commencing any exercise regimen. Notably, in 2019, the European Commission's Digital Economy and Society Index (DESI) identified Spain as the third-ranking country within the European Union in eHealth utilization [61]. This statistical revelation reveals Spain's prior commitment to eHealth solutions, even preceding the global pandemic, underscoring the compelling prospects that future research should explore in harnessing these digital tools to enhance the welfare of HF patients.

5. Conclusions

Our findings revealed that regardless of age, HF patients experienced reduced walking and total PA levels during the lockdown, while quality of life and sleep remained relatively stable. Age-wise, both younger and older patients showed decreased PA levels during lockdown, with older patients also reporting reduced quality of life during this period. Sex-based comparisons indicated that men and women experienced declines in PA, while women reported decreased quality of life. Sleep quality, however, exhibited no significant sex-based differences. These results highlight the need for innovative strategies to boost PA and promote healthier lifestyles, particularly during public health crises like the COVID-19 lockdown. Implementing eHealth services and telerehabilitation programs could be valuable solutions to support patients. Engaging HF patients in PA-based initiatives elevates their PA levels and enhances their overall quality of life. It is especially critical when reduced PA may heighten the risk of disease exacerbation and increased patient vulnerability, especially when healthcare resources are constrained. These policies should extend beyond the HF population to encompass the entire community, contributing to maintaining a healthier population and reducing the strain on healthcare resources during health system stress.

Author Contributions: Conceptualization, E.M.-S., L.A.-B., R.L.-V. and J.L.S.-G.; methodology, J.L.S.-G., N.M.-S., A.S.-S., H.A. and R.J.-V.; software, F.G.-Á.; formal analysis, F.G.-Á.; investigation, N.M.-S., A.S.-S. and H.A.; resources, E.M.-S., H.A. and A.S.-S.; data curation, J.L.S.-G. and F.G.-Á.; writing—original draft preparation, J.L.S.-G. and F.G.-Á.; writing—review and editing, E.M.-S., N.M.-S., H.A., A.S.-S., L.A.-B. and R.J.-V.; supervision, E.M.-S., L.A.-B., H.A., A.S.-S. and I.S.-A.; project administration, E.M.-S., L.A.-B. and C.I.T.-G. All authors H.A. All authors have read and agreed to the published version of the manuscript.

Funding: This research received no external funding.

Institutional Review Board Statement: This study was conducted in accordance with the Declaration of Helsinki and approved by the Institutional Review Board of the Regional Ethics Committee (no. IE1529273).

Informed Consent Statement: Informed consent was obtained from all subjects involved in the study.

Data Availability Statement: Data will be provided upon request to the corresponding author.

Conflicts of Interest: The authors declare no conflict of interest.

References

1. Ploumpidis, D. Living with COVID-19. *Psychiatriki* **2020**, *31*, 197–200. [CrossRef] [PubMed]
2. Vetrovsky, T.; Frybova, T.; Gant, I.; Semerad, M.; Cimler, R.; Bunc, V.; Siranec, M.; Miklikova, M.; Vesely, J.; Griva, M.; et al. The detrimental effect of COVID-19 nationwide quarantine on accelerometer-assessed physical activity of heart failure patients. *ESC Heart Fail.* **2020**, *7*, 2093–2097. [CrossRef] [PubMed]
3. Brooks, S.K.; Webster, R.K.; Smith, L.E.; Woodland, L.; Wessely, S.; Greenberg, N.; Rubin, G.J. The psychological impact of quarantine and how to reduce it: A Rapid review of the evidence. *Lancet* **2020**, *395*, 912–920. [CrossRef] [PubMed]
4. Srivastav, A.K.; Sharma, N.; Samuel, A.J. Impact of Coronavirus disease-19 (COVID-19) lockdown on physical activity and energy expenditure among physiotherapy professionals and students using web-based open E-survey sent through WhatsApp, Facebook and Instagram messengers. *Clin. Epidemiol. Glob. Health* **2020**, *9*, 78–84. [CrossRef]
5. Chen, P.; Mao, L.; Nassis, G.P.; Harmer, P.; Ainsworth, B.E.; Li, F. Coronavirus disease (COVID-19): The need to maintain regular physical activity while taking precautions. *J. Sport Health Sci.* **2020**, *9*, 103–104. [CrossRef]

6. Sell, N.M.; Silver, J.K.; Rando, S.; Draviam, A.C.; Mina, D.S.; Qadan, M. Prehabilitation Telemedicine in Neoadjuvant Surgical Oncology Patients During the Novel COVID-19 Coronavirus Pandemic. *Ann. Surg.* **2020**, *272*, e81–e83. [CrossRef]
7. Lippi, G.; Henry, B.M.; Sanchis-Gomar, F. Physical inactivity and cardiovascular disease at the time of coronavirus disease 2019 (COVID-19). *Eur. J. Prev. Cardiol.* **2020**, *27*, 906–908. [CrossRef]
8. Chu, D.-T.; Ngoc, S.-M.V.; Thi, H.V.; Thi, Y.-V.N.; Ho, T.-T.; Hoang, V.-T.; Singh, V.; Al-Tawfiq, J.A. COVID-19 in Southeast Asia: Current status and perspectives. *Bioengineered* **2022**, *13*, 3797–3809. [CrossRef]
9. Schwalb, A.; Armyra, E.; Méndez-Aranda, M.; Ugarte-Gil, C. COVID-19 in Latin America and the Caribbean: Two years of the pandemic. *J. Intern. Med.* **2022**, *292*, 409–427. [CrossRef]
10. American Heart Association. What Is Heart Failure. 2023. Available online: https://www.heart.org/en/health-topics/heart-failure/what-is-heart-failure (accessed on 4 November 2023).
11. Schmitt, J.; Wenzel, B.; Brüsehaber, B.; Anguera, I.; de Sousa, J.; Nölker, G.; Bulava, A.; Marques, P.; Hatala, R.; Golovchiner, G.; et al. Impact of lockdown during COVID-19 pandemic on physical activity and arrhythmia burden in heart failure patients. *Pacing Clin. Electrophysiol.* **2022**, *45*, 471–480. [CrossRef]
12. Harrison, S.L.; Buckley, B.J.R.; Rivera-Caravaca, J.M.; Zhang, J.; Lip, G.Y.H. Cardiovascular risk factors, cardiovascular disease, and COVID-19: An umbrella review of systematic reviews. *Eur. Heart J.—Qual. Care Clin. Outcomes* **2021**, *7*, 330–339. [CrossRef] [PubMed]
13. Bhaskarabhatla, K.V.; Birrer, R. Physical Activity and Diabetes Mellitus. *Compr. Ther.* **2005**, *31*, 291–298. [CrossRef] [PubMed]
14. Sanchis-Gomar, F.; Lucia, A.; Yvert, T.; Ruiz-Casado, A.; Pareja-Galeano, H.; Santos-Lozano, A.; Fiuza-Luces, C.; Garatachea, N.; Lippi, G.; Bouchard, C.; et al. Physical Inactivity and Low Fitness Deserve More Attention to Alter Cancer Risk and Prognosis. *Cancer Prev. Res.* **2015**, *8*, 105–110. [CrossRef] [PubMed]
15. Castrogiovanni, P.; Trovato, F.M.; Szychlinska, M.A.; Nsir, H.; Imbesi, R.; Musumeci, G. The importance of physical activity in osteoporosis. From the molecular pathways to the clinical evidence. *Histol. Histopathol.* **2016**, *31*, 1183–1194. [CrossRef] [PubMed]
16. Vasankari, V.; Husu, P.; Vähä-Ypyä, H.; Suni, J.H.; Tokola, K.; Borodulin, K.; Wennman, H.; Halonen, J.; Hartikainen, J.; Sievänen, H.; et al. Subjects with cardiovascular disease or high disease risk are more sedentary and less active than their healthy peers. *BMJ Open Sport Exerc. Med.* **2018**, *4*, e000363. [CrossRef] [PubMed]
17. Van Bakel, B.M.; Bakker, E.A.; de Vries, F.; Thijssen, D.H.; Eijsvogels, T.M. Changes in Physical Activity and Sedentary Behaviour in Cardiovascular Disease Patients during the COVID-19 Lockdown. *Int. J. Environ. Res. Public Health* **2021**, *18*, 11929. [CrossRef]
18. Van Bakel, B.M.A.; Bakker, E.A.; de Vries, F.; Thijssen, D.H.J.; Eijsvogels, T.M.H. Impact of COVID-19 lockdown on physical activity and sedentary behaviour in Dutch cardiovascular disease patients. *Neth. Heart J.* **2021**, *29*, 273–279. [CrossRef]
19. Brasca, F.M.A.; Casale, M.C.; Canevese, F.L.; Tortora, G.; Pagano, G.; Botto, G.L. Physical Activity in Patients with Heart Failure During and After COVID-19 Lockdown: Single-Center Observational Retrospective Study. *JMIR Cardio* **2022**, *6*, e30661. [CrossRef]
20. Cunha, P.M.; Ribeiro, A.S.; Tomeleri, C.M.; Schoenfeld, B.J.; Silva, A.M.; Souza, M.F.; Nascimento, M.A.; Sardinha, L.B.; Cyrino, E.S. The effects of resistance training volume on osteosarcopenic obesity in older women. *J. Sports Sci.* **2018**, *36*, 1564–1571. [CrossRef]
21. Hwang, S.; Liao, W.; Huang, T. Predictors of quality of life in patients with heart failure. *Jpn. J. Nurs. Sci.* **2014**, *11*, 290–298. [CrossRef]
22. Sang, X.; Menhas, R.; Saqib, Z.A.; Mahmood, S.; Weng, Y.; Khurshid, S.; Iqbal, W.; Shahzad, B. The Psychological Impacts of COVID-19 Home Confinement and Physical Activity: A Structural Equation Model Analysis. *Front. Psychol.* **2021**, *11*, 614770. [CrossRef] [PubMed]
23. Dai, J.; Sang, X.; Menhas, R.; Xu, X.; Khurshid, S.; Mahmood, S.; Weng, Y.; Huang, J.; Cai, Y.; Shahzad, B.; et al. The Influence of COVID-19 Pandemic on Physical Health–Psychological Health, Physical Activity, and Overall Well-Being: The Mediating Role of Emotional Regulation. *Front. Psychol.* **2021**, *12*, 667461. [CrossRef] [PubMed]
24. Voitsidis, P.; Gliatas, I.; Bairachtari, V.; Papadopoulou, K.; Papageorgiou, G.; Parlapani, E.; Syngelakis, M.; Holeva, V.; Diakogiannis, I. Insomnia during the COVID-19 pandemic in a Greek population. *Psychiatry Res.* **2020**, *289*, 113076. [CrossRef] [PubMed]
25. Falkingham, J.; Evandrou, M.; Vlachantoni, A.; Qin, M. Sleep Problems and New Occurrence of Chronic Conditions during the COVID-19 Pandemic in the UK. *Int. J. Environ. Res. Public Health* **2022**, *19*, 15664. [CrossRef] [PubMed]
26. Gualano, M.R.; Lo Moro, G.; Voglino, G.; Bert, F.; Siliquini, R. Effects of COVID-19 Lockdown on Mental Health and Sleep Disturbances in Italy. *Int. J. Environ. Res. Public Health* **2020**, *17*, 4779. [CrossRef]
27. Silva, P.C.; Neto, O.P.d.A.; Resende, E.S. Epidemiological profile, cardiopulmonary fitness and health-related quality of life of patients with heart failure: A longitudinal study. *Health Qual. Life Outcomes* **2021**, *19*, 129. [CrossRef]
28. Peng, M.; Mo, B.; Liu, Y.; Xu, M.; Song, X.; Liu, L.; Fang, Y.; Guo, T.; Ye, J.; Yu, Z.; et al. Prevalence, risk factors and clinical correlates of depression in quarantined population during the COVID-19 outbreak. *J. Affect. Disord.* **2020**, *275*, 119–124. [CrossRef]
29. Martínez-Quintana, E.; Vega-Acedo, L.d.C.; Santana-Herrera, D.; Pérez-Acosta, C.; Medina-Gil, J.M.; Muñoz-Díaz, E.; Rodríguez-González, F. Mental well-being among patients with congenital heart disease and heart failure during the COVID-19 pandemic. *Am. J. Cardiovasc. Dis.* **2021**, *11*, 618–623.
30. Faulkner, J.; O'brien, W.J.; McGrane, B.; Wadsworth, D.; Batten, J.; Askew, C.D.; Badenhorst, C.; Byrd, E.; Coulter, M.; Draper, N.; et al. Physical activity, mental health and well-being of adults during initial COVID-19 containment strategies: A multi-country cross-sectional analysis. *J. Sci. Med. Sport* **2020**, *24*, 320–326. [CrossRef]
31. Beck, F.; Léger, D.; Fressard, L.; Peretti-Watel, P.; Verger, P. The Coconel Group COVID-19 health crisis and lockdown associated with high level of sleep complaints and hypnotic uptake at the population level. *J. Sleep Res.* **2021**, *30*, e13119. [CrossRef]

32. Craig, C.L.; Marshall, A.L.; Sjöström, M.; Bauman, A.E.; Booth, M.L.; Ainsworth, B.E.; Pratt, M.; Ekelund, U.L.; Yngve, A.; Sallis, J.F.; et al. International Physical Activity Questionnaire: 12-Country Reliability and Validity. *Med. Sci. Sports Exerc.* **2003**, *35*, 1381–1395. [CrossRef] [PubMed]
33. Hurtig-Wennlöf, A.; Hagströmer, M.; Olsson, L.A. The International Physical Activity Questionnaire modified for the elderly: Aspects of validity and feasibility. *Public Health Nutr.* **2010**, *13*, 1847–1854. [CrossRef] [PubMed]
34. Castañeda, F.J.R. Medición de la Actividad Física en Personas Mayores de 65 Años Mediante El Ipaq-E: Validez de Contenido, Fiabilidad y Factores Asociados. *Rev. Esp. Salud. Pública.* **2017**, *91*, e1–e12.
35. Cantril, H. *The Pattern of Human Concerns*; Rutgers University: New Brunswick, NJ, USA, 1965.
36. Jaarsma, T.; Kastermans, M.C. Recovery and Quality of Life One Year after Coronary Artery Bypass Grafting. *Scand. J. Caring Sci.* **1997**, *11*, 67–72. [CrossRef] [PubMed]
37. Jenkins, L.S.; Brodsky, M.; Schron, E.; Chung, M.; Rocco, T.; Lader, E.; Constantine, M.; Sheppard, R.; Holmes, D.; Mateski, D.; et al. Quality of life in atrial fibrillation: The Atrial Fibrillation Follow-up Investigation of Rhythm Management (AFFIRM) study. *Am. Heart J.* **2005**, *149*, 112–120. [CrossRef]
38. Senten, M.C. The Well-Being of Patients Having Coronary Artery Bypass Surgery: A Test of Orem's Self-Care Nursing Theory. Ph.D. Thesis, Maastricht University, Maastricht, The Netherlands, 1991.
39. Jaarsma, T.; Halfens, R.; Abu-Saad, H.H.; Dracup, K.; Stappers, J.; van Ree, J. Quality of life in older patients with systolic and diastolic heart failure. *Eur. J. Heart Fail.* **1999**, *1*, 151–160. [CrossRef]
40. Levin, K.A.; Currie, C. Reliability and Validity of an Adapted Version of the Cantril Ladder for Use with Adolescent Samples. *Soc. Indic. Res.* **2014**, *119*, 1047–1063. [CrossRef]
41. Czapinski, J. Illusions and Biases in Psychological Well Being: An "Onion" Theory of Happiness. In *Working Meeting of ISR and ISS*; Institute for Social Studies, University of Warsaw: Warsaw, Poland, 2001.
42. Hellström, A.; Hagell, P.; Fagerström, C.; Willman, A. Measurement properties of the Minimal Insomnia Symptom Scale (MISS) in an elderly population in Sweden. *BMC Geriatr.* **2010**, *10*, 84. [CrossRef]
43. Broman, J.-E.; Smedje, H.; Mallon, L.; Hetta, J. The Minimal Insomnia Symptom Scale (MISS). *Upsala J. Med. Sci.* **2008**, *113*, 131–142. [CrossRef]
44. Tison, G.H.; Avram, R.; Kuhar, P.; Abreau, S.; Marcus, G.M.; Pletcher, M.J.; Olgin, J.E. Worldwide Effect of COVID-19 on Physical Activity: A Descriptive Study. *Ann. Intern. Med.* **2020**, *173*, 767–770. [CrossRef]
45. Kirsch, M.; Vitiello, D. The COVID-19 Pandemic Lowers Active Behavior of Patients with Cardiovascular Diseases, Healthy Peoples and Athletes. *Int. J. Environ. Res. Public Health* **2022**, *19*, 1108. [CrossRef]
46. Kim, K.; Zhang, S.; Ding, P.; Wang, Y.; Yim, B.H.; Hu, Z.; Sui, S. Changes in Physical Activity and Health Indicators among Koreans during the COVID-19 Pandemic: Comparison between 2019 and 2020. *Healthcare* **2022**, *10*, 2549. [CrossRef] [PubMed]
47. Rees-Punia, E.; Newton, C.C.; Rittase, M.H.; Hodge, R.A.; Nielsen, J.; Cunningham, S.; Teras, L.R.; Patel, A. Prospective changes in physical activity, sedentary time and sleep during the COVID-19 pandemic in a US-based cohort study. *BMJ Open* **2021**, *11*, e053817. [CrossRef] [PubMed]
48. Van Erck, D.; Dolman, C.D.; Snaterse, M.; Tieland, M.; Driessen, A.H.G.; Weijs, P.J.M.; Reimer, W.J.M.S.O.; Henriques, J.P.; Schoufour, J.D. Physical activity, dietary intake and quality of life during COVID-19 lockdown in patients awaiting transcatheter aortic valve implantation. *Neth. Heart J.* **2021**, *29*, 460–467. [CrossRef] [PubMed]
49. Banerjee, S.; Mukherjee, A.; Bhattacharyya, B.; Mohanakumar, K.; Biswas, A. Quality of life and concerns of parkinson's disease patients and their caregivers during COVID-19 pandemic: An indian study. *Ann. Indian Acad. Neurol.* **2022**, *25*, 676. [CrossRef] [PubMed]
50. Constandt, B.; Thibaut, E.; De Bosscher, V.; Scheerder, J.; Ricour, M.; Willem, A. Exercising in Times of Lockdown: An Analysis of the Impact of COVID-19 on Levels and Patterns of Exercise among Adults in Belgium. *Int. J. Environ. Res. Public Health* **2020**, *17*, 4144. [CrossRef]
51. Okely, J.A.; Corley, J.; Welstead, M.; Taylor, A.M.; Page, D.; Skarabela, B.; Redmond, P.; Cox, S.R.; Russ, T.C. Change in Physical Activity, Sleep Quality, and Psychosocial Variables during COVID-19 Lockdown: Evidence from the Lothian Birth Cohort 1936. *Int. J. Environ. Res. Public Health* **2020**, *18*, 210. [CrossRef] [PubMed]
52. Dobler, C.L.; Krüger, B.; Strahler, J.; Weyh, C.; Gebhardt, K.; Tello, K.; Ghofrani, H.A.; Sommer, N.; Gall, H.; Richter, M.J.; et al. Physical Activity and Mental Health of Patients with Pulmonary Hypertension during the COVID-19 Pandemic. *J. Clin. Med.* **2020**, *9*, 4023. [CrossRef] [PubMed]
53. Kite, C.; Atkinson, L.; McGregor, G.; Clark, C.C.T.; Brown, J.E.; Kyrou, I.; Randeva, H.S. Sleep Disruption and Depression, Stress and Anxiety Levels in Women with Polycystic Ovary Syndrome (PCOS) During the Lockdown Measures for COVID-19 in the UK. *Front. Glob. Women's Health* **2021**, *2*, 649104. [CrossRef]
54. ElHafeez, S.A.; Cruz, M.M.E.; Gouda, S.; Nofal, M.; Fayed, A.; Ghazy, R.M.; Mekky, J. Sleep quality and anxiety among Egyptian population during COVID-19 pandemic. *Sleep Sci.* **2022**, *15*, 8–16. [CrossRef]
55. Doukky, R.; Mangla, A.; Ibrahim, Z.; Poulin, M.-F.; Avery, E.; Collado, F.M.; Kaplan, J.; Richardson, D.; Powell, L.H. Impact of Physical Inactivity on Mortality in Patients with Heart Failure. *Am. J. Cardiol.* **2016**, *117*, 1135–1143. [CrossRef] [PubMed]
56. Akar, J.G.; Bao, H.; Jones, P.W.; Wang, Y.; Varosy, P.D.; Masoudi, F.A.; Stein, K.M.; Saxon, L.A.; Normand, S.-L.T.; Curtis, J.P.; et al. Use of Remote Monitoring Is Associated with Lower Risk of Adverse Outcomes Among Patients With Implanted Cardiac Defibrillators. *Circ. Arrhythmia Electrophysiol.* **2015**, *8*, 1173–1180. [CrossRef] [PubMed]

57. Jensen, M.T.; Treskes, R.W.; Caiani, E.G.; Casado-Arroyo, R.; Cowie, M.R.; Dilaveris, P.; Duncker, D.; Di Rienzo, M.; Frederix, I.; De Groot, N.; et al. ESC working group on e-cardiology position paper: Use of commercially available wearable technology for heart rate and activity tracking in primary and secondary cardiovascular prevention—In collaboration with the European Heart Rhythm Association, European Association of Preventive Cardiology, Association of Cardiovascular Nursing and Allied Professionals, Patient Forum, and the Digital Health Committee. *Eur. Heart J.—Digit. Health* **2021**, *2*, 49–59. [CrossRef] [PubMed]
58. Shakhovska, N.; Fedushko, S.; Greguš ml., M.; Melnykova, N.; Shvorob, I.; Syerov, Y. Big Data analysis in development of personalized medical system. *Procedia Comput. Sci.* **2019**, *160*, 229–234. [CrossRef]
59. Scherrenberg, M.; Wilhelm, M.; Hansen, D.; Völler, H.; Cornelissen, V.; Frederix, I.; Kemps, H.; Dendale, P. The future is now: A call for action for cardiac telerehabilitation in the COVID-19 pandemic from the secondary prevention and rehabilitation section of the European Association of Preventive Cardiology. *Eur. J. Prev. Cardiol.* **2021**, *28*, 524–540. [CrossRef]
60. Arnett, D.K.; Blumenthal, R.S.; Albert, M.A.; Buroker, A.B.; Goldberger, Z.D.; Hahn, E.J.; Himmelfarb, C.D.; Khera, A.; Lloyd-Jones, D.; McEvoy, J.W.; et al. 2019 ACC/AHA Guideline on the primary prevention of cardiovascular disease: A report of the american college of cardiology/American heart association task force on clinical practice guidelines. *Circulation* **2019**, *140*, e596–e646. [CrossRef]
61. European Commission. *The Digital Economy and Society Index (DESI)*; European Commission: Brussels, Belgium, 2022.

Disclaimer/Publisher's Note: The statements, opinions and data contained in all publications are solely those of the individual author(s) and contributor(s) and not of MDPI and/or the editor(s). MDPI and/or the editor(s) disclaim responsibility for any injury to people or property resulting from any ideas, methods, instructions or products referred to in the content.

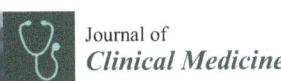

Article

The Impact of Previous Comorbidities on New Comorbidities and Medications after a Mild SARS-CoV-2 Infection in a Lithuanian Cohort

Dovilė Važgėlienė [1,2], Raimondas Kubilius [1,2] and Indre Bileviciute-Ljungar [3,4,*]

1. Department of Physical Rehabilitation Medicine, Kaunas Clinic of the Lithuanian University of Health Sciences, 50161 Kaunas, Lithuania; raimondas.kubilius@lsmuni.lt (R.K.)
2. Department of Nursing, Lithuanian University of Health Sciences, 44307 Kaunas, Lithuania
3. Department of Clinical Sciences, Karolinska Institute, Danderyd University Hospital, 182 57 Stockholm, Sweden
4. Multidisciplinary Pain Clinic, Capio St. Göran Hospital, 112 19 Stockholm, Sweden
* Correspondence: indre.ljungar@ki.se

Abstract: This cross-sectional study investigates new comorbidities and new medications after a mild SARS-CoV-2 infection. Data were collected after an acute SARS-CoV-2 infection by online survey in a Lithuanian cohort. Sociodemographic data, SARS-CoV-2-related symptoms, previous and new comorbidities, and medications were analysed. The results of 895 participants (mean age: 44 years) show that 91% were women, 58% had higher education, and 84% were working. Among those, 473 (52.8%) answered being "healthy" before infection; 823 (92%) indicated being positive on diagnostic tests; and 841 (94%) were non-hospitalized. Asymptomatic infection was reported by 17 participants (1.9%). Participants reporting any comorbidity before a SARS-CoV-2 infection reported more frequently having remaining symptoms compared to those who were "healthy", particularly in relation to neurological symptoms. Thirteen percent of participants reported new comorbidities, and thirty-five percent started new medication. Among new medications, an intake of vitamins/supplements (21%) and anti-inflammatory drugs (4%) was more often reported by "unhealthy" participants. Regression analysis revealed that new cardiovascular and pulmonary diagnoses predicted each other. Participants reporting prior neurological disorders tended to have an increased risk of intaking new vitamins/supplements and anti-inflammatory drugs after infection. The results indicate a significantly increased consumption of medication, particularly unprescribed substances, after SARS-CoV-2, indicating a need of more research in this area.

Keywords: SARS-CoV-2 virus; medication; comorbidities; post-COVID-19 condition; vitamins/supplements

Citation: Važgėlienė, D.; Kubilius, R.; Bileviciute-Ljungar, I. The Impact of Previous Comorbidities on New Comorbidities and Medications after a Mild SARS-CoV-2 Infection in a Lithuanian Cohort. *J. Clin. Med.* **2024**, *13*, 623. https://doi.org/10.3390/jcm13020623

Academic Editors: Domingo Palacios-Ceña and César Fernández De Las Peñas

Received: 26 December 2023
Revised: 17 January 2024
Accepted: 18 January 2024
Published: 22 January 2024

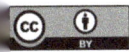

Copyright: © 2024 by the authors. Licensee MDPI, Basel, Switzerland. This article is an open access article distributed under the terms and conditions of the Creative Commons Attribution (CC BY) license (https://creativecommons.org/licenses/by/4.0/).

1. Introduction

Ailments that linger longer than three months after a SARS-CoV-2 infection and affect daily life activities are known as a post-COVID-19 condition, according to World Health Organization (WHO) [1]. According to WHO, approximately 10% of all infected people may suffer from a post-COVID-19 condition [1]. However, the epidemiological data are not clear. In Sweden, a study analysing data from the health care system for the period 2021–2022 found that approximately 2% of population of 4.1 million have been diagnosed with a post-COVID-19 condition after an acute SARS-CoV-2 infection [2] Among them, the majority were non-hospitalised inhabitants.

Theoretically, previous comorbidities might increase the severity of a post-COVID-19 condition, although studies examining this particular risk factor are few, especially after a mild SARS-CoV-2 infection. In 2021, Kayaaslan et al. have already reported that persistent symptoms in both inpatients and outpatients after SARS-CoV-2 were predicted by previous comorbidities [3]; however, they were not confirmed by others [4]. In a large cohort including mainly females and health care workers, previous mental distress was reported to be a risk factor for those with a post-COVID-19 condition [5]. Moreover, a recent systemic review and meta-analysis revealed several risk factors, i.e., demographic (age, sex), higher body mass index, smoking, and comorbidities such as depression, cardiovascular, pulmonary, endocrine, and immune suppression diseases, while vaccination lowered the risk by approximately at 40% [6]. Recently, we reported data from the first survey (first pandemic wave) of a Lithuanian cohort showing that both previous comorbidities and medication increased symptomatology during an acute infection and after 28 days [7].

The aim of this study was to study further previous and new comorbidities as well as previous and new medications after a SARS-CoV-2 infection in mainly non-hospitalized persons in a Lithuanian cohort during the pandemic's second wave in 2021–2022. The hypothesis was that participants with previous comorbidities will report more remaining symptoms and more new comorbidities and medication use.

2. Materials and Methods

This study was performed by inviting participants to answer anonymously an Internet-based questionnaire, created by D.V. via Google Drive (Alphabet Inc., Googleplex, Mountain View, CA, USA). The questionnaire was distributed in the Lithuanian language through Lithuanian websites, including private/public Facebook groups, city/town/district hospitals, and media outlets (Supplementary Material S1). Study encouraged participation independent of the presence or absence of persistent symptoms. Ethical approval was obtained from the Kaunas Regional Ethics Committee for Biomedical Research on the 11th of May 2021 (approval number: BE-2-65). This study has been registered with ClinicalTrials.gov (ID: NCT05000229). Informed consent was obtained from each participant. The study protocol, materials concerning ethical permission, and consent information provided to participants are available at the university's website (https://lsmu.lt/en/about-lsmu/structure/medical-academy/faculty-of-nursing/projektine-veikla/, accessed on 22 December 2021). Questions were formulated to gather information regarding sociodemographic characteristics, the data of acute SARS-CoV-2 infection, including diagnostics tests, information related to comorbidities, and the daily use of medication before and after an infection, remaining symptoms after the infection, and attitudes regarding the need for rehabilitation. The questions were of exploratory nature with free or predefined answers. Here, we present a second collection of the survey (from 10 August 2021 to 31 December 2022), excluding questions related to the need for rehabilitation.

Inclusion criteria for participation were as follows: (1) age of 18 years or older, (2) known SARS-CoV-2 infection with or without specific diagnostic tests (PCR, antigen test, antibodies), and (3) a post-infection period of at least 28 days before participating in the survey.

Exclusion criteria were as follows: hospitalized patients still receiving treatment or rehabilitation after a SARS-CoV-2 infection, unstable or untreated comorbidities, or the ongoing stabilisation of comorbidities. None of the participants indicated the presence of exclusion criteria in the questionnaire.

For persistent symptoms, we created 64 preselected answers as well as the possibility to leave free comments regarding other symptoms. Persistent symptoms were formed into major groups as indicated in Supplementary Material S2.

For comorbidities, the participants were asked to answer the presence of any chronic disease prior to and after a SARS-CoV-2 infection. In cases of previous and recent disease, the participant was asked to specify the ailment. Furthermore, the comorbidities could be selected from 21 preselected disorders as well as the possibility to leave free comments regarding other diseases. For medication, the participants were asked for the presence of any daily medication before and after a SARS-CoV-2 infection. In cases with previous and recent medication, the participant was asked to specify the medication. Both comorbidities and medications were grouped as indicated in the respective Supplements (see Methods).

Statistics

Results from the survey were analysed with SPSS version 29 (Statistical Package for the Social Sciences, IBM, New York, NY, USA) after downloading into a Microsoft Excel 2019 file (Microsoft Corporation, Washington, DC, USA). A major part of data was nominal in nature, and therefore, presented as a number of participants and as a percentage of the whole cohort. Nominal data were compared using two-tailed Chi-square test. For parametric data (the duration of symptoms), an independent t-test was applied between the groups ("healthy" vs. "unhealthy"). The predictors of new comorbidities and new medications were analysed with separate binary logistic regression models for those dependent variables, showing significant differences between the groups and even including sex as an additional covariate. Statistical significance was considered as $p < 0.05$.

3. Results

3.1. Participants and Persistent Symptoms in Relation to Previous Health Status

The survey of participants is presented in Supplementary Material S1. The final data analysis included 895 participants with a mean age of 44 years (SD: 12.54 years, range: 18–79 years). Nearly 90% of participants were females and younger than 60 years (Table 1). Approximately 65% participants were from the three biggest cities in Lithuania, including Kaunas (the second-largest city in Lithuania, 27.6%), Vilnius (the capital of Lithuania, 26.3%), and Klaipėda (11.8%); therefore 72.0% participants were living in an urban environment (Table 1). Diagnostic testing was reported by 92.0% of participants, and an asymptomatic infection by approximately 2%. Approximately 71% of participants reported being vaccinated, with no difference observed between "healthy" and "unhealthy" participants (Chi-Square test, $p = 0.47$). The median duration after a SARS-CoV-2 infection and the responding survey was 27 weeks (range: 4–129 weeks, mean: 30 weeks, and SD: 22 weeks), with no difference found between "healthy" and "unhealthy" participants (independent t-test, $p = 0.36$). Approximately 61% of participants reported to be "officially" healthy from the acute SARS-CoV-2 infection within 2 weeks, 27% within 2–4 weeks, and 10% after 4 weeks.

The majority od participants (94.0%) reported being non-hospitalized, whereas 5% reported being hospitalized during an acute SARS-CoV-2 infection. The results show that "unhealthy" participants were older, among them many were retired and unemployed, see Table 1. No statistical difference was revealed regarding sex for "healthy" and "unhealthy" participants.

Approximately 92.2% of participants reported persistent symptoms with a total number ranging from 0 to 45 (median 7 symptoms). All 64 symptoms are presented in Supplementary Material S2. The most frequently reported remaining symptoms were related to the nervous system and chronic pain, followed by symptoms of the upper respiratory tract, see Table 2. Thereafter, symptoms related to the cardiovascular system, skin, mood/emotions, the lower respiratory tract, the endocrine system, vision, and the gastrointestinal tract were reported. Participants reporting any comorbidity before SARS-CoV-2 infection ("unhealthy") mentioned all remaining symptoms more frequently compared to those who did not report any symptoms ("healthy"), except for psychological symptoms, Table 2.

Table 1. The socioeconomic data of participants presented as numbers and percentages of a whole cohort and among those reported as "healthy" and "unhealthy" prior to the infection.

		All N = 895 (100%)	"Healthy" N = 473 (52.8%)	"Unhealthy" N = 422 (47.2%)	Statistics
Sex	Female	816 (91.2%)	431 (48.2%)	385 (43.0%)	0.524
	Male	79 (8.8%)	42 (4.7%)	37 (4.1%)	
Age group	Younger than 40 years	373 (41.7%)	269 (30.1%)	104 (11.6%)	<0.001
	41–60 years	418 (46.7%)	187 (20.9%)	231 (25.8%)	
	61–80 years	104 (11.6%)	17 (1.9%)	87 (9.7%)	

Table 1. Cont.

		All N = 895 (100%)	"Healthy" N = 473 (52.8%)	"Unhealthy" N = 422 (47.2%)	Statistics
Education	Primary/secondary Higher non-university Higher university Other	106 (11.8%) 266 (29.7%) 520 (58.1%) 3 (0.3%)	49 (5.5%) 129 (14.4%) 294 (32.8%) 1 (0.1%)	57 (6.4%) 137 (15.53%) 226 (25.3%) 2 (0.2%)	0.066
Socioeconomic situation	Employed/working Temporary unemployed Unemployed Retired Student	749 (83.7%) 30 (3.4%) 55 (6.0%) 52 (5.8%) 9 (1.0%)	426 (47.6%) 10 (1.1%) 26 (2.9%) 7 (0.8%) 5 (0.6%)	323 (36.1%) 20 (2.2%) 29 (3.2%) 45 (5.0%) 4 (0.4%)	<0.001
Region of Residence in Lithuania	Kaunas Vilnius Klaipėda Šiauliai Panevėžys Telšiai Marijampolė Alytus Utena Tauragė	247 (27.6%) 236 (26.3%) 106 (11.8%) 75 (8.3%) 73 (8.2%) 40 (4.5%) 36 (4.0%) 33 (3.7%) 31 (3.5%) 18 (2.0%)	140 (15.6%) 126 (14.1%) 52 (5.8%) 42 (4.7%) 33 (3.7%) 22 (2.5%) 16 (1.8%) 16 (1.8%) 20 (2.2%) 6 (0.7%)	107 (12.0%) 110 (12.3%) 54 (6.0%) 33 (3.7%) 40 (4.5%) 18 (2.0%) 20 (2.2%) 17 (1.9%) 11 (1.2%) 12 (1.3%)	0.359
Living area	Settlement Village City Suburbs	41 (4.6%) 101 (11.3%) 644 (72.0%) 109 (12.2%)	17 (1.9%) 51 (5.7%) 340 (38.0%) 65 (7.3%)	24 (2.7%) 50 (5.6%) 304 (34.0%) 44 (4.9%)	0.224

Table 2. Groups according to remaining symptoms presented as the number and percentage of a whole cohort and among those reported as "healthy" and "unhealthy" prior to the infection. Differences between these two latter groups are presented as p-values. Originally marked symptoms are presented in Supplementary Material S2.

Symptoms Related to	All N = 895 (100%)	"Healthy" N = 473 (52.8%)	"Unhealthy" N = 422 (47.2%)	Statistics
Nervous system	739 (82.6%)	370 (41.3%)	369 (42.2%)	$p < 0.001$
Chronic pain	477 (53.3%)	219 (24.5%)	258 (28.8%)	$p < 0.001$
Throat, nose, and ear	420 (46.9%)	203 (22.7%)	217 (24.2.6%)	$p = 0.007$
Heart	364 (40.7%)	156 (17.4%)	208 (23.2%)	$p < 0.001$
Skin	335 (37.4%)	149 (16.6%)	186 (20.8%)	$p < 0.001$
Mood and emotions	307 (34.3)	165 (18.4%)	142 (15.9%)	$p = 0.375$
Lung	258 (28.8%)	116 (13.0%)	142 (15.9%)	$p = 0.002$
Endocrine	254 (28.4%)	117 (13.1%)	137 (15.3%)	$p = 0.006$
Vision and eyes	246 (27.5%)	103 (11.5%)	143 (16.0%)	$p < 0.001$
Gastrointestinal tract	165 (18.4%)	73 (8.2%)	92 (10.3%)	$p = 0.009$
Other	601 (67.2%)	291 (32.5%)	310 (34.6%)	$p < 0.001$

3.2. Comorbidities and Medications Prior to SARS-CoV-2 Infection

Approximately 53% of participants reported being "healthy" prior to their SARS-CoV-2 infection. Comorbidities were grouped according to major disease groups and presented in Table 3. High blood pressure dominated among cardiovascular diseases ($N = 172$ or 19.2%); obesity among endocrine diseases ($N = 90$ or 10.1%); sleep disorders among neurological diseases ($N = 62$ or 6.9%); anxiety among psychiatric diseases ($N = 43$ or 4.8%); thereafter unspecified diseases of the gastrointestinal tract ($N = 68$ or 7.6%); unspecified allergic diseases ($N = 49$ or 5.5%); unspecified rheumatic diseases ($N = 49$ or 5.5%); asthma among pulmonary diseases ($N = 37$ or 4.1%); unspecified kidney diseases ($N = 18$ or 2%);

unspecified oncological diseases ($N = 17$ or 1.9%); unspecified immunodeficiency diseases ($N = 7$ or 0.8%); and others ($N = 22$ or 2.5%) (Table 3).

Of those with comorbidities, the greatest portion had one comorbidity (20.1%), and only two (0.2%) participants reported nine comorbidities. The total number of comorbidities varied from zero to nine, with a median of two comorbidities.

Table 3. Grouped comorbidities in "unhealthy" participants are presented as a number and a percentage of a whole cohort. Originally marked comorbidities and groupings are presented in Supplementary Material S3.

Disorders	All $N = 895$ (100%)	"Healthy" $N = 473$ (52.8%)	"Unhealthy" $N = 422$ (47.2%)	Statistics
Cardiovascular	209 (23.4%)	0	209 (23.4%)	$p < 0.001$
Endocrine	158 (17.7%)	0	158 (17.7%)	$p < 0.001$
Neurological	111 (12.4%)	0	111 (12.4%)	$p < 0.001$
Gastrointestinal	68 (7.6%)	0	68 (7.6%)	$p < 0.001$
Psychiatric	63 (7.0%)	0	63 (7.0%)	$p < 0.001$
Skin	49 (5.5%)	0	49 (5.5%)	$p < 0.001$
Inflammatory rheumatic	49 (5.5%)	0	49 (5.5%)	$p < 0.001$
Pulmonary	49 (5.5%)	0	49 (5.5%)	$p < 0.001$
Renal	18 (2.0%)	0	18 (2.0%)	$p < 0.001$
Oncological	17 (1.9%)	0	17 (1.9%)	$p < 0.001$
Immunodeficiency	7 (0.8%)	0	7 (0.8%)	$p = 0.005$
Others	22 (2.5%)	0	22 (2.5%)	$p < 0.001$

Approximately 68% of participants reported not taking any medication before a SARS-CoV-2 infection. Among those reporting medication, the cardiovascular system-modulating drugs were consumed by 12% of participants, followed by hormones (7%) and "other" drugs (12%). Psychopharmacological, anti-allergic, anti-inflammatory/anti-bacterial, and supplements/vitamins were taken by certain percentages of participants in the whole cohort, see Table 4. As expected, "unhealthy" participants more often reported a daily pharmacological treatment before an acute infection.

Table 4. Grouped medications before a SARS-CoV-2 infection presented as a number and a percentage in a whole cohort and among those reported as "healthy" and "unhealthy" prior to the infection. Differences between these two latter groups are presented as p-values. Originally marked medications and groupings are presented in Supplementary Material S4.

Drug Regulating	All $N = 895$ (100%)	"Healthy" $N = 473$ (52.8%)	"Unhealthy" $N = 422$ (47.2%)	Statistics
The cardiovascular system	109 (12.2%)	11 (2.3%)	98 (10.9%)	$p < 0.001$
The endocrine system	61 (6.8%)	10 (1.1%)	51 (5.7%)	$p < 0.001$
Psychological functions (psychopharmacology)	23 (2.6%)	0 (0.0)	23 (2.6%)	$p < 0.001$
Inflammation (nonsteroidal anti-inflammatory drugs and antibiotics)	13 (1.5%)	2 (0.2%)	11 (1.2%)	$p = 0.006$
The immune system (antiallergic and anti-asthmatic)	10 (1.1%)	0 (0.0)	10 (1.1%)	$p < 0.001$
Gastrointestinal tract	10 (1.1%)	0 (0.0)	10 (1.1%)	$p < 0.001$
Supplements/vitamins	9 (1.0%)	2 (0.2%)	7 (0.8%)	$p = 0.064$
Other	105 (11.7%)	9 (1.0%)	96 (10.7%)	$p < 0.001$

3.3. New Comorbidities and Medications after SARS-CoV-2 Infection

One hundred and fourteen participants reported new diagnoses. Among them, 82 participants received one new diagnosis, 25 participants received two new diagnoses, 4 participants received three new diagnoses, and 3 participants received four new diagnoses. Cardiovascular, neurological, and pulmonary diagnoses were new diagnoses reported by 3.5%, 2.6%, and 1.8% of participants, respectively, see Table 5. "Other" diagnoses were reported by 3.1% participants, and the remaining diagnoses (gastrointestinal, endocrine, inflammatory/rheumatic, renal, dermatological, psychiatric, and gynaecological) were reported by approximately 1% or less of participants per each diagnosis, see Table 5. A significant difference was found between "healthy" and "unhealthy" participants regarding new cardiovascular and pulmonary diagnoses, which were more often reported by "unhealthy" participants, see Table 2.

Table 5. New diagnoses after a SARS-CoV-2 infection are presented as a number and a percentage in a whole cohort and among those reported as "healthy" and "unhealthy" prior to the infection. Differences between these two latter groups are presented as p-values. Originally marked comorbidities and groupings are presented in Supplementary Material S3.

	All N = 895 (100%)	"Healthy" N = 473 (52.8%)	"Unhealthy" N = 422 (47.2%)	Statistics
Cardiovascular	31 (3.5%)	9 (1.0%)	22 (2.5%)	$p = 0.006$
Neurological	23 (2.6%)	9 (1.0%)	14 (1.6%)	$p = 0.131$
Pulmonary	16 (1.8%)	4 (0.4%)	12 (1.3%)	$p = 0.022$
Gastrointestinal	12 (1.3%)	6 (0.7%)	6 (0.7%)	$p = 0.534$
Endocrine	11 (1.2%)	3 (0.3%)	8 (0.9%)	$p = 0.079$
Inflammatory rheumatic	8 (0.9%)	2 (0.2%)	6 (0.7%)	$p = 0.109$
Renal	6 (0.7%)	1 (0.1%)	5 (0.6%)	$p = 0.084$
Dermatological	6 (0.7%)	3 (0.3%)	3 (0.3%)	$p = 0.602$
Psychiatric	5 (0.6%)	2 (0.2%)	3 (0.3%)	$p = 0.447$
Gynaecological	1 (0.1%)	1 (0.1%)	0 (0%)	$p = 0.528$
Others	28 (3.1%)	13 (1.5%)	15 (1.7%)	$p = 0.308$

Three hundred and thirteen participants started new medications. Among them, 228 participants started one new medication, 74 started two, 10 started three, and 1 started four medications/supplements/vitamins. The results show that supplements and vitamins were most frequently reported as new medications (by almost 21% of participants), followed by "other" drugs (reported by approximately 11% of participants) and cardiovascular drugs (reported by approximately 6% of participants), see Table 6. Less than 5% of participants reported new anti-inflammatory and psychopharmacological drugs, while new endocrine- and/or immune system-regulating drugs were consumed by less than 1% of the cohort. Statistical analysis revealed that "unhealthy" participants more often reported taking supplements and vitamins and anti-inflammatory/antibacterial drugs compared to "healthy" ones, see Table 6.

3.4. Regression Analysis for Predictors of New Comorbidities and New Medications after SARS-CoV-2 Infection

The predictors of new comorbidities and new medications were analysed with separate binary logistic regression models for the dependent variables, showing significant differences between the groups. Sex was an additional covariate in the analysis since women were overrepresented in the study cohort. To analyse the predictors for new cardiovascular and pulmonary diagnoses, we chose the following covariates: age group, sex, socioeconomic situation, new daily intake of vitamins/supplements, anti-inflammatory drugs, and all three major prior comorbidities (cardiovascular, endocrine, and neurological). To analyse the predictors for new daily intake of vitamins/supplements and anti-inflammatory drugs, we choose the following covariates: age group, sex, socioeconomic situation, new cardiovascular and pulmonary diagnoses, and all three major prior comorbidities (cardiovascular, endocrine, and neurological). Table 7 summarises the un-adjusted regression coefficients, showing that new cardiovascular diseases were predicted due to new pulmonary diseases and vice versa with odds of up to 5.1–5.2 (95% CI: 1.3–20).

Table 6. New medications after a SARS-CoV-2 infection presented as a number and a percentage in a whole cohort and among those reported as "healthy" and "unhealthy" prior to the infection. Differences between these two latter groups are presented as *p*-values. Originally marked medications and groupings are presented in Supplementary Material S4.

Drugs Regulating:	All N = 895 (100%)	"Healthy" N = 473 (52.8%)	"Unhealthy" N = 422 (47.2%)	Statistics
Supplements/vitamins	187 (20.9%)	82 (9.2%)	105 (11.7%)	$p = 0.004$
The cardiovascular system	55 (6.1%)	26 (2.9%)	29 (3.2%)	$p = 0.237$
Inflammation (nonsteroidal anti-inflammatory drugs and antibiotics)	38 (4.2%)	11 (1.2%)	27 (3.0%)	$p = 0.002$
Psychological functions (psychopharmacology)	22 (2.5%)	8 (0.9%)	14 (1.6%)	$p = 0.127$
The immune system (antiallergic and anti-asthmatic)	6 (0.7%)	2 (0.2%)	4 (0.4%)	$p = 0.291$
The endocrine system	8 (0.9%)	2 (0.4%)	6 (0.5%)	$p = 0.151$
Other	96 (10.7%)	43 (4.8%)	53 (5.9%)	$p = 0.059$

Table 7. Regressors predicting new diagnoses and medication after a SARS-CoV-2 infection.

Regressors	New Cardiovascular Disease OR (95% CI), *p*-Value	New Pulmonary Disease OR (95% CI), *p*-Value	New Vitamins/Supplements OR (95% CI), *p*-Value	New Anti-Inflammatory Drugs OR (95% CI), *p*-Value
Age group	n.s.	n.s.	n.s.	n.s.
Sex	n.s.	n.s.	0.33 (0.15–0.74), $p = 0.007$	n.s.
Sociodemographic characteristics	n.s.	n.s.	n.s.	n.s.
Prior cardiovascular diseases	n.s.	n.s.	n.s.	n.s.
Prior endocrine diseases	n.s.	n.s.	n.s.	n.s.
Prior nervous system diseases	n.s.	n.s.	n.s.	n.s.
New cardiovascular disease	-	5.24 (1.33–20.55), 0.018	n.s.	n.s.
New pulmonary disease	5.1 (1.3–19.76), 0.02	-	n.s.	n.s.
New vitamins/supplements	n.s.	n.s.	-	n.s.
New anti-inflammatory drugs	n.s.	n.s.	n.s.	-

Abbreviations: n.s. = not significant.

The intake of new vitamins/supplements was slightly predicted by sex with odds of up to 0.33 (95% CI 0.15–0.74). A previous neurological disease also showed a tendency to predict the intake of new vitamins/supplements with odds up of up to 1.6 (95% CI: 1.0–2.6, $p = 0.059$).

We did not find any significant predictors for new anti-inflammatory drugs, except for a prior neurological disease showing a tendency with odds of up to 2.2 (95% CI: 0.9–5.1, $p = 0.074$).

4. Discussion

The results of the second survey confirm that neurological symptoms (fatigue, neurocognitive issues, sleep-related symptoms, and pain) were the most reported by participants during the second wave of pandemics. Among comorbidities prior to SARS-CoV-2 infection, cardiovascular, endocrine, and neurological diseases dominated, even among the middle-aged population, mostly employed women. As expected, and as reported previously [7], those with any chronic disease prior to an infection ("unhealthy") more often reported persistent symptoms and took daily medication. Those categorised as "unhealthy" also more frequently reported new diagnoses and new medications after an infection. Among new diagnoses, cardiovascular issues were the most frequent, having been reported by 3.5% of participants. In the present study population, cardiovascular comorbidities already dominated prior to a SARS-CoV-2 infection, which could naturally result in more frequent new cardiovascular diagnoses after an infection. Alternatively, 6.1% of participants reported new cardiovascular drugs without a statistically significant difference between the "healthy" vs. "unhealthy" participants. Studies regarding an increased risk for acute myocardial infarction and ischaemic stroke following COVID infection have been published [8], whereas postural orthostatic tachycardia syndrome (POTS) as a sign of dysregulation in the autonomic nervous system has been reported as a symptom of the post-COVID-19 condition [9]. The molecular mechanisms behind cardiovascular symptoms in a post-COVID-19 condition are unknown, but recently, the dysregulation of the proteome, cytokines, chemokines, and sphingolipid levels has been reported [10]. Another study reveals a prevalence of low vitamin D among 447 post-COVID-19 patients but did not find any difference in the prevalence of symptoms or symptom severity between low and normal vitamin D groups [11].

Unexpectedly, we found an increase from 1% to almost 21% in the consumption of unprescribed vitamins/supplements after a SARS-CoV-2 infection, which was very slightly influenced by the female sex. Self-medication, including supplements and vitamins, have been studied mostly during an acute COVID infection [12]. Carrasco-Garrido and colleagues reported an increased consumption of psychopharmacological substances in the anonymously collected data of Spanish participants with post-COVID-19 symptoms [13], where almost 45% of 391 participants reported taking benzodiazepines and Z-hypnotics; however, the study did not report if it was a new medication or an already established intake before a SARS-CoV-2 infection. Another study reported an increased burden on the health care system at six months after a SARS-CoV-2 infection, where the prescription of medication(s) was a part of the burden but was not analysed in detail [14]. To our knowledge, there is no study examining the patterns of the consumption of prescribed and unprescribed drugs, including vitamins and supplements, related to a post-COVID-19 condition. Some studies investigated the effects of supplements/vitamins, for example, reporting the positive effects of 1-arginine plus vitamin C supplementation [15] and fermented tropical fruits [16] in randomised controlled trials in participants with a post-COVID-19 condition. However, a recent systematic review of 39 randomised controlled studies on eight dietary supplements protecting the immune system against stressors in healthy individuals did not show conclusive results [17]. Therefore, a careful anamnesis of unprescribed medication should be included in clinical practice for patients with a post-COVID-19 condition, especially for female patients with previous comorbidities related to the nervous system.

The daily intake of new anti-inflammatory substances was reported by 4.2% of participants, more often by "unhealthy" participants. We hypothesize that an increased intake of new medications might be rather predicted by the remaining symptoms than comorbidities and needs further exploration. Taken together, prior neurological disorders were reported by approximately 12% of the study cohort and tended to be associated with an increased intake of vitamins/supplements and anti-inflammatory drugs (non-steroidal anti-inflammatory drugs or antibiotics) after an infection. Both vitamins and supplements, but not antibiotics, could be obtained as over-the-counter medications, which indicates an increased consumption of unprescribed drugs in people with persistent post-infectious symptoms. Therefore, in the next step, we will analyse a consumption of new medications in terms of symptomatology since neurological symptoms were predominant in the study cohort.

This study has several limitations: (1) the generalizability is limited by recruitment through social media and the representation of mainly middle-aged women; (2) the limited control of gathered data due to anonymity and self-reported data; (3) the absence of information if medication was prescribed or obtained over-the-counter and the reason for the prescription; and (4) the retrospective collection of data regarding previous medications and comorbidities. The present study was started prior to WHO defining a post-COVID-19 condition [1]. Therefore, it reports rather on the health status of participants after a SARS-CoV-2 infection than on a post-COVID-19 condition.

Following are the strengths of the study: (1) the questionnaire covered a broad spectrum of comorbidities and medications both before and after an infection and (2) the expanded analysis of comorbidities and medications was performed by three independent clinicians.

5. Conclusions

In conclusion, the results of this study revealed that previous comorbidities are associated with more persistent symptoms, increased new comorbidities, and new prescribed and unprescribed medications after a SARS-CoV-2 infection. Particularly, unprescribed vitamins/supplements and anti-inflammatory drugs should be inquired about during the clinical evaluations of patients with a post-COVID-19 condition, especially when involving female patients. Since the clinical value of unprescribed medications used for a post-COVID-19 condition is not yet known, more research in this area is warranted.

Supplementary Materials: The following supporting information can be downloaded at: https://www.mdpi.com/article/10.3390/jcm13020623/s1, Supplementary Materials S1 includes links to websites for study dissemination and flow figure of survey. Supplementary Materials S2 includes all persistent symtoms of the study cohort and grouping of symptoms. Supplementary Materials S3 includes grouping of comorbidities and Supplementary Materials S4 includes grouping of medication.

Author Contributions: Conceptualization, D.V., R.K. and I.B.-L.; methodology, D.V. and I.B.-L.; software, D.V. and I.B.-L.; validation, D.V., R.K. and I.B.-L.; formal analysis, D.V., R.K. and I.B.-L.; investigation, D.V.; resources, I.B.-L. and R.K.; data curation, D.V. and I.B.-L.; writing—original draft preparation, D.V. and I.B.-L.; writing—review and editing, D.V., R.K. and I.B.-L.; visualization, I.B.-L.; supervision, R.K. and I.B.-L.; project administration, R.K. and I.B.-L.; funding acquisition, D.V. and R.K. All authors have read and agreed to the published version of the manuscript.

Funding: This research was funded by Department of Nursing, Lithuanian University of Health Sciences, Kaunas, Lithuania.

Institutional Review Board Statement: The study was approved by the Kaunas Regional Ethics Committee for Biomedical Research (approval number: BE-2-65) and is registered on ClinicalTrials.gov (Identifier: NCT05000229).

Informed Consent Statement: Informed consent was obtained from all subjects involved in the study.

Data Availability Statement: The data that support the findings of this study are available from the first author (D.V.) upon reasonable request.

Conflicts of Interest: The authors declare that they have no financial disclosures or conflicts of interest.

References

1. World Health Oranizatio (WHO). A Clinical Case Definition of Post COVID-19 Condition by a Delphi Consensus. 6 October 2021. Available online: https://www.who.int/publications/i/item/WHO-2019-nCoV-Post_COVID-19_condition-Clinical_case_definition-2021.1 (accessed on 25 December 2023).
2. Bygdell, M.; Leach, S.; Lundberg, L.; Gyll, D.; Martikainen, J.; Santosa, A.; Li, H.; Gisslen, M.; Nyberg, F. A comprehensive characterisation of patients diagnosed with post-COVID-19 condition in Sweden 16 months after the introduction of the ICD-10 diagnosis code (U09.9): A population-based cohort study. *Int. J. Infect. Dis.* **2022**, *126*, 104–113. [CrossRef] [PubMed]
3. Kayaaslan, B.; Eser, F.; Kalem, A.K.; Kaya, G.; Kaplan, B.; Kacar, D.; Hasanoglu, I.; Coskun, B.; Guner, R. Post-COVID syndrome: A single-center questionnaire study on 1007 participants recovered from COVID-19. *J. Med. Virol.* **2021**, *93*, 6566–6574. [CrossRef]
4. Moreno-Perez, O.; Merino, E.; Leon-Ramirez, J.M.; Andres, M.; Ramos, J.M.; Arenas-Jimenez, J.; Asensio, S.; Sanchez, R.; Ruiz-Torregrosa, P.; Galan, I.; et al. Post-acute COVID-19 syndrome. Incidence and risk factors: A Mediterranean cohort study. *J. Infect.* **2021**, *82*, 378–383. [CrossRef]
5. Wang, S.; Quan, L.; Chavarro, J.E.; Slopen, N.; Kubzansky, L.D.; Koenen, K.C.; Kang, J.H.; Weisskopf, M.G.; Branch-Elliman, W.; Roberts, A.L. Associations of Depression, Anxiety, Worry, Perceived Stress, and Loneliness Prior to Infection with Risk of Post-COVID-19 Conditions. *JAMA Psychiatry* **2022**, *79*, 1081–1091. [CrossRef] [PubMed]
6. Tsampasian, V.; Elghazaly, H.; Chattopadhyay, R.; Debski, M.; Naing, T.K.P.; Garg, P.; Clark, A.; Ntatsaki, E.; Vassiliou, V.S. Risk Factors Associated with Post-COVID-19 Condition: A Systematic Review and Meta-analysis. *JAMA Intern. Med.* **2023**, *183*, 566–580. [CrossRef] [PubMed]
7. Vazgeliene, D.; Kubilius, R.; Bileviciute-Ljungar, I. Do Comorbidities and Daily Medication before SARS-CoV-2 Infection Play a Role in Self-Reported Post-Infection Symptoms? *J. Clin. Med.* **2022**, *11*, 6278. [CrossRef] [PubMed]
8. Katsoularis, I.; Fonseca-Rodriguez, O.; Farrington, P.; Lindmark, K.; Fors Connolly, A.M. Risk of acute myocardial infarction and ischaemic stroke following COVID-19 in Sweden: A self-controlled case series and matched cohort study. *Lancet* **2021**, *398*, 599–607. [CrossRef] [PubMed]
9. Bisaccia, G.; Ricci, F.; Recce, V.; Serio, A.; Iannetti, G.; Chahal, A.A.; Stahlberg, M.; Khanji, M.Y.; Fedorowski, A.; Gallina, S. Post-Acute Sequelae of COVID-19 and Cardiovascular Autonomic Dysfunction: What Do We Know? *J. Cardiovasc. Dev. Dis.* **2021**, *8*, 156. [CrossRef] [PubMed]
10. Mahdi, A.; Zhao, A.; Fredengren, E.; Fedorowski, A.; Braunschweig, F.; Nygren-Bonnier, M.; Runold, M.; Bruchfeld, J.; Nickander, J.; Deng, Q.; et al. Dysregulations in hemostasis, metabolism, immune response, and angiogenesis in post-acute COVID-19 syndrome with and without postural orthostatic tachycardia syndrome: A multi-omic profiling study. *Sci. Rep.* **2023**, *13*, 20230. [CrossRef] [PubMed]
11. Hikmet, R.G.; Wejse, C.; Agergaard, J. Effect of Vitamin D in Long COVID Patients. *Int. J. Environ. Res. Public. Health* **2023**, *20*, 7058. [CrossRef] [PubMed]
12. Krupa-Kotara, K.; Grajek, M.; Murzyn, A.; Sloma-Krzeslak, M.; Sobczyk, K.; Bialek-Dratwa, A.; Kowalski, O. Proper Dietary and Supplementation Patterns as a COVID-19 Protective Factor (Cross-Sectional Study-Silesia, Poland). *Life* **2022**, *12*, 1976. [CrossRef] [PubMed]
13. Carrasco-Garrido, P.; Fernandez-de-Las-Penas, C.; Hernandez-Barrera, V.; Palacios-Cena, D.; Jimenez-Trujillo, I.; Gallardo-Pino, C. Benzodiazepines and Z-hypnotics consumption in long-COVID-19 patients: Gender differences and associated factors. *Front. Med.* **2022**, *9*, 975930. [CrossRef] [PubMed]
14. Xie, Y.; Bowe, B.; Al-Aly, Z. Burdens of post-acute sequelae of COVID-19 by severity of acute infection, demographics and health status. *Nat. Commun.* **2021**, *12*, 6571. [CrossRef] [PubMed]
15. Tosato, M.; Calvani, R.; Picca, A.; Ciciarello, F.; Galluzzo, V.; Coelho-Junior, H.J.; Di Giorgio, A.; Di Mario, C.; Gervasoni, J.; Gremese, E.; et al. Effects of l-Arginine Plus Vitamin C Supplementation on Physical Performance, Endothelial Function, and Persistent Fatigue in Adults with Long COVID: A Single-Blind Randomized Controlled Trial. *Nutrients* **2022**, *14*, 4984. [CrossRef] [PubMed]
16. Kharaeva, Z.; Shokarova, A.; Shomakhova, Z.; Ibragimova, G.; Trakhtman, P.; Trakhtman, I.; Chung, J.; Mayer, W.; De Luca, C.; Korkina, L. Fermented *Carica papaya* and *Morinda citrifolia* as Perspective Food Supplements for the Treatment of Post-COVID Symptoms: Randomized Placebo-Controlled Clinical Laboratory Study. *Nutrients* **2022**, *14*, 2203. [CrossRef] [PubMed]
17. Crawford, C.; Brown, L.L.; Costello, R.B.; Deuster, P.A. Select Dietary Supplement Ingredients for Preserving and Protecting the Immune System in Healthy Individuals: A Systematic Review. *Nutrients* **2022**, *14*, 4604. [CrossRef] [PubMed]

Disclaimer/Publisher's Note: The statements, opinions and data contained in all publications are solely those of the individual author(s) and contributor(s) and not of MDPI and/or the editor(s). MDPI and/or the editor(s) disclaim responsibility for any injury to people or property resulting from any ideas, methods, instructions or products referred to in the content.

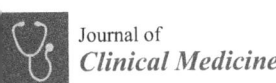

Article

Impact of the COVID-19 Pandemic on Obesity, Metabolic Parameters and Clinical Values in the South Korean Adult Population

Anna Kim [1,†], Eun-yeob Kim [2,†] and Jaeyoung Kim [2,3,*]

1. Department of Dermatology, College of Medicine, Korea University, Seoul 02841, Republic of Korea; annaykim31@gmail.com
2. Research Institute for Skin Image, Korea University College of Medicine, Seoul 08308, Republic of Korea; key0227@korea.ac.kr
3. Department of Convergence Medicine, College of Medicine, Korea University, Seoul 02841, Republic of Korea
* Correspondence: jaykim830@gmail.com
† These authors contributed equally to this work.

Abstract: This study aimed to evaluate the effects of the COVID-19 pandemic on obesity, metabolic parameters, and clinical values in the South Korean population. Data from the seventh and eighth National Health and Nutrition Examination Surveys were analyzed, comprising 3560 participants in 2018 (pre-COVID-19) and 3309 participants in 2021 (post-COVID-19). The study focused on adults aged 19 years and older who were overweight (BMI $\geq$ 25 kg/m^2). The results showed a significant increase in waist circumference (approximately 2 cm), BMI (approximately 0.11 kg/m^2), systolic blood pressure, fasting blood sugar (1.76 mg/dL higher), and glycated hemoglobin (0.14% higher) in the post-COVID-19 group compared to the pre-COVID-19 group. Additionally, the prevalence of hypercholesterolemia increased by 4% after the COVID-19 pandemic. These findings suggest an increased risk of obesity, abdominal obesity, and metabolic disorders, such as blood sugar disorders, in the post-COVID-19 period. Urine analysis revealed abnormal findings, including occult blood, urobilinogen, hematuria, proteinuria, ketone urea, glycosuria, and bacteriuria. The study highlights the negative impact of lifestyle changes, such as reduced physical activity and social gatherings, on physical vital signs and clinical values during the COVID-19 pandemic.

Keywords: COVID-19 pandemic; obesity; metabolic parameters; clinical values; population health

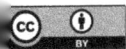

1. Introduction

The COVID-19 pandemic, also referred to as the "COVID-19 crisis", had a sudden and massive impact on daily life, politics, economics, society, and culture [1,2]. However, three years after the global outbreak that originated in Wuhan, China, the incidence rate has decreased, but the pandemic has not yet ended [3]. The most significant changes resulting from this health crisis were not limited to the healthcare sector alone; the event led to a restructuring of the socioeconomic order and a fundamental transformation of the social system [4]. Due to the outbreak of the novel infectious disease COVID-19, human physiology has undergone many alterations [1,4]. Additionally, efforts have been made to prevent the spread of the infectious disease by imposing restrictions on global transportation [5]. Furthermore, social and personal activities have been forcibly reduced and prohibited [6,7]. Unlike previous outbreaks, such as those of SARS and MERS, COVID-19 has had a significant impact on politics, economics, society, and culture [8]. The Ministry of Culture, Sports, and Tourism in South Korea conducted a survey in 2020 on the public's perception of COVID-19 quarantine measures. The survey revealed that 84.3% of respondents took the situation seriously, while 55.8% expressed concern and worry about the possibility of infection [9].

In 2018, the Korean Diabetes Association (KDA) estimated that between 13.8% and 26.9% of adults over the age of 30 in South Korea are expected to have impaired fasting glucose, and that 35% of diabetic patients have not yet been diagnosed with diabetes [10]. South Korea is experiencing a significant prevalence of diabetes, with 53.2% of individuals with diabetes also having hypertension, and 72% having hypercholesterolemia, necessitating urgent and systematic management strategies for this patient population [10–12].

In this study, we investigated the alterations in physical vital signs, blood tests, and urine tests among overweight and obese adults aged 19 years and above in South Korea, before and after the onset of the COVID-19 pandemic. To achieve our objective, we aimed to examine the variations in physical vital signs, blood tests, and urine test values from the data collected by national institutions. Additionally, we aimed to assess how the risk of developing adverse health conditions changed. Based on these findings, we intended to provide a foundation for research aimed at identifying, managing, and preventing factors that can have adverse effects on both mental and physical health during and after the COVID-19 pandemic. Furthermore, we believe that this research will provide essential data for managing the health of individuals in the event of future infectious disease outbreaks, similar to that of COVID-19.

2. Materials and Methods

2.1. Study Designs and Sampling

This study utilized raw public data from the seventh and eighth National Health and Nutrition Examination Surveys, which are nationally approved statistical sources (No. 117002), for the second time. Out of a total of 15,082 participants, only individuals with a body mass index (BMI) classified as overweight or obese (BMI ≥ 25) and aged 19 years or older were included in the study. Participants under the age of 19 were excluded. The final study sample comprised 3560 participants from 2018 and 3309 participants from 2021. Data were obtained through the online distribution procedure of the relevant institution, utilizing national open data. The two groups were designated as pre-COVID-19 and post-COVID-19, respectively. The study focused on overweight and obese adults aged 19 years and older, with a BMI of 25 or higher (Figure 1).

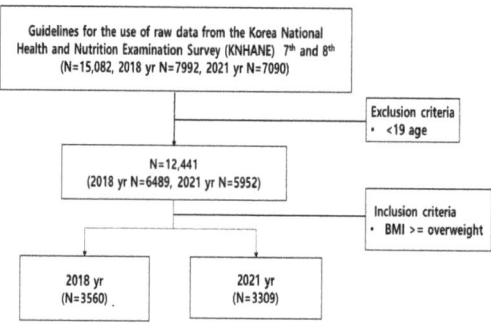

Figure 1. Data cleaning process flow. (The year 2018 was a year before the COVID-19 outbreak, and 2021 was the year after the COVID-19 outbreak.)

2.2. Data Variables

The variables examined in this study include the following: (1) physical characteristics, such as gender, age, height, weight, waist circumference, body mass index (BMI) based on Asian standards, pulse rate, and blood pressure (average of two measurements); (2) blood test parameters, including fasting blood glucose, glycated hemoglobin (HbA1c), total cholesterol, high-density lipoprotein (HDL) cholesterol, triglycerides, low-density lipoprotein (LDL) cholesterol, the prevalence of hypercholesterolemia, the prevalence of hypertriglyceridemia, aspartate aminotransferase (AST), alanine aminotransferase (ALT), hepatitis B surface antigen positivity, hepatitis C antibody positivity, hemoglobin, hematocrit, the prevalence of anemia, blood urea nitrogen, serum creatinine, white blood cell (WBC) count, red blood cell (RBC) count, and platelet count; and (3) urine test parameters, including uric acid, urine pH, nitrite, urine protein, urine glucose, and urine ketone. Additionally, participants underwent tests for urine bilirubin, urine occult blood, urobilinogen, urine creatinine, and urine bilirubin, as well as measurements of sodium, potassium, and cotinine levels in urine.

2.3. Data Analysis

The study variables were categorized as being either categorical or continuous variables. Categorical variables were presented as frequencies and percentages, while continuous variables were reported as means and standard deviations after assessing the normality of their distributions. Differences between the groups were analyzed by using the Mann–Whitney U test for continuous variables and Fisher's exact test or the chi-square test for categorical variables, as appropriate. Multiple regression analysis was performed to identify variables associated with the severity of the COVID-19 outbreak, with a significance level criterion of 0.10 for input variable selection. All statistical analyses were conducted using IBM SPSS software (version 25.0, IBM Corp., Armonk, NY, USA), with a significance level of 0.05.

3. Results

3.1. Blood Pressure Changes in Overweight/Obese Adults Pre-/Post-COVID-19

Changes in the general characteristics of the overweight group before and after the COVID-19 outbreak are presented in Table 1. A significant difference was observed in systolic blood pressure (122.12 ± 16.29 mmHg vs. 123.32 ± 15.12 mmHg) and diastolic blood pressure (77.39 ± 10.45 mmHg vs. 75.56 ± 9.60 mmHg) between the group classified as obese (BMI ≥ 30 kg/m^2, 13.4%) and the non-obese group (BMI 25–29.9 kg/m^2, 16.7%) (Table 1).

Table 1. General characteristics of the overweight group before and after the COVID-19 outbreak.

Characteristic			Before the COVID-19 Outbreak (2018)		After the COVID-19 Outbreak (2021)		$Z^2/{}^4X^2$	p-Value [3]
			N [5]/Mean [1]	% [5]/SD [1]	N/Mean	%/SD		
Sex [4]		Male	1817	51.0	1687	51.0	0.002	0.962
		Female	1743	49.0	1622	49.0		
	Age [1]		53.54	15.97	54.73	16.39	−3.382	0.001
	Height (cm) [1]		163.81	9.85	163.97	10.03	−0.501	0.617
	Weight (kg) [1]		70.79	11.58	71.26	12.02	−1.363	0.173
	Waist circumference [1]		88.41	7.95	90.35	8.20	−9.694	<0.001
	Body mass index (BMI) [1]		26.28	2.77	26.39	2.88	−1.499	0.134
	Pulse (60 s) [1]		56.68	10.60	57.62	13.00	−0.711	0.477
	Systole [1,6]		122.12	16.29	123.32	15.12	−3.593	<0.001
	Diastole [1,6]		77.39	10.45	75.56	9.60	−8.255	<0.001
BMI [4] (weight control for 1 year)	BMI 23.0~24.9 (overweight)	Loss effort	545	39.0	529	41.6	3.908	0.272
		Maintenance effort	313	22.4	299	23.5		
		Gain effort	28	2.0	23	1.8		
		Never effort	510	36.5	420	33.0		
	BMI 25.0~29.9 (obesity)	Loss effort	992	55.3	931	55.8	10.432	0.015
		Maintenance effort	241	13.4	279	16.7		
		Gain effort	6	0.3	5	0.3		
		Never effort	554	30.9	453	27.2		
	BMI 30.0 over (high obesity)	Loss effort	219	64.4	228	65.3	0.249	0.883
		Maintenance effort	32	9.4	35	10.0		
		Gain effort	0	0.0	0	0.0		
		Never effort	89	26.2	86	24.6		

[1] M: average; SD: standard deviation; [2] Mann–Whitney test; [3] $p < 0.05$; [4] X^2: chi-square test; [5] N: frequency; %: percentage; and [6] average of two measurements.

3.2. Blood Test Changes in Overweight/Obese Adults Pre-/Post-COVID-19

The differences in blood test values before and after the COVID-19 outbreak are presented in Table 2. Significant differences were observed in fasting blood glucose levels (104.84 ± 24.24 mg/dL vs. 106.60 ± 25.98 mg/dL), glycated hemoglobin (HbA1c) levels (5.83 ± 0.84% vs. 5.97 ± 0.90%), total cholesterol levels (193.81 ± 39.21 mg/dL vs. 189.07 ± 40.17 mg/dL), high-density lipoprotein (HDL) cholesterol levels (48.02 ± 11.26 mg/dL vs. 49.17 ± 11.66 mg/dL), and triglyceride levels (154.60 ± 118.50 mg/dL vs. 141.33 ± 106.48 mg/dL) between the pre-COVID-19 and post-COVID-19 groups (Table 2).

Table 2. Blood test values before and after the COVID-19 outbreak.

Characteristic		Before the COVID-19 Outbreak (2018)		After the COVID-19 Outbreak (2021)		$Z^2/{}^4X^2$	p-Value [3]
		N [5]/Mean [1]	% [5]/SD [1]	N/Mean	%/SD		
Fasting blood sugar (FBS) [1]		104.84	24.24	106.60	25.98	−4.508	<0.001
HbA1c [1]		5.83	0.84	5.97	0.90	−9.984	<0.001
Total cholesterol [1]		193.81	39.21	189.07	40.17	−4.845	<0.001
HDL cholesterol [1]		48.02	11.26	49.17	11.66	−4.114	<0.001
Triglycerides [1]		154.60	118.50	141.33	106.48	−6.643	<0.001
LDL cholesterol [1]		115.86	33.96	116.24	35.98	−0.075	0.940
Hypercholesterolemia [4]	No	2370	70.6	2092	66.6	12.557	<0.001
	Yes	985	29.4	1051	33.4		
Hypertriglyceridemia [4]	No	2233	79.8	2388	84.5	21.389	<0.001
	Yes	566	20.2	438	15.5		
AST(SGOT) [1]		25.23	14.37	26.41	12.88	−5.977	<0.001
ALT(SGPT) [1]		26.40	19.20	27.45	21.28	−2.622	0.009
Hepatitis B surface antigen [4]	Negative	3354	97.1	3141	97.1	0.002	0.966
	Positive	101	2.9	94	2.9		
Hepatitis C antibody [4]	Negative	3429	99.2	3203	99.0	1.089	0.297
	Positive	26	0.8	32	1.0		
Hemoglobin [1]		14.37	1.60	14.03	1.58	−8.663	<0.001
Hematocrit [1]		43.00	4.30	42.56	4.28	−4.074	<0.001
Anemia [4]	Negative	3234	93.8	2906	89.9	33.283	<0.001
	Positive	215	6.2	326	10.1		
Blood urea nitrogen [1]		15.74	4.89	15.25	4.73	−4.590	<0.001
Blood creatinine [1]		0.83	0.21	0.82	0.22	−1.650	0.099
WBC [1]		6.35	1.74	6.26	1.66	−2.205	0.027
RBC [1]		4.66	0.50	4.63	0.51	−2.563	0.010
Platelets [1]		262.32	64.45	253.84	62.79	−5.251	<0.001

[1] M: average; SD: standard deviation; [2] Mann–Whitney test; [3] $p < 0.05$; [4] X^2: chi-square test; [5] N: frequency; and %: percentage.

3.3. Urinalysis Changes in Overweight/Obese Adults Pre/Post-COVID-19

The results of the differences in urine test values before and after the COVID-19 outbreak are presented in Table 3. Significant differences were observed in the percentage of participants with negative results for urinary protein (80.2% vs. 90.9%), negative urinary glucose (94.7% vs. 91.9%), negative urinary ketone (98.5% vs. 98.9%), negative urinary bilirubin (99.3% vs. 100.0%), negative urinary occult blood (82.8% vs. 93.5%), negative urobilinogen (99.5% vs. 99.3%), as well as in urine creatinine levels (147.08 ± 80.10 mg/dL vs. 125.89 ± 74.77 mg/dL), urine sodium levels (116.79 ± 48.09 mmol/L vs. 113.66 ± 47.75 mmol/L), urine potassium levels (52.66 ± 23.22 mmol/L vs. 41.51 ± 20.75 mmol/L), and urine cotinine levels (346.22 ± 718.56 ng/mL vs. 783.69 ± 826.45 ng/mL) between the pre-COVID-19 and post-COVID-19 groups (Table 3).

Table 3. Urine test before and after the COVID-19 outbreak.

Characteristic		Before the COVID-19 Outbreak (2018)		After the COVID-19 Outbreak (2021)		$Z^{2/4}X^2$	p-Value [3]
		N/Mean [1]	%/SD [1]	N/Mean	%/SD		
Uric acid [1]		5.44	1.41	5.47	1.43	−0.970	0.332
Uric acidity [1]		5.87	0.74	5.90	0.77	−0.940	0.347
Nitrate [4]	No	3334	97.5	3172	97.7	0.490	0.484
	Yes	87	2.5	74	2.3		
Urine protein [4]	Negative	2743	80.2	2950	90.9	171.090	<0.001
	Trace	510	14.9	197	6.1		
	1+	131	3.8	65	2.0		
	2+	33	1.0	28	0.9		
	3+	1	0.0	4	0.1		
	4+	3	0.1	2	0.1		
Urine glucose [4]	Negative	3241	94.7	2984	91.9	40.045	<0.001
	Trace	44	1.3	66	2.0		
	1+	23	0.7	35	1.1		
	2+	33	1.0	25	0.8		
	3+	38	1.1	33	1.0		
	4+	42	1.2	103	3.2		
Urine ketone [4]	Negative	3370	98.5	3209	98.9	20.122	<0.001
	Trace	17	0.5	0	0.0		
	1+	20	0.6	28	0.9		
	2+	12	0.4	9	0.3		
	3+	2	0.1	-	-		
	4+	-	-	-	-		
Urine bilirubin [4]	Negative	3397	99.3	3246	100.0	22.855	<0.001
	trace	-	-	-	-		
	1+	24	0.7	-	-		
	2+	-	-	-	-		
	3+	-	-	-	-		
	4+	-	-	-	-		
Urine occult blood [4]	Negative	2831	82.8	3034	93.5	191.933	<0.001
	trace	336	9.8	122	3.8		
	1+	138	4.0	32	1.0		
	2+	67	2.0	30	0.9		
	3+	43	1.3	28	0.9		
	4+	6	0.2	-	-		
Urine bilinogen [4]	Negative	3405	99.5	3222	99.3	8.533	0.014
	trace	4	0.1	-	-		
	1+	12	0.4	23	0.7		
	2+	-	-	1	0.0		
	3+	-	-	-	-		
	4+	-	-	-	-		
Urine creatinine [1]		147.08	80.10	125.89	74.77	−11.726	0.000
Urine sodium [1]		116.79	48.09	113.66	47.75	−3.212	0.001
Urine potassium [1]		52.66	23.22	41.51	20.75	−19.034	0.000
Urine cotinine [1]		346.22	718.56	783.69	826.45	−23.264	0.000

[1] M: average; SD: standard deviation; [2] Mann–Whitney test; [3] $p < 0.05$; [4] X^2: chi-square test; [5] N: frequency; %: percentage.

3.4. Multivariate Analysis of Blood Test Changes Pre-/Post-COVID-19

The results of the multivariate analysis on changes in blood test values before and after the COVID-19 outbreak are presented in Table 4. The analysis revealed that systolic blood pressure was significantly higher after the COVID-19 outbreak ($\beta = 0.964$, 95% CI: 0.956–0.972, $p < 0.001$). The results of the study showed significant associations between various health indicators and the outcome variable. Specifically, diastolic blood pressure ($\beta = 0.964$, 95% CI: 0.956–0.972, $p < 0.001$), high-density lipoprotein (HDL) cholesterol ($\beta = 1.010$, 95% CI: 1.004–1.016, $p = 0.001$), hemoglobin ($\beta = 0.280$, 95% CI: 0.240–0.326, $p < 0.001$), hematocrit ($\beta = 1.476$, 95% CI: 1.386–1.572, $p < 0.001$), blood urea nitrogen ($\beta = 0.963$, 95% CI: 0.950–0.975, $p < 0.001$), red blood cell (RBC) count ($\beta = 1.352$, 95% CI: 1.016–1.801, $p = 0.039$), and platelet count ($\beta = 0.996$, 95% CI: 0.995–0.997, $p < 0.001$) were significantly associated with the outcome variable (Table 4).

Table 4. Blood and urine test values before and after the COVID-19 outbreak.

	Blood Test *				Urine Test *			
	ORs	95% CI		p-Value		ORs	95% CI	p-Value
Systole	1 + 0.019	1.014	1.024	<0.001	Systole	1.018	1.010 1.025	<0.001
					Diastole	0.958	0.948 0.969	<0.001
Diastole	0.964	0.956	0.972	<0.001	Protein No			<0.001
					Ttrace	0.385	0.276 0.537	<0.001
FBS	1.000	0.995	1.004	0.910	Protein [1+]	0.597	0.340 1.049	0.073
HbA1c	1.062	0.934	1.206	0.359	Protein [2+]	1.281	0.487 3.371	0.616
					Protein [3+]	5.83×10^9	0.000	0.999
Total cholesterol	0.999	0.997	1.001	0.201	Protein [4+]	0.000	0.000	0.999
					Glucose No			0.001
HDL cholesterol	1.010	1.004	1.016	0.001	Trace	1.832	0.980 3.425	0.058
					Glucose [1+]	1.949	0.807 4.710	0.138
Triglycerides	1.000	0.999	1.000	0.322	Glucose [2+]	0.420	0.171 1.028	0.057
					Glucose [3+]	0.630	0.280 1.415	0.263
Hypercholesterolemia, yes	1.131	0.993	1.287	0.063	Glucose [4+]	2.311	1.350 3.955	0.002
					Ketone No			0.699
Hypertriglyceridemia, yes	0.917	0.741	1.134	0.422	Trace	0.000	0.000	0.998
					Ketone [1+]	1.460	0.556 3.829	0.442
AST (SGOT)	1.004	0.998	1.011	0.189	Ketone [2+]	1.861	0.498 6.945	0.355
					Urine bilirubin Trace	0.000	0.000	0.999
ALT (SGPT)	1.003	0.998	1.008	0.245	Urine occult blood No			<0.001
					Trace	0.374	0.246 0.568	<0.001
Hemoglobin	0.280	0.240	0.326	<0.001	Occult blood [1+]	0.203	0.085 0.481	<0.001
					Occult blood [2+]	0.477	0.193 1.178	0.108
Hematocrit	1.476	1.386	1.572	<0.001	Occult blood [3+]	0.963	0.408 2.274	0.931
					Occult blood [4+]	0.000	0.000	0.999
Blood urea nitrogen	0.963	0.950	0.975	<0.001	Urobilinogen No	-	-	0.660
					Trace	0.000	0.000	0.999
WBC	0.964	0.928	1.001	0.056	Urobilinogen [1+]	1.584	0.589 4.261	0.362
					Urine creatinine	1.003	1.001 1.005	<0.001
RBC	1.352	1.016	1.801	0.039	Urine sodium	1.000	0.998 1.002	0.776
					Urine potassium	0.973	0.968 0.977	<0.001
Platelets	0.996	0.995	0.997	<0.001	Urine cotinine	1.001	1.001 1.001	<0.001

[1] M: average; SD: standard deviation; [2] Mann–Whitney test; [3] $p < 0.05$; [4] X^2: chi-square test; [5] N: frequency; and %: percentage. * Multi-variable regression analysis adjusted for age, waist circumference, and BMI.

3.5. Multivariate Analysis of Urine Test Changes Pre-/Post-COVID-19

The results of the multivariate analysis on the changes in urine test values before and after the COVID-19 outbreak are presented in Table 4. After the COVID-19 outbreak, compared to the pre-COVID-19 period, there was a significant increase in trace urinary protein levels (β = 0.385, 95% CI: 0.208–0.486, p < 0.001), urinary glucose levels of +++ or higher (β = 2.311, 95% CI: 1.350–3.955, p = 0.002), trace urinary occult blood levels (β = 0.374, 95% CI: 0.246–0.568, p < 0.001), urinary occult blood levels of + or higher (β = 0.203, 95% CI: 0.085–0.481, p < 0.001), urine creatinine levels (β = 1.003, 95% CI: 1.001–1.005, p < 0.001), urine potassium levels (β = 0.973, 95% CI: 0.968–0.977, p < 0.001), and urine cotinine levels (β = 1.001, 95% CI: 1.001–1.001, p < 0.001) (Table 4).

4. Discussion

This study analyzed changes in blood and urine test results among adults aged 19 years and older who were overweight before and after the outbreak of COVID-19, an emerging infectious disease. The COVID-19 pandemic imposed significant lifestyle changes and various restrictions on daily activities. It was deemed necessary to monitor the impact of these changes on physical health indicators.

This study found that participants' mean waist circumference increased by approximately 2 cm, and that their mean body mass index (BMI) increased by approximately 0.11 compared to pre-pandemic measurements. Additionally, their mean systolic blood pressure was higher than pre-COVID-19 levels. An increase in blood pressure is known to correlate with a higher incidence of hypertension. Previous studies have reported an association between the prevalence of hypertension and the incidence of kidney disease. Research indicates that maintaining appropriate blood pressure levels can reduce the risk of kidney disease by an odds ratio (OR) of 0.42 [13].

The COVID-19 pandemic imposed limitations on daily activities and reduced in-person interactions, which may have negatively impacted physical well-being. Adolescence is a critical period for developing lifelong health habits, both mentally and physically [14–17]. It is noteworthy that individuals over 19 years of age made efforts to sustain their weight during the pandemic, as evidenced by this study. When assessing disease risk, there was an OR of 1.019 for increased systolic blood pressure, an OR of 0.964 for increased diastolic blood pressure, and an OR of 0.999 for increased high-density lipoprotein (HDL) cholesterol levels.

For diabetes, fasting blood glucose and glycated hemoglobin are recognized as important diagnostic factors [18,19]. In clinical practice, risk factors related to diabetes, such as genetics and lifestyle, are considered important, along with disease risk factors associated with obesity. In this study, the mean fasting blood glucose was 1.76 mg/dL higher, and mean glycated hemoglobin was 0.14% higher than pre-pandemic levels. The pandemic led to an increased risk of diabetes due to restrictions on physical activity and sudden lifestyle changes [18,20–22].

The prevalence of hypercholesterolemia has increased by 4% since the start of the COVID-19 pandemic. According to the 2010 National Health and Nutrition Examination Survey, the prevalence of hypercholesterolemia increased significantly from 8.0% in 2005 to 11.5% in 2009 among individuals aged 30 years and older [23]. In 2016, the prevalence rose to 14.4% among those over 30 years of age [24]. These findings suggest an ongoing increase in the prevalence of dyslipidemia. The present study revealed a mean increase of 0.38 mg/dL in high-density lipoprotein (HDL) cholesterol levels. Dyslipidemia is characterized by decreased HDL cholesterol concentration [25–27]. Low HDL cholesterol levels are specifically linked to cardiovascular disease risk. The Framingham Study by Gordon et al. (1977) found that, among adults aged 49–82 years, individuals with low HDL cholesterol levels had a higher incidence of cardiovascular disease, even with low low-density lipoprotein (LDL) cholesterol [28].

Additionally, low HDL cholesterol levels have been associated with abdominal adiposity [29], metabolic syndrome [30], cognitive impairment and dementia [31], impaired fasting glucose [32], and diabetes [33]. Therefore, managing obesity and daily lifestyle habits is crucial for maintaining healthy HDL cholesterol levels, which are strongly linked to adult diseases like cardiovascular disease [34,35]. The observed changes were likely due to decreased physical activity, the adoption of a Westernized diet, and pandemic-related lifestyle restrictions. These factors can lead to increased obesity, abdominal obesity, and a risk of conditions such as dysglycemia. In modern society, various home-based training programs can increase aerobic and resistance exercise, which is particularly important during periods of restricted movement due to infectious diseases like COVID-19. Appropriate physical activity can also aid weight management and reduce the risk of dysglycemia that may be exacerbated by frequent alcohol consumption. Furthermore, if hepatocellular injury is severe, aspartate aminotransferase (AST) levels rise more than those of alanine aminotransferase (ALT). When the hepatocyte membrane is damaged, both AST and ALT enzymes are released into the bloodstream, causing an increase [36]; however, elevated AST and ALT levels do not always indicate the extent of hepatocyte necrosis or injury. Levels exceeding five times the upper limit are considered indicative of impaired liver function [36]. In this study, mean AST levels increased by 1.18 U/L and mean ALT levels increased by 1.05 U/L compared to pre-pandemic levels.

Anemia is a condition that often coexists with various diseases and is particularly prevalent in chronic conditions such as infectious diseases, autoimmune disorders, chronic kidney disease, and cancer [37]. The prevalence of anemia was 3.9% higher in this study, with a mean decrease of $0.03 \times 10^6/\mu L$ in red blood cells and a mean decrease of $0.09 \times 10^3/\mu L$ in white blood cells. Anemia is characterized by a lower-than-normal number of red blood cells, which are responsible for oxygen transport, leading to an increased risk of tissue hypoxia. During a recent study on COVID-19, mean hemoglobin levels decreased by 0.34 g/dL. This decrease has been linked to hemoglobinopathies and hypoxic damage, potentially leading to the development of hypoxemic blood disorders due to dysregulated iron metabolism [38]. The emergence of novel infectious and inflammatory viral diseases poses unknown outbreak risks [39].

Urinalysis can detect abnormalities such as occult blood, urobilinogen, hematuria, proteinuria, ketonuria, glycosuria, and bacteriuria. It is primarily performed to detect and manage diseases of the kidneys and urinary tract [40]. In this study, the prevalence of proteinuria was 10.7%, and glycosuria was 2.8%. The prevalence of ketonuria was 0.4%, and urobilinogen was 0.7%. The prevalence of hematuria was 10.7%, while mean urobilinogen levels decreased by 0.2 mg/dL. Mean urea nitrogen decreased by 21.19 mg/dL, while mean sodium increased by 3.13 mmol/L. Mean potassium decreased by 11.51 mmol/L. The presence of proteinuria was significant, with an odds ratio (OR) of 0.385. Similarly, the presence of glycosuria and hematuria was significant, with ORs of 0.374 and 0.203 for trace and gross hematuria, respectively. Urinalysis indicated that mean hemoglobin was likely to decrease by 0.280 g/dL, while mean hematocrit was likely to increase by 1.746%. Blood urea nitrogen was likely to decrease by 0.963 mg/dL and mean red blood cell as well as platelet counts were likely to decrease by factors of 1.352 and 0.966, respectively.

5. Conclusions

COVID-19 is a novel infectious disease unprecedented in modern times. Unlike past epidemics, it has resulted in widespread restrictions at the individual, societal, and national levels, with significant global economic impacts. The ongoing nature of the COVID-19 situation, rather than it being a short-term crisis, has underscored the importance of maintaining mental and physical health. The pandemic has necessitated a shift towards reduced in-person interaction, with restrictions on activities such as dining out and social gatherings; however, this study confirms that such lifestyle changes have had negative impacts on physical vital signs and clinical laboratory values.

This study examined the pre- and post-COVID-19 outbreak situations; however, caution is needed in interpreting the following results. A nationwide survey of living conditions was conducted at a time when social and economic facilities were completely suspended or restricted due to the widespread occurrence of the pandemic and national-level disease control measures; however, there are limitations to extrapolating these findings to the direct impact of COVID-19. Additionally, although age, regional, and other stratified surveys were conducted by national research institutions, attention is needed due to the small sample size of this study. Finally, there is a need to directly investigate the impact of COVID-19 on individuals by examining factors such as their physical condition, blood, and urine.

Future research should continue to investigate the impact of COVID-19 on dental practices and explore innovative strategies with which to optimize patient care while ensuring the safety of both patients and dental professionals. Additionally, studies examining the psychological impact of the pandemic on dental professionals and effective interventions to promote their well-being are warranted [41,42].

Author Contributions: Conceptualization, A.K., E.-y.K. and J.K.; data curation, A.K. and E.-y.K.; formal analysis, A.K., E.-y.K. and J.K.; funding acquisition, J.K.; investigation, E.-y.K. and J.K.; methodology, A.K., E.-y.K. and J.K.; project administration, J.K.; resources, E.-y.K. and J.K.; software, E.-y.K.; supervision, J.K.; validation, E.-y.K. and J.K.; visualization, E.-y.K.; writing—original draft, A.K. and E.-y.K.; writing—review and editing, J.K. All authors have read and agreed to the published version of the manuscript.

Funding: This study was supported by the Korea University Grant, Basic Science Research Program through the National Research Foundation of Korea (NRF), funded by the Ministry of Education, Science, and Technology (NRF-2022R1I1A1A01071220).

Institutional Review Board Statement: Not applicable.

Informed Consent Statement: Not applicable.

Data Availability Statement: Data are contained within the article.

Acknowledgments: The authors gratefully acknowledge the valuable support provided by the Boeun Forum, which facilitated this research.

Conflicts of Interest: The authors declare no conflicts of interest.

References

1. Afonso, P. The impact of the COVID-19 pandemic on mental health. *Acta Medica Port.* **2020**, *33*, 356–357. [CrossRef] [PubMed]
2. Ministry of Culture, Sports and Tourism. Public Perception Survey Regarding COVID-19 Self-Isolation. 2020. Available online: http://www.mcst.go.kr/english/ (accessed on 10 May 2023).
3. Park, M.G. Corona 19 Crisis' and Seeking Socio-Economic Transformation. *Labor Rev.* **2020**, *187*, 19–40.
4. Korea Disease Control and Prevention Agency. Press Release. Korea Disease Control and Prevention Agency: Cheongju-si, Republic of Korea, 2020. Available online: https://www.kdca.go.kr/board/board.es?mid=a30402000000&bid=0030 (accessed on 10 May 2023).
5. Kim, E.Y.; Kim, J.Y. Adult's Perception of Every Day Life Change After COVID-19. *J. Korea Acad.-Ind. Coop. Soc.* **2022**, *23*, 377–385.
6. Rotter, M.; Brandmaier, S.; Prehn, C.; Adam, J.; Rabstein, S. Stability of targeted metabolite profiles of urine samples under different storage conditions. *Metabolomics* **2017**, *13*, 4. [CrossRef]
7. Ministry of Health and Welfare. (2.23) Briefing on the Pan-Governmental Meeting for COVID-19. Ministry of Health and Welfare: Sejong, Republic of Korea, 2020. Available online: https://www.mohw.go.kr/board.es?mid=a20401000000&bid=0032&tag=&act=view&list_no=353124 (accessed on 11 May 2023).
8. World Health Organization. *WHO Coronavirus (COVID-19) Dashboard*; World Health Organization: Geneva, Switzerland, 2021; [cited 18 October 2021]; Available online: https://covid19.who.int/ (accessed on 11 May 2023).
9. Park, S.M. The impact of the COVID-19 pandemic on mental health among population. *J. Health Educ. Promot.* **2020**, *37*, 83–91. [CrossRef]
10. Ministry of Health and Welfare. *COVID-19 Pan-Government Preparedness Conference Briefing*; Ministry of Health and Welfare: Sejong, Republic of Korea, 2020. Available online: http://www.mohw.go.kr/react/al/sal0301vw.jsp?PARMENU_ID=04&MENU_ID=0403&page=2&CONT_SEQ=353064&SEARCHKEY=TITLE&SEARCHVALUE=23%EC%9D%BC (accessed on 11 May 2023).
11. Jung, C.H.; Son, J.W.; Kang, S.; Kim, W.J.; Kim, H.S.; Kim, H.S.; Seo, M.; Shin, H.-J.; Lee, S.-S.; Jeong, S.J.; et al. Diabetes fact sheets in Korea, 2020: An appraisal of current status. *J. Diabetes Metab.* **2021**, *45*, 1–10. [CrossRef] [PubMed]
12. Korean Diabetes Association. *Diabetes Fact Sheet in Korea*; Korean Diabetes Association: Seoul, Republic of Korea, 2020.
13. Kim, H.S. Importance of Target Blood Pressure Management in Diabetic Kidney Disease. *J. Korea Contents Assoc.* **2019**, *19*, 461–470.

14. Kim, J.Y. The Study of Physical Activity Level on Serum BDNF and Cognitive Function in Adolescence. *J. Growth Dev.* **2014**, *22*, 119–125.
15. Oh, J.W.; Woo, S.S.; Kwon, H.J.; Kim, Y.S. Examining the Association of Physical Activity and PAPS Health-related Physical Fitness on the Physical Self-Description of a Specialized Male Highschool Students. *J. Phys. Educ.* **2013**, *52*, 97–108.
16. Lee, B.S. A Comparative Study on Dietary Life and Recognition of Diet Related Factors in Elementary, Middle and High School Students. *Korean J. Diet. Assoc.* **2004**, *10*, 364–374.
17. Lee, A.; Tsang, C.K. Youth risk behavior in a Chinese population: A territory wide youth risk behavioral surveillance in Hong Kong. *J. Public Health* **2004**, *118*, 88–95. [CrossRef] [PubMed]
18. Lee, Y.J.; Kim, J.H. A Study Analyzing the Relationship among Impaired Fasting Glucose (IFG), Obesity Index, Physical Activity, and Beverage and Alcohol Consumption Frequency in 20s and 30s: The Korea National Health and Nutrition Examination Survey (KNHANES) 2013–2015. *J. Community Living Sci.* **2022**, *33*, 19–38. [CrossRef]
19. Korea Diabetes Association (KDA). *Clinical Practice Guidelines for Diabetes*, 7th ed.; Korea Diabetes Association: Seoul, Republic of Korea, 2021; pp. 8–10.
20. Blair, S.N.; Broney, S. Effects of physical inactivity and obesity on morbidity and mortality: Current evidence and research issues. *Med. Sci. Sports Exerc.* **1999**, *31*, S646. [CrossRef] [PubMed]
21. Jekal, Y.; Lee, M.K.; Kim, E.S.; Park, J.H.; Lee, H.J.; Han, S.J.; Kang, E.S.; Lee, H.C.; Kim, S.Y.; Jeon, J.Y. Effects of walking and physical activity on glucose regulation among type 2 diabetics. *J. Korean Diabetes* **2008**, *2*, 60–67. [CrossRef]
22. Singh, G.M.; Micha, R.; Khatibzadeh, S.; Lim, S.; Ezzati, M.; Mozaffarian, D. Chronic Diseases Expert G (2015) Estimated global, regional, and national disease burdens related to sugarsweetened beverage consumption in 2010. *Circulation* **2015**, *132*, 639–666. [CrossRef] [PubMed]
23. Kim, Y.; Park, S.; Oh, K.; Choi, H.; Jeong, E.K. Changes in the management of hypertension, diabetes mellitus, and hypercholesterolemia in Korean adults before and during the coronavirus disease 2019 pandemic: Data from the 2010–2020 Korea National Health and Nutrition Examination Survey. *Epidemiol. Health* **2023**, *45*, e2023014. [CrossRef] [PubMed]
24. Han, I.H.; Chong, M.Y. The Study on the Difference of Blood Level of HDL-Cholesterol by Obesity and Health Behavior from the Seventh (2016) Korea National Health and Nutrition Examination Survey. *Korean Soc. Food Sci. Nutr.* **2020**, *49*, 1377–1388. [CrossRef]
25. Committee for Guidelines for Management of Dyslipidemia. Korean guidelines for management of dyslipidemia. *J. Lipid Atheroscler.* **2015**, *4*, 61–92. [CrossRef]
26. Dichtl, W.; Nilsson, L.; Goncalves, I.; Ares, M.; Banfi, C.; Calara, F.; Hamsten, A.; Erilsson, P.; Nilsson, J. Very low-density lipoprotein activates nuclear factor-κB in endothelial cells. *Circ. Res.* **1999**, *84*, 1085–1094. [CrossRef]
27. Lutgens, E.; Van Suylen, R.J.; Faber, B.C.; Gijbels, M.J.; Eurlings, P.M.; Bijnens, A.P.; Cleutjens, K.B.; Heeneman, S.; Daemen, M. Atherosclerotic plaque rupture: Local or systemic process? *Arterioscler. Thromb. Vasc. Biol.* **2003**, *23*, 2123–2130. [CrossRef]
28. Gordon, T.; Castelli, W.P.; Hjortland, M.C.; Kannel, W.B.; Dawber, T.R. High density lipoprotein as a protective factor against coronary heart disease. The Framingham Study. *Am. J. Med.* **1977**, *62*, 707–714. [CrossRef] [PubMed]
29. Song, S.O.; Hwang, Y.C.; Kahn, S.E.; Leonetti, D.L.; Fujimoto, W.Y.; Boyko, E.J. Intra-abdominal fat and high density lipoprotein cholesterol are associated in a non-linear pattern in Japanese Americans. *Diabetes Metab. J.* **2020**, *44*, 277–285. [CrossRef]
30. de Melo, L.G.P.; Nunes, S.O.V.; Anderson, G.; Vargas, H.O.; Barbosa, D.S.; Galecki, P.; Carvalho, A.F.; Maes, M. Shared metabolic and immune-inflammatory, oxidative and nitrosative stress pathways in the metabolic syndrome and mood disorders. *Prog. Neuro-Psychopharmacol. Biol. Psychiatry* **2017**, *78*, 34–50. [CrossRef] [PubMed]
31. Atti, A.R.; Valente, S.; Iodice, A.; Caramella, I.; Ferrari, B.; Albert, U.; Mandelli, L.; De Ronchi, D. Metabolic syndrome, mild cognitive impairment, and dementia: A meta-analysis of longitudinal studies. *Am. J. Geriatr. Psychiatry* **2019**, *27*, 625–637. [CrossRef]
32. Jin, S.H. The Relation of Impaired Fasting Glucose and HDL-Cholesterol by Gender and Body Mass Index. *J. Health Inform. Stat.* **2019**, *44*, 8–13. [CrossRef]
33. Pal, K.; Mukadam, N.; Petersen, I.; Cooper, C. Mild cognitive impairment and progression to dementia in people with diabetes, prediabetes and metabolic syndrome: A systematic review and meta-analysis. *Soc. Psychiatry Psychiatr. Epidemiol.* **2018**, *53*, 1149–1160. [CrossRef] [PubMed]
34. Rashid, S.; Genest, J. Effect of obesity on high-density lipoprotein metabolism. *Obesity* **2007**, *15*, 2875–2888. [CrossRef]
35. Seo, J.B.; Chung, W.Y. The importance of treatment of low HDL cholesterolemia in cardiovascular disease. *J. Lipid Atheroscler.* **2008**, *18*, 270–276.
36. Dufour, D.R.; Lott, J.A.; Nolte, F.S.; Gretch, D.R.; Koff, R.S.; Seeff, L.B. Diagnosis and monitoring of hepatic injury. II. recommendations for use of laboratory tests in screening, diagnosis, and monitoring. *Clin. Chem.* **2000**, *46*, 2050–2068. [CrossRef]
37. Weiss, G.; Goodnough, L.T. Anemia of chronic disease. *N. Engl. J. Med.* **2005**, *352*, 1011–1023. [CrossRef]
38. Sharrett, A.R.; Ballantyne, C.M.; Coady, S.A.; Heiss, G.; Sorlie, P.D.; Catellier, D.; Patsch, W. Coronary heart disease prediction from lipoprotein cholesterol levels, triglycerides, lipoprotein(a), apolipoproteins A-I and B, and HDL density subfractions: The Atherosclerosis Risk in Communities (ARIC) study. *Circulation* **2001**, *104*, 1108–1113. [CrossRef] [PubMed]
39. Cavezzi, A.; Emidio, T.; Salvatore, C. COVID-19: Hemoglobin, iron, and hypoxia beyond inflammation. A narrative review. *Clin. Pract.* **2020**, *10*, 1271. [PubMed]

40. Medical Information on the National Health Information Portal. Available online: https://health.kdca.go.kr/healthinfo/ (accessed on 21 May 2023).
41. Paolone, G.; Mazzitelli, C.; Formiga, S.; Kaitsas, F.; Breschi, L.; Mazzoni, A.; Tete, G.; Polizzi, E.; Gherlone, E.; Cantatore, G. One-year impact of COVID-19 pandemic on Italian dental professionals: A cross-sectional survey. *Minerva Dent. Oral. Sci.* **2022**, *71*, 212–222. [CrossRef] [PubMed]
42. Gherlone, E.; Polizzi, E.; Tete, G.; Cappare, P. Dentistry and Covid-19 pandemic: Operative indications post-lockdown. *New Microbiol.* **2021**, *44*, 1–11. [PubMed]

Disclaimer/Publisher's Note: The statements, opinions and data contained in all publications are solely those of the individual author(s) and contributor(s) and not of MDPI and/or the editor(s). MDPI and/or the editor(s) disclaim responsibility for any injury to people or property resulting from any ideas, methods, instructions or products referred to in the content.

MDPI AG
Grosspeteranlage 5
4052 Basel
Switzerland
Tel.: +41 61 683 77 34

Journal of Clinical Medicine Editorial Office
E-mail: jcm@mdpi.com
www.mdpi.com/journal/jcm

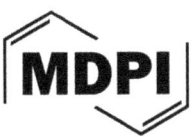

Disclaimer/Publisher's Note: The statements, opinions and data contained in all publications are solely those of the individual author(s) and contributor(s) and not of MDPI and/or the editor(s). MDPI and/or the editor(s) disclaim responsibility for any injury to people or property resulting from any ideas, methods, instructions or products referred to in the content.

www.ingramcontent.com/pod-product-compliance
Lightning Source LLC
LaVergne TN
LVHW070643100526
838202LV00013B/871